Congenital Anomalies of the Kidney and Urinary Tract

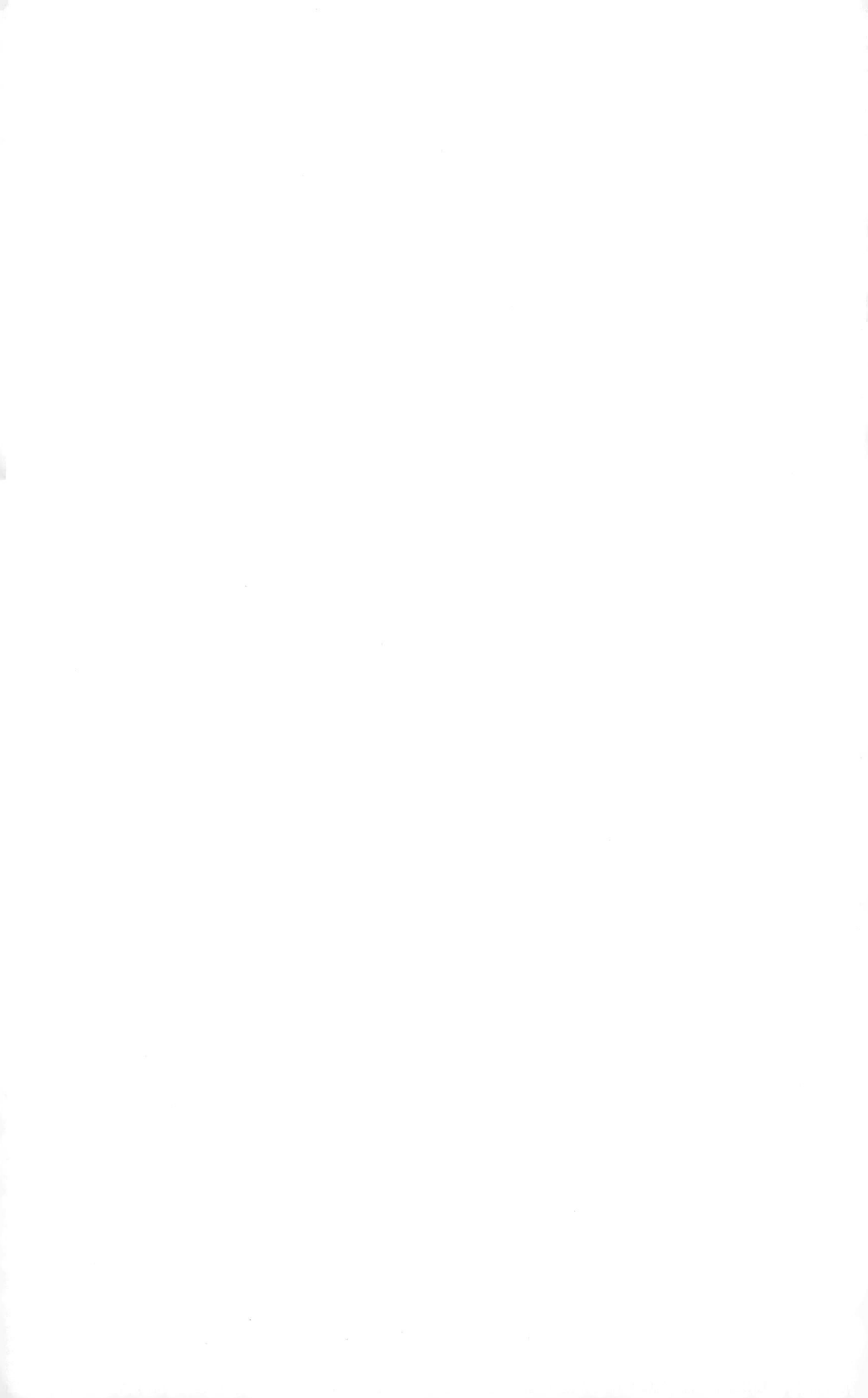

Amin J. Barakat • H. Gil Rushton

Editors

Congenital Anomalies of the Kidney and Urinary Tract

Clinical Implications in Children

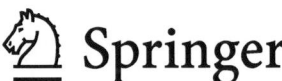 Springer

Editors
Amin J. Barakat
Department of Pediatrics
Georgetown University Medical Center
Washington, DC, USA

H. Gil Rushton
Division of Pediatric Urology
Children's National Medical Center
Departments of Urology and Pediatrics
George Washington University School
    of Medicine
Washington, DC, USA

ISBN 978-3-319-29217-5   ISBN 978-3-319-29219-9   (eBook)
DOI 10.1007/978-3-319-29219-9

Library of Congress Control Number: 2016941057

This Springer imprint is published by Springer Nature
The registered company is Springer International Publishing AG Switzerland

To our families and the families of our patients
who inspire us to further our knowledge

Foreword

We are now seeing an increasing number of children and young adults with congenital anomalies of the kidney and urinary tract. Many of these conditions are diagnosed in the prenatal period. Although there has been a significant improvement in the imaging, genetics, and treatment of these anomalies, their overall diagnosis and management can be very challenging. Thus the need for such a comprehensive book could not be more timely.

This is a very impressive reference book written by an outstanding group of internationally recognized pediatric nephrologists and urologists. The editors, Drs. Barakat and Rushton, are well-known leaders in the field. Although the book is meant to be a desk reference to aid physicians to diagnose, manage, and refer children with various congenital anomalies of the kidney and urinary tract, it is certainly a very comprehensive one. This book will also serve as a guide for medical students, house officers in training, and other healthcare professionals.

Each chapter is very well organized and discusses clinical presentation, workups, laboratory testing including imaging and treatment as well as surgery. The genetics of many of these conditions is also discussed as well as the prenatal diagnosis and subsequent postnatal management.

Controversies in management of various conditions, e.g., vesicoureteral reflux, are discussed in a very objective and fair manner.

The last chapter of the book stresses the association of congenital anomalies of the kidney and urinary tract with those of other organ systems and is an important reference guide. The appendix is very well organized and includes various syndromes associated with congenital anomalies of the kidney and urinary tract.

In summary, this book is a very important and comprehensive reference guide for all physicians and health professionals dealing with congenital anomalies of the kidney and urinary tract.

Alan B. Retik, M.D.
Urologist-in-Chief Emeritus
Boston Children's Hospital
Professor of Surgery
Harvard Medical School
Boston, MA, USA

Preface

Congenital anomalies of the kidney and urinary tract (CAKUT) are a major cause of morbidity in children. They occur in 5–10 % of the population and represent 25 % of sonographically diagnosed fetal malformations. In addition, these anomalies occur in about a quarter of patients with chromosomal aberrations and two-thirds of patients with abnormalities of other organ systems. Some CAKUT are minor; others are major leading to obstruction, urinary tract infection, renal scarring, and chronic kidney disease (CKD). In fact, CAKUT is responsible for most cases of CKD in children.

Knowledge concerning terminology, pathogenesis, and treatment of CAKUT has improved significantly over the past two decades. Also, there have been significant advances in the prenatal diagnosis of these anomalies. Improved technology has contributed to better knowledge of the fetal renal function, renal cortex volume and corticomedullary differentiation, as well as prenatal treatment options. A unified position on prenatal urinary tract dilatation was recently adopted by a consortium of healthcare providers with a consensus on terminology, prenatal follow-up, and post-natal recommendations for imaging and institution of prophylactic antibiotics.

Although the great majority of CAKUT are sporadic and their causes are still unknown, genetic and environmental factors seem to play a major role in their etiology. Based on animal studies, it is believed that genetic mutations may emerge as the main etiologic cause of CAKUT. Mutations in several renal development genes produce defects in the morphogenesis of the kidney and urinary tract causing CAKUT. Molecular analysis of CAKUT-causing genes is now available for clinicians. In spite of continued technical and ethical issues, genetic testing has improved our diagnostic capabilities, allowing the prenatal diagnosis of certain renal diseases in at-risk fetuses, and identifying potential renal disease before it has become manifest. Identification of a specific gene mutation also holds the possibility of correction through gene therapy, although this remains experimental at the present time.

Advances in genetic testing, prenatal diagnosis, fetal surgery, organ transplantation, and surgical treatment of CAKUT have improved the prognosis and quality of life of affected patients. CAKUT have significant impact in clinical medicine and across various specialties, making the book an important reference to pediatricians, primary care physicians, urologists, pediatric nephrologists, residents, medical students, and healthcare professionals who deal with children. The book is not meant to be a textbook, but rather a concise, easy-to-use clinical reference to help physicians diagnose and manage children with CAKUT and to advise them when to refer patients to the pediatric urologist or nephrologist.

To this end, we have assembled a panel of leading authorities in pediatric urology and nephrology to cover a complete scope of CAKUT and its clinical implications in children. The book stresses clinical presentation of various anomalies, workup, interpretation of imaging studies, genetics, prenatal diagnosis, and treatment. Pathogenesis, etiology, pathology, and surgical management are discussed briefly to help the reader understand the scope of the problem. Other system abnormalities associated with CAKUT are also discussed. Tables, figures, algorithms, and images are provided to assist physicians in the differential diagnosis and workup of different conditions. An extensive appendix listing conditions and syndromes associated with CAKUT is also provided.

We thank our distinguished authors for their authoritative contributions. We are also thankful to Elektra McDermott for her outstanding editorial assistance and to the publishing and editorial staff of Springer for their help and support. We sincerely hope that this book will help our readers to understand, diagnose, and manage CAKUT in children.

Washington, DC, USA   Amin J. Barakat
                                                                     H. Gil Rushton

Contents

Contributors

Ardalan E. Ahmad, M.D. Division of Urology, University of Toronto, Toronto, ON, Canada

Angela M. Arlen, M.D. Department of Urology, University of Iowa Hospitals and Clinics, University of Iowa Carver College of Medicine, Iowa City, IA, USA

Amin J. Barakat, M.D., F.A.A.P. Department of Pediatrics, Georgetown University Medical Center, Washington, DC, USA

Stuart B. Bauer, M.D. Department of Urology (Surgery), Harvard Medical School, Boston Children's Hospital, Boston, MA, USA

Patrick C. Cartwright, M.D. Division of Urology, University of Utah Primary Children's Hospital, Salt Lake City, UT, USA

Donna Claes, M.D., M.S., B.S.Pharm. Division of Pediatric Nephrology and Hypertension, Cincinnati Children's Hospital Medical Center, Cincinnati, OH, USA

Andrew J. Combs, P.A.-C. Division of Urology, Weill Cornell Medical College, New York, NY, USA

Christopher S. Cooper, M.D., F.A.C.S., F.A.A.P. Department of Urology, University of Iowa Hospitals and Clinics, University of Iowa Carver College of Medicine, Iowa City, IA, USA

Prasad Devarajan, M.D., F.A.A.P. Division of Nephrology and Hypertension, Cincinnati Children's Hospital Medical Center, University of Cincinnati College of Medicine, Cincinnati, OH, USA

Orchid Djahangirian, M.D. Department of Urology, University of California, Irvine, CA, USA

Department of Urology, Children's Hospital of Orange County, Orange, CA, USA

Kenneth I. Glassberg, M.D. Department of Urology, Columbia University Medical Center, New York, NY, USA

Amnah Al-Harbi, Ph.D. Nephrology Group, Developmental Biology and Cancer Programme (DBCP), Institute of Child Health (ICH), London, UK

C.D. Anthony Herndon, M.D., F.A.C.S., F.A.A.P. Departments of Urology and Pediatrics, University of Virginia School of Medicine, Charlottesville, VA, USA

Friedhelm Hildebrandt, M.D. Division of Nephrology, Boston Children's Hospital, Boston, MA, USA

Division of Nephrology, Harvard Medical School, Boston, MA, USA

Division of Nephrology, Howard Hughes Medical Institute, Boston, MA, USA

David B. Joseph, M.D., F.A.C.S., F.A.A.P. Department of Urology, The University of Alabama at Birmingham, Birmingham, AL, USA

Antoine Khoury, M.D., F.R.C.S.C., F.A.A.P. Department of Urology, University of California, Irvine, CA, USA

Children's Hospital of Orange County, Orange, CA, USA

Barry A. Kogan, M.D. Division of Urology, Departments of Surgery and Pediatrics, Albany Medical College, Albany, NY, USA

Nora G. Lee, M.D. Department of Urology, University of Virginia Health System, Charlottesville, VA, USA

John H. Makari, M.D., F.A.A.P., F.A.C.S. Departments of Urology and Pediatrics, University of Connecticut School of Medicine, Farmington, CT, USA

Connecticut Children's Medical Center, Hartford, CT, USA

Matthew D. Mason, M.D. Division of Pediatric Urology, Upstate Medical University, Syracuse, NY, USA

Rosalia Misseri, M.D. Department of Urology, Riley Hospital for Children, Indianapolis, IN, USA

Department of Urology, Indiana University School of Medicine, Indianapolis, IN, USA

John C. Pope, IV, M.D. Division of Pediatric Urologic Surgery, Vanderbilt University Medical Center, Nashville, TN, USA

Norman D. Rosenblum, M.D., F.R.C.P.C. Departments of Pediatrics, Nephrology, Physiology, Laboratory Medicine and Pathobiology, The Hospital for Sick Children, University of Toronto, Toronto, ON, Canada

Sherry S. Ross, M.D. Department of Urology, The University of North Carolina at Chapel Hill, Chapel Hill, NC, USA

H. Gil Rushton, M.D., F.A.A.P. Division of Pediatric Urology, Children's National Medical Center, and Departments of Urology and Pediatrics, The George Washington University School of Medicine, Washington, DC, USA

Paul H. Smith, III, M.D. Division of Urology, University of Connecticut School of Medicine, Farmington, CT, USA

Division of Urology, Connecticut Children's Medical Center, Hartford, CT, USA

Jason P. Van Batavia, M.D. Division of Urology, Children's Hospital of Philadelphia, Philadelphia, PA, USA

Asaf Vivante, M.D., Ph.D. Division of Nephrology, Boston Children's Hospital, Boston, MA, USA

Paul Winyard, B.M., B.Ch., Ph.D. Nephrology Section, Developmental Biology and Cancer Programme (DBCP), UCL Institute of Child Health (ICH), London, UK

Division of Pediatric Nephrology, Great Ormond Street Hospital for Children, Great Ormond Street, London, UK

Rebecca S. Zee, M.D., Ph.D. Department of Urology, University of Virginia School of Medicine, Charlottesville, VA, USA

Chapter 1
Congenital Anomalies of the Kidney and Urinary Tract: An Overview

Norman D. Rosenblum

Abbreviations

CAKUT   Congenital anomalies of the kidney and urinary tract
CKD   Chronic kidney disease
ESRD   End-stage renal disease
VCUG   Voiding cystourethrogram
VUR   Vesicoureteral reflux

Introduction

Congenital anomalies of the kidney and urinary tract (CAKUT) are the most common cause of all birth defects, constituting 23 % of all such defects [1]. As a group, CAKUT are the cause of 30–50 % of all cases of end-stage renal disease (ESRD) in children [2]. Further, they are the most frequent malformations detected by ultrasound in utero [3]. Lower urinary tract abnormalities can be identified in approximately 50 % of affected patients and include vesicoureteral reflux (VUR) (25 %), ureteropelvic junction obstruction (11 %), and ureterovesical junction obstruction (11 %) [4]. Renal malformations, other than mild antenatal pelviectasis, occur in association with non-renal malformations in about 30 % of cases [3]. This chapter is an overview of issues related to the etiology, pathobiology, diagnosis, and clinical management of CAKUT and serves as a foundation for more detailed presentation in subsequent chapters.

N.D. Rosenblum, M.D., F.R.C.P.C. (✉)
Departments of Pediatrics, Nephrology, Physiology, Laboratory Medicine and Pathobiology, The Hospital for Sick Children, University of Toronto, 686 Bay Street, 16th Floor, Room 16.9706, Toronto, ON, Canada, M5G0A4
e-mail: norman.rosenblum@sickkids.ca

© Springer International Publishing Switzerland 2016   1
A.J. Barakat, H. Gil Rushton (eds.), *Congenital Anomalies of the Kidney and Urinary Tract*, DOI 10.1007/978-3-319-29219-9_1

Clinical Classification

Renal–urinary tract malformations are classified under the rubric congenital anomalies of the kidney and urinary tract (CAKUT). An overarching classification for these malformations was proposed due to recognition that (1) multiple structures within one or both kidney–urinary tract units may be affected within any given affected individual, (2) mutation in a particular gene is associated with different urinary tract anomalies in different affected individuals, and (3) mutations in different genes give rise to similar renal and lower urinary tract phenotypes. Within the CAKUT rubric, a spectrum of phenotypes exist ranging from aplasia (agenesis), defined as congenital absence of kidney tissue; to simple hypoplasia, defined as renal length <2 s.d. below the mean for age and normal renal architecture; dysplasia±cysts, defined as malformation of tissue elements; and isolated dilatation of the renal pelvis±ureters (collecting system). Any malformation phenotype can be observed for a kidney in an orthotopic (normal) position or an ectopic kidney.

Pathogenesis of CAKUT

Genetic Mechanisms

The genetics of CAKUT are complex (Refer to Chap. 15). The incidence of gene mutations in patients with CAKUT is unknown since population-based genome-wide sequencing studies are only now being performed. In the majority of affected patients, congenital renal malformations occur as sporadic events. In approximately 30 % of affected individuals, CAKUT occurs as part of a multiorgan genetic syndrome. Over 200 distinct genetic syndromes feature some type of kidney and urinary tract malformation. More than 30 genes have been identified as mutant in multiorgan syndromes with CAKUT (Table 1.1). Incomplete penetrance with variable expressivity is frequent in affected families. Studies of patients with CAKUT but without evidence of a multiorgan syndrome indicate that a minority of such patients will manifest mutations in genes which have been associated with genetic syndromes. For example, a study in which a small number of genes were examined in 100 patients with renal hypodysplasia and renal insufficiency demonstrated a gene mutation in genes including *TCF2* and *PAX2* in 16 % of affected individuals [5]. Some of the mutations were de novo mutations, explaining the sporadic appearance of CAKUT. Careful clinical analysis of patients with *TCF2* and *PAX2* mutations revealed the presence of extrarenal symptoms in only 50 %, supporting previous reports that *TCF2* and *PAX2* mutations can be responsible for isolated renal tract anomalies or at least CAKUT malformations with minimal extrarenal features [6, 7]. It is not uncommon for first-degree relatives of individuals with bilateral renal agenesis or bilateral renal dysgenesis and without evidence of a genetic syndrome or a family history to have ultrasound evidence of a renal–urinary tract malformation of some type. Studies have suggested an incidence ranging from 9 to 23 % [8, 9].

Table 1.1 Human gene mutations associated with syndromic CAKUT

Primary disease	Gene	Kidney phenotype
Alagille syndrome	*JAGGED1*	Cystic dysplasia
Apert syndrome	*FGFR2*	Hydronephrosis
Beckwith–Wiedemann syndrome	*p57^{KIP2}*	Medullary dysplasia
Branchio-oto-renal (BOR) syndrome	*EYA1, SIX1, SIX5*	Unilateral or bilateral agenesis/ dysplasia, hypoplasia, collecting system anomalies
Campomelic dysplasia	*SOX9*	Dysplasia, hydronephrosis
Duane-radial ray (Okihiro) syndrome	*SALL4*	UNL agenesis, VUR, malrotation, cross-fused ectopia, pelviectasis
Fraser syndrome	*FRAS1*	Agenesis, dysplasia
Isolated renal hypoplasia	*BMP4, RET*	Hypoplasia, VUR
Hypoparathyroidism, sensorineural deafness and renal disease (HDR) syndrome	*GATA3*	Dysplasia
Kallmann syndrome	*KAL1, FGFR1, PROK2, PROK2R*	Agenesis
Mammary–ulnar syndrome	*TBX3*	Dysplasia
Meckel-Gruber syndrome	*MKS1, MKS3, NPHP6, NPHP8*	Dysplasia
Nephronophthisis	*CEP290, GL1S2, RPGR1P1L, NEK8, SDCCAG8, TMEM67, TTC21B*	Dysplasia
Pallister–Hall syndrome	*GLI3*	Agenesis, dysplasia, hydronephrosis
Renal coloboma syndrome	*PAX2*	Hypoplasia, vesicoureteral reflux
Renal tubular dysgenesis	*RAS* components	Tubular dysplasia
Renal cysts and diabetes syndrome	*HNF1b (TCF2)*	Dysplasia, hypoplasia
Rubinstein–Taybi syndrome	*CREBBP*	Agenesis, hypoplasia
Simpson–Golabi–Behmel syndrome	*GPC3*	Medullary dysplasia
Smith–Lemli–Opitz syndrome	*7-Hydroxy-cholesterol reductase*	Agenesis, dysplasia
Townes–Brock syndrome	*SALL1*	Hypoplasia, dysplasia, VUR
Ulnar–mammary syndrome	*TBX3*	Hypoplasia
Zellweger syndrome	*PEX1*	VUR, cystic dysplasia

Embryologic Mechanisms

CAKUT arises from disrupted renal development. Formation of renal–urinary tract structures is initiated at 5-week gestation and concludes by about 34-week gestation. Here, the morphologic and genetic events that control kidney development are summarized. At 5-week gestation in humans, the ureteric duct is induced to undergo lateral outgrowth from the Wolffian duct and to invade the adjacent metanephric mesenchyme. After invading the metanephric mesenchyme, the ureteric bud then undergoes repetitive branching events, so termed because each event consists of expansion of the advancing ureteric bud branch at its leading tip and division of the ampulla, resulting in formation of new branches and elongation of the newly formed branches. This process results in formation of approximately 65,000 collecting ducts. During the latter stages of kidney development, tubular segments formed from the first five generations of ureteric bud branching undergo remodeling to form the kidney pelvis and calyces [10].

Identification of genes mutated in humans with CAKUT coupled with analyses of genes expressed in the developing kidney and urinary tract has provided critical insights into the mechanisms that govern mammalian renal–urinary tract morphogenesis in health and disease. Here, examples of how the study of genes mutated in human CAKUT has informed our understanding of renal development are discussed as a framework for a more detailed discussion of such studies elsewhere in this book.

Outgrowth of a single ureteric bud in the correct position is a critical initial stage of renal development. Without this process, induction of the metanephric mesenchyme does not occur. The budding process is dependent on a signaling axis comprised of *Ret,* a proto-oncogene and tyrosine kinase receptor, and its ligand, *Gdnf.* RET is expressed on the surface of ureteric cells [11], while GDNF is expressed by metanephric mesenchyme cells [12]. Homozygous deletion of either *Ret* or *Gdnf* in mice causes failure of ureteric outgrowth and renal agenesis. Patients with CAKUT have mutations in the RET/GDNF signaling pathway [13–16]. A study of 122 patients with CAKUT identified heterozygous deleterious sequence variants in *GDNF* or *RET* in 6/122 patients, 5 %, while another group screened 749 families from all over the world and identified three families with heterozygous mutations in RET [13]. Similar findings have been reported in studies of fetuses with bilateral or unilateral renal agenesis [14, 16].

The site of ureteric bud outgrowth from the Wolffian duct is normally invariant and the number of outgrowths is limited to one. Outgrowth of more than one ureteric bud can result in renal malformations including a double collecting system and duplication of the ureter. The position at which the ureteric bud arises from the Wolffian duct relative to the metanephric mesenchyme influences the interactions between the ureteric bud and the metanephric mesenchyme; ectopic positioning of the ureteric bud is associated with renal dysplasia and is also thought to contribute to the integrity of the ureterovesical junction. Mackie and Stephens postulated [17] that an abnormal position of the ureteral orifice in the bladder is associated with vesicoureteral reflux in humans. This hypothesis is supported by the discovery that mutations in *ROBO2*, a cell surface receptor expressed in the metanephric mesenchyme, are associated with vesicoureteral reflux in humans [18, 19]. Mice deficient in *Robo2* exhibit ectopic ureteric bud formation, multiple ureters, and hydroureter [20].

Branching of the ureteric bud is initiated immediately following invasion of the metanephric mesenchyme by the ureteric bud. The number of ureteric bud branches elaborated is considered to be a major determinant of final nephron number since each ureteric bud branch tip induces a discrete subset of metanephric mesenchyme cells to undergo nephrogenesis. Regulation of ureteric branch number has been informed by complementary studies in humans and mice. Mutations in *PAX2* cause renal coloboma syndrome (also named papillo-renal syndrome), an autosomal dominant disorder characterized by the association of renal hypoplasia, vesicoureteric reflux, and optic nerve coloboma [21]. During renal development, *Pax2* is expressed in the Wolffian duct, the ureteric bud, and the metanephric mesenchyme. Studies in the *1Neu* mouse strain, which is characterized by a *Pax2* mutation, demonstrated decreased ureteric branching in association with decreased nephron number. Decreased ureteric branch number and nephron number are rescued by inhibition of apoptosis in the ureteric lineage [22, 23]. Studies in normal term newborns suggest that loss of PAX2 function may also contribute to generating a lower number of nephrons within the range of nephron number (approximately 250,000–1,600,000) observed in humans [24]. Goodyer hypothesized that gene polymorphisms that generate loss of PAX2 function could contribute to mild reductions in nephron number and discovered that a *PAX2* haplotype (*PAX2^{AAA}*) is associated with an approximately 10 % decrease in kidney volume in a cohort of newborn infants [25].

As discussed above, GDNF expression by metanephric mesenchyme cells is critical to ureteric branching. In the metanephric mesenchyme, *Sall1*, *Eya1*, and *Six1* positively control *Gdnf* expression. *Sall1*, a member of the Spalt family of transcriptional factors [26], is expressed in the metanephric mesenchyme prior to and during ureteric bud invasion. Mutational inactivation of *Sall1* in mice causes renal agenesis or severe dysgenesis and a marked decrease in GDNF expression [27]. Mutations in *SALL1* are associated with Townes–Brock syndrome, an autosomal dominant malformation syndrome characterized by imperforate anus, preaxial polydactyly and/or triphalangeal thumbs, external ear defects, sensorineural hearing loss, and, less frequently, kidney, urogenital, and heart malformations [28, 29]. EYA1, a DNA-binding transcription factor, is expressed in metanephric mesenchyme cells in the same spatial and temporal pattern as GDNF. EYA1 functions in a molecular complex with SIX1 [30] to control expression of *Gdnf* [31]. Both EYA1 and SIX1 are also expressed in developing otic and branchial tissues [32, 33]. Mice with EYA1 deficiency demonstrate renal agenesis and failure of GDNF expression [32]. Mutations in *EYA1* and *SIX1* occur in humans with branchio-oto-renal (BOR) syndrome [30, 34], which consists, in its classic form, of conductive and/or sensorineural hearing loss, branchial defects, ear pits, and renal anomalies [35, 36]. Renal malformations include unilateral or bilateral renal agenesis, hypodysplasia, as well as malformation of the lower urinary tract including vesicoureteral reflux, pyeloureteral obstruction, and ureteral duplication.

While the genome was originally conceived as consisting of two copies of each gene, the situation is more complex. Within the genome, there exist stretches of DNA that exist in less than or more than two copies. These genomic regions are termed copy number variants (CNV) and are defined as stretches of DNA that are larger than 1kb in length. Rare CNVs, that is, CNVs that are detected with a very low frequency in a human population, have recently been implicated in syndromes with CAKUT [37, 38]. For example, Sanna-Cherchi et al. examined the frequency of rare CNVs in individuals with CAKUT and identified such variants in 10 % of affected individuals compared to 0.2 % of population controls [38]. Deletions at the *HNF1* locus (chromosome 17q12) and the locus for DiGeorge syndrome (chromosome 22q11) were most frequently identified, suggesting these are "hotspots" for copy number variation. Interestingly, 90 % of the CNVs associated with congenital renal malformations were previously reported to predispose to developmental delay or neuropsychiatric disease, suggesting that there are shared pathways implicated in renal and central nervous system development. Similarly, Handrigan et al. demonstrated that copy number variants at chromosome 16q24.2 are associated with autism spectrum disorder, intellectual disability, and congenital renal malformations [37].

Mechanisms Related to the Environment and Exposures in Utero

A substantial body of evidence, derived from human epidemiological studies and animal models, demonstrates an important role for the intrauterine environment in the pathogenesis of renal hypoplasia and predisposition to later kidney disease (reviewed in [39]). Renal hypoplasia with low nephron number is associated with low birth weight or intrauterine growth retardation (IGUR) and maternal undernutrition in animals [40, 41]. While the underlying mechanisms are not well defined, there is some evidence suggesting that the maternal diet programs the expression of critical genes required for embryonic kidney development, cell survival, and renal function [42–44].

Maternal diabetes is associated with renal hypoplasia in the absence of reduced birth weight. In animal models, offspring of hyperglycemic or diabetic mothers demonstrate a significant nephron deficit [45]. In utero exposure to drugs and alcohol has also been associated with renal hypoplasia. Maternal intake of angiotensin-converting enzyme inhibitors during the first trimester in humans is associated with an increased risk of renal dysplasia as well as cardiovascular and central nervous system malformations [46]. Human infants exposed to cocaine in utero have an increased risk of renal tract anomalies [47]. Similarly, infants with fetal alcohol syndrome have a higher incidence of CAKUT [48].

Diagnosis of CAKUT in Utero

The human kidney does not exhibit a capacity to accelerate the rate of nephron formation in children born prematurely or to extend the period of nephrogenesis beyond the equivalent of 34-week gestation [49]. Thus, the integrity of nephron formation in utero is absolutely critical to postnatal life. The number of functional nephrons formed by 32–34-week gestation has been implicated in short- and long-term renal function. Infants with a moderate to severe degree of hypodysplasia exhibit renal insufficiency. A more subtle deficiency in nephron number has been associated with adult-onset hypertension [50], consistent with the "Barker hypothesis," which is based on epidemiologic evidence showing a correlation between birth weight and the incidence of cardiovascular diseases and proposes that adult-onset diseases such as hypertension have a fetal origin [51, 52]. Growth of renal tubules and expansion of glomerular cross-sectional area in utero and after birth is critical to renal functional capacity. The observation in animal models that tubule number, cross-sectional area, and cellular maturation are abnormal in renal dysgenesis is consistent with clinical observations that infants with moderate to severe renal hypoplasia or dysplasia demonstrate a limitation of GFR and tubular function.

The widespread use and 80 % sensitivity of fetal ultrasound in identifying renal–urinary tract anomalies has led to the frequent diagnosis of these anomalies in utero [53]. The fetal kidney can be visualized at 12–15 weeks of human gestation. Corticomedullary differentiation is distinct by 25 weeks of gestation and sometimes earlier. The fetal ureters are not normally detected by ultrasound. Visualization of ureters may be indicative of ureteric or bladder obstruction, or VUR. A urine-filled bladder is normally identified at 13–15-week gestation [54]. Development of the kidney in utero is commonly assessed using fetal renal length standardized for gestational age as a surrogate marker [55]. The volume of amniotic fluid is a surrogate measure of renal function. Fetal urine production begins at 9 weeks of gestation. By 20-week gestation and thereafter, fetal urine is the primary source of amniotic fluid volume [56]. A decrease in amniotic fluid volume, termed oligohydramnios, at or beyond the 20th week of gestation is an excellent indicator of a critical defect in both kidneys, for example, bilateral renal dysplasia (or a critical defect in one kidney where a solitary kidney exists), bilateral ureteral obstruction, or obstruction of the bladder outlet. Severe oligohydramnios in the second trimester can result in lung hypoplasia since an adequate amniotic fluid volume is critical for lung development [57].

Fetal urine is also used as a marker of kidney function in utero and after birth. Levels of sodium and beta-2-microglobulin in fetal urine decrease with increasing gestational age, while urine osmolality increases [58, 59]. Impaired resorption occurs in fetuses with bilateral renal dysplasia or severe bilateral obstructive uropathy, resulting in abnormal high urine levels of sodium and beta 2 microglobulin and high urine osmolality [60]. In general, sodium and chloride concentration greater than 90 meq/l (90 mmol/l), urinary osmolality greater than 210 mosmol/kg H_2O (210 mmol/kg H_2O), and urinary beta-2-microglobulin levels >6 mg/l raise concern as to postnatal renal prognosis [61, 62]. However, the predictive value of these indices is by no means 100 %, providing motivation for the development of other biomarkers to predict renal function. A recent study of fetuses with posterior urethral values demonstrates the promise of such approaches. Analysis of the fetal urine proteome in affected fetuses vs. controls generated a peptide profile that correctly predicted postnatal renal function with 88 % sensitivity and 95 % specificity in affected fetuses and was superior to fetal urine biochemistry and fetal ultrasound in this group of patients [63].

Clinical Sequelae and Management of CAKUT

Because CAKUT play a causative role in 30–50 % of cases of CKD in children [64], it is important to diagnose and initiate therapy to minimize renal damage, prevent or delay the onset of ESRD, and provide supportive care to avoid complications of ESRD. Counseling of families during pregnancy is a key element in the management of CAKUT. Coordinated consultation among professionals in the disciplines of obstetrics, pediatric nephrology, pediatric urology, and neonatology is critical. Consistent and clear clinical information regarding diagnosis and prognosis should be provided during pregnancy and after birth. The level of certainty regarding the severity of the diagnosis and prognosis has a major impact on decision-making during pregnancy and in the immediate postnatal period. To date, little evidence exists that relief of urinary tract obstruction in utero prevents the development of associated renal dysplasia or renal scarring. In contrast, insertion of a bladder–amniotic cavity shunt in the fetus with obstruction below the bladder neck can rescue oligohydramnios and pulmonary hypoplasia [65, 66]. Diagnostic and therapeutic management after birth should be anticipated via the coordinated actions of obstetricians, neonatologists, pediatric nephrologists, and pediatric urologists and should include an immediate assessment in the postnatal period of the need for specialized imaging, assessment of renal function, and management of nutrition and electrolytes.

After delivery, a detailed history and careful physical examination should be performed in all infants with an antenatally detected renal malformation. The examination should include the respiratory system to assess the presence of pulmonary insufficiency; the abdomen to detect the presence of a mass that could represent an enlarged kidney due to obstructive uropathy or multicystic dysplastic kidney or a palpable enlarged bladder, which could suggest posterior urethral valves; the ears, since outer ear abnormalities are associated with an increased risk of CAKUT; and the umbilicus, since a single umbilical artery is also associated with an increased risk of CAKUT.

In newborns with bilateral renal malformation, a solitary malformed kidney, or a history of oligohydramnios, an abdominal ultrasound is recommended within the first 24 h of life since an intervention such as decompression of the bladder with a transurethral catheter may be required. Newborn infants with unilateral involvement do not need immediate attention. In these infants, a renal ultrasound is generally performed after 72 h of age and within the first week of life. Ultrasound examination before 72 h of age may not detect collecting system dilatation since a newborn is relatively volume contracted during this period of time [67]. The serum creatinine estimates the extent of renal impairment and should be utilized when there is bilateral renal disease or an affected solitary kidney. The serum creatinine concentration at birth is similar to that in the mother (usually ≤ 1.0 mg/dl [88 μmol/l]). Thus, serum creatinine should be measured after the first 24 h of life. It declines to normal values (serum creatinine 0.3–0.5 mg/dl [27–44 μmol/l]) within approximately 1 week in term infants and 2–3 weeks in preterm infants.

Management of CAKUT is further guided by the characteristics of specific phenotypes.

Renal anomalies are frequently associated with collecting system abnormalities including VUR. Because of the frequent association of upper urinary tract anomalies including dysplasia and ectopy with a collecting system anomaly in the affected and in an apparently normal contralateral renal unit, a VCUG should be considered in such patients. A DMSA radionuclide scan can provide further information on the differential function of each kidney, which may be useful in management decisions regarding surgical interventions. Also refer to Chap. 14.

Clinical Outcomes of CAKUT

Clinical outcomes in CAKUT vary widely from no symptoms whatsoever to CKD, resulting in a need for renal replacement during a period ranging from the newborn period to the 4th and 5th decades of life. Risk factors for mortality during infancy and early childhood include coexistence of renal and nonrenal disease, prematurity, low birth weight, oligohydramnios, and severe forms of CAKUT (agenesis, hypodysplasia) [68]. In a case series of 822 children with prenatally detected CAKUT that were followed for a median time of 43 months, Quirino et al. reported a mortality of 1.5 % and morbidities including urinary tract infection, hypertension, and CKD in 29, 2.7, and 6 % of surviving children, respectively [69]. A faster rate of decline of renal function in patients with CAKUT and CKD has been associated with a urine albumin to creatinine ratio greater than 200 mg/mmol compared to less than 50 mg/mmol (eGFR: -6.5 ml/min/1.73 m^2/year vs. -1.5 ml/min/1.73 m^2/year), and with more than two (vs. <2) febrile urinary tract infections (eGFR -3.5 ml/min/1.73m^2 vs. -2 ml/min/1.73 m^2 year). A greater decline in eGFR occurs during puberty (eGFR: -4 ml/min/1.73 m^2/year vs. -1.9 ml/min/1.73m^2/year) [70]. A study examining the risk for dialysis in patients with CAKUT demonstrated a significantly higher risk for patients with a solitary kidney compared to non-disease controls [71]. These results raise the possibility that the prognosis for a solitary apparently normal kidney may not be as "normal" as previously thought. Finally, a study of CAKUT patients receiving some form of replacement therapy and registered within the European Dialysis and Transplant Association Registry showed that some of these patients only require renal replacement in the 3rd, 4th, or 5th decade of life. The finding that the mean age at which patients with CAKUT require dialysis and/or transplantation is 31 years indicates that children with CAKUT are at risk of developing a requirement for dialysis and/or transplantation as adults [72].

Conclusions

A majority of CAKUT can be identified in utero. However, the ability to predict the natural history of particular phenotypes is limited, and therapies, beyond surgical correction that treats the primary cause of these disorders, are nonexistent. New developments in human genetics and rapid evolution of DNA sequencing technology provide a basis to identify genetic variants in affected individuals using tools such as next-generation genomic sequencing. The knowledge gained will inform new genotype–phenotype correlation and natural history studies and the development of nongenetic disease biomarkers. This, in turn, can provide a basis for biological signatures that inform the pathobiology of specific disorders, predict their natural history, and guide personalized therapy. Further, with such knowledge, it may be possible to design new interventions to extend the current repertoire of interventions which can be used to relieve or correct urinary tract obstruction but are otherwise limited in their ability to address tissue malformation at more fundamental level using regenerative medicine strategies.

References

1. Loane M, Dolk H, Kelly A, Teljeur C, Greenlees R, Densem J, et al. Paper 4: EUROCAT statistical monitoring: identification and investigation of ten year trends of congenital anomalies in Europe. Birth Defects Res A Clin Mol Teratol. 2011;91 Suppl 1:S31–43.
2. Ardissino G, Dacco V, Testa S, Bonaudo R, Claris-Appiani A, Taioli E, et al. Epidemiology of chronic renal failure in children: data from the ItalKid project. Pediatrics. 2003;111(4 Pt 1):e382–7. Epub 2003/04/03.eng.
3. Wiesel A, Queisser-Luft A, Clementi M, Bianca S, Stoll C. Prenatal detection of congenital renal malformations by fetal ultrasonographic examination: an analysis of 709,030 births in 12 European countries. Eur J Med Genet. 2005;48:131–44.
4. Piscione TD, Rosenblum ND. The malformed kidney: disruption of glomerular and tubular development. Clin Genet. 1999;56:343–58.
5. Weber S, Moriniere V, Knuppel T, Charbit M, Dusek J, Ghiggeri GM, et al. Prevalence of mutations in renal developmental genes in children with renal hypodysplasia: results of the ESCAPE study. J Am Soc Nephrol. 2006;17:2864–70.
6. Salomon R, Tellier AL, Attie-Bitach T, Amiel J, Vekemans M, Lyonnet S, et al. PAX2 mutations in oligomeganephronia. Kidney Int. 2001;59:457–62.
7. Ulinski T, Lescure S, Beaufils S, Guigonis V, Decramer S, Morin D, et al. Renal phenotypes related to hepatocyte nuclear factor-1beta (TCF2) mutations in a pediatric cohort. J Am Soc Nephrol. 2006;17:497–503.
8. Roodhooft AM, Jason MD, Birnholz JC, Holmes LB. Familial nature of congenital absence and severe dysgenesis of both kidneys. N Eng J Med. 1984;310:1341–4.
9. Bulum B, Ozcakar ZB, Ustuner E, Dusunceli E, Kavaz A, Duman D, et al. High frequency of kidney and urinary tract anomalies in asymptomatic first-degree relatives of patients with CAKUT. Pediatr Nephrol. 2013;28:2143–7.
10. Rosenblum ND. Developmental biology of the human kidney. Semin Fetal Neonatal Med. 2008;13:125–32. Epub 2007/12/22.eng.
11. Pachnis V, Mankoo B, Constantini F. Expression of the *c-ret* proto-oncogene during mouse embryogenesis. Development. 1993;119:1005–17.
12. Hellmich HL, Kos L, Cho ES, Mahon KA, Zimmer A. Embryonic expression of glial cell-line derived neurotrophic factor (GDNF) suggests multiple developmental roles in neural differentiation and epithelial-mesenchymal interactions. Mech Dev. 1996;54:95–105.
13. Chatterjee R, Ramos E, Hoffman M, VanWinkle J, Martin DR, Davis TK, et al. Traditional and targeted exome sequencing reveals common, rare and novel functional deleterious variants in RET-signaling complex in a cohort of living US patients with urinary tract malformations. Hum Genet. 2012;131:1725–38. Pubmed Central PMCID: 3551468, Epub 2012/06/26. eng.

14. Skinner MA, Safford SD, Reeves JG, Jackson ME, Freemerman AJ. Renal aplasia in humans is associated with RET mutations. Am J Hum Genet. 2008;82:344–51.
15. Yang D, Zhang J, Chen C, Xie M, Sperling S, Fang F, et al. BMPR IA downstream genes related to VSD. Pediatr Res. 2008;63:602–6.
16. Jeanpierre C, Mace G, Parisot M, Moriniere V, Pawtowsky A, Benabou M, et al. RET and GDNF mutations are rare in fetuses with renal agenesis or other severe kidney development defects. J Med Genet. 2011;48:497–504. Epub 2011/04/15.eng.
17. Mackie GG, Stephens FD. Duplex kidneys: a correlation of renal dysplasia with position of the ureteral orifice. J Urol. 1975;114:274–80.
18. Bertoli-Avella AM, Conte ML, Punzo F, de Graaf BM, Lama G, La Manna A, et al. ROBO2 gene variants are associated with familial vesicoureteral reflux. J Am Soc Nephrol. 2008;19:825–31.
19. Piper M, Georgas K, Yamada T, Little M. Expression of the vertebrate Slit gene family and their putative receptors, the Robo genes, in the developing murine kidney. Mech Dev. 2000;94:213–7.
20. Grieshammer U, Le M, Plump AS, Wang F, Tessier-Lavigne M, Martin GR. SLIT2-mediated ROBO2 signaling restricts kidney induction to a single site. Dev Cell. 2004;6:709–17.
21. Weaver RG, Cashwell LF, Lorentz W, Whiteman D, Geisinger KR, Ball M. Optic nerve coloboma associated with renal disease. Am J Med Genet. 1988;29:597–605.
22. Porteous S, Torban E, Cho N-P, Cunliffe H, Chua L, McNoe L, et al. Primary renal hypoplasia in humans and mice with PAX2 mutations: evidence of increased apoptosis in fetal kidneys of Pax2^{1Neu} +/− mutant mice. Hum Mol Genet. 2000;9:1–11.
23. Dziarmaga A, Eccles M, Goodyer P. Suppression of ureteric bud apoptosis rescues nephron endowment and adult renal function in Pax2 mutant mice. J Am Soc Nephrol. 2006;17:1568–75.
24. Nyengaard JR, Bendtsen TF. Glomerular number and size in relation to age, kidney weight, and body surface in normal man. Anat Rec. 1992;232:194–201.
25. Quinlan J, Lemire M, Hudson T, Qu H, Benjamin A, Roy A, et al. A common variant of the PAX2 gene is associated with reduced newborn kidney size. J Am Soc Nephrol. 2007;18:1915–21.
26. Kohlhase J, Wischermann A, Reichenbach H, Froster U, Engel W. Mutations in the SALL1 putative transcription factor gene cause Townes-Brocks syndrome. Nat Genet. 1998;18:81–3.
27. Nishinakamura R, Matsumoto Y, Nakao K, Nakamura K, Sato A, Copeland NG, et al. Murine homolog of SALL1 is essential for ureteric bud invasion in kidney development. Development. 2001;128:3105–15.
28. Townes PL, Brocks ER. Hereditary syndrome of imperforate anus with hand, foot, and ear anomalies. J Pediatr. 1972;81:321–6.
29. O'Callaghan M, Young ID. The Townes-Brocks syndrome. J Med Genet. 1990;27:457–61.
30. Ruf RG, Xu PX, Silvius D, Otto EA, Beekmann F, Muerb UT, et al. SIX1 mutations cause branchio-oto-renal syndrome by disruption of EYA1-SIX1-DNA complexes. Proc Natl Acad Sci U S A. 2004;101:8090–5.
31. Sajithlal G, Zou D, Silvius D, Xu PX. Eya1 acts as a critical regulator for specifying the metanephric mesenchyme. Dev Biol. 2005;284:323–36.
32. Xu PX, Adams J, Peters H, Brown MC, Heaney S, Maas R. Eya1-deficient mice lack ears and kidneys and show abnormal apoptosis of organ primordia. Nat Genet. 1999;23:113–7. Epub 1999/09/02.eng.
33. Ozaki H, Watanabe Y, Ikeda K, Kawakami K. Impaired interactions between mouse Eya1 harboring mutations found in patients with branchio-oto-renal syndrome and Six, Dach, and G proteins. J Hum Genet. 2002;47:107–16. Epub 2002/04/13.eng.
34. Abdelhak S, Kalatzis V, Heilig R, Compain S, Samson D, Vincent C, et al. A human homologue of the *Drosophila eyes absent* gene underlies Branchio-Oto-Renal (BOR) syndrome and identifies a novel gene family. Nat Gen. 1997;15:157–64.
35. Chen A, Francis M, Ni L, Cremers CW, Kimberling WJ, Sato Y, et al. Phenotypic manifestations of branchio-oto-renal syndrome. Am J Med Genet. 1995;58:365–70.

36. Chang EH, Menezes M, Meyer NC, Cucci RA, Vervoort VS, Schwartz CE, et al. Branchio-oto-renal syndrome: the mutation spectrum in EYA1 and its phenotypic consequences. Hum Mutat. 2004;23:582–9.

37. Handrigan GR, Chitayat D, Lionel AC, Pinsk M, Vaags AK, Marshall CR, et al. Deletions in 16q24.2 are associated with autism spectrum disorder, intellectual disability and congenital renal malformation. J Med Genet. 2013;50:163–73. Epub 2013/01/22.eng.

38. Sanna-Cherchi S, Kiryluk K, Burgess KE, Bodria M, Sampson MG, Hadley D, et al. Copy-number disorders are a common cause of congenital kidney malformations. Am J Hum Genet. 2012;91:987–97. Pubmed Central PMCID: 3516596, Epub 2012/11/20. eng.

39. Denton KM. Can adult cardiovascular disease be programmed in utero? J Hypertens. 2006;24:1245–7. Epub 2006/06/24.eng.

40. Wlodek ME, Mibus A, Tan A, Siebel AL, Owens JA, Moritz KM. Normal lactational environment restores nephron endowment and prevents hypertension after placental restriction in the rat. J Am Soc Nephrol. 2007;18:1688–96.

41. Zohdi V, Moritz KM, Bubb KJ, Cock ML, Wreford N, Harding R, et al. Nephrogenesis and the renal renin-angiotensin system in fetal sheep: effects of intrauterine growth restriction during late gestation. Am J Physiol Regul Integr Comp Physiol. 2007;293:R1267–73. Epub 2007/06/22.eng.

42. Abdel-Hakeem AK, Henry TQ, Magee TR, Desai M, Ross MG, Mansano RZ, et al. Mechanisms of impaired nephrogenesis with fetal growth restriction: altered renal transcription and growth factor expression. Am J Obstet Gynecol. 2008;199:252 e1–7. Epub 2008/07/22. eng.

43. Gilbert JS, Lang AL, Grant AR, Nijland MJ. Maternal nutrient restriction in sheep: hypertension and decreased nephron number in offspring at 9 months of age. J Physiol. 2005;565:137–47. Epub 2005/03/26. eng.

44. Welham SJ, Riley PR, Wade A, Hubank M, Woolf AS. Maternal diet programs embryonic kidney gene expression. Physiol Genomics. 2005;22:48–56. Epub 2005/04/14. eng.

45. Amri K, Freund N, Vilar J, Merlet-Benichou C, Lelievre-Pegorier M. Adverse effects of hyperglycemia on kidney development in rats: in vivo and in vitro studies. Diabetes. 1999;48:2240–5. Epub 1999/10/27.eng.

46. Cooper WO, Hernandez-Diaz S, Arbogast PG, Dudley JA, Dyer S, Gideon PS, et al. Major congenital malformations after first-trimester exposure to ACE inhibitors. N Engl J Med. 2006;354:2443–51.

47. Battin M, Albersheim S, Newman D. Congenital genitourinary tract abnormalities following cocaine exposure in utero. Am J Perinatol. 1995;12:425–8. Epub 1995/11/01.eng.

48. Taylor CL, Jones KL, Jones MC, Kaplan GW. Incidence of renal anomalies in children prenatally exposed to ethanol. Pediatrics. 1994;94:209–12. Epub 1994/08/01.eng.

49. Potter EL. Normal and abnormal development of the kidney. Chicago: Year Book Medical Publishers Inc; 1972. 305 p.

50. Keller G, Zimmer G, Mall G, Ritz E, Amann K. Nephron number in patients with primary hypertension. New Engl J Med. 2003;348:101–8.

51. Barker DJ, Osmond C, Golding J, Kuh D, Wadsworth ME. Growth in utero, blood pressure in childhood and adult life, and mortality from cardiovascular disease. BMJ. 1989;298:564–7. Epub 1989/03/04. eng.

52. Barker DJ, Bagby SP, Hanson MA. Mechanisms of disease: in utero programming in the pathogenesis of hypertension. Nat Clin Pract Nephrol. 2006;2:700–7.

53. Vanderheyden T, Kumar S, Fisk NM. Fetal renal impairment. Semin Neonatol. 2003;8:279–89. Epub 2004/03/06.eng.

54. Cohen HL, Kravets F, Zucconi W, Ratani R, Shah S, Dougherty D. Congenital abnormalities of the genitourinary system. Semin Roentgenol. 2004;39:282–303. Epub 2004/05/18.eng.

55. Cohen HL, Cooper J, Eisenberg P, Mandel FS, Gross BR, Goldman MA, et al. Normal length of fetal kidneys: sonographic study in 397 obstetric patients. Am J Roentgenol. 1991;157:545–8. Epub 1991/09/01.eng.

56. Gilbert WM, Brace RA. Amniotic fluid volume and normal flows to and from the amniotic cavity. Semin Perinatol. 1993;17:150–7. Epub 1993/06/01.eng.
57. Potter EL. Bilateral renal agenesis. J Pediatr. 1946;29:68–76. Epub 1946/07/01.eng.
58. Nicolini U, Fisk NM, Rodeck CH, Beacham J. Fetal urine biochemistry: an index of renal maturation and dysfunction. Br J Obstet Gynecol. 1992;99:46–50.
59. Muller F, Dommergues M, Bussieres L, Lortat-Jacob S, Loirat C, Oury JF, et al. Development of human renal function: reference intervals for 10 biochemical markers in fetal urine. Clin Chem. 1996;42:1855–60. Epub 1996/11/01.eng.
60. Muller F, Dommergues M, Mandelbrot L, Aubry MC, Nihoul-Fekete C, Dumez Y. Fetal urinary biochemistry predicts postnatal renal function in children with bilateral obstructive uropathies. Obstet Gynecol. 1993;82:813–20.
61. Glick PL, Harrison MR, Golbus MS, Adzick NS, Filly RA, Callen PW, et al. Management of the fetus with congenital hydronephrosis II: prognostic criteria and selection for treatment. J Pediatr Surg. 1985;20:376–87. Epub 1985/08/01.eng.
62. Morris RK, Quinlan-Jones E, Kilby MD, Khan KS. Systematic review of accuracy of fetal urine analysis to predict poor postnatal renal function in cases of congenital urinary tract obstruction. Prenat Diagn. 2007;27:900–11. Epub 2007/07/05.eng.
63. Klein J, Lacroix C, Caubet C, Siwy J, Zurbig P, Dakna M, et al. Fetal urinary peptides to predict postnatal outcome of renal disease in fetuses with posterior urethral valves (PUV). Sci Transl Med. 2013;5:198ra06.
64. Seikaly MG, Ho PL, Emmett L, Fine RN, Tejani A. Chronic renal insufficiency in children: the 2001 Annual Report of the NAPRTCS. Pediatr Nephrol. 2003;18:796–804.
65. Elder JS, Duckett Jr JW, Snyder HM. Intervention for fetal obstructive uropathy: has it been effective? Lancet. 1987;2(8566):1007–10. Epub 1987/10/31.eng.
66. Freedman AL, Johnson MP, Smith CA, Gonzalez R, Evans MI. Long-term outcome in children after antenatal intervention for obstructive uropathies. Lancet. 1999;354(9176):374–7.
67. Bueva A, Guignard JP. Renal function in preterm neonates. Pediatr Res. 1994;36:572–7.
68. Melo BF, Aguiar MB, Bouzada MC, Aguiar RL, Pereira AK, Paixao GM, et al. Early risk factors for neonatal mortality in CAKUT: analysis of 524 affected newborns. Pediatr Nephrol. 2012;27:965–72. Epub 2012/03/10.eng.
69. Quirino IG, Diniz JS, Bouzada MC, Pereira AK, Lopes TJ, Paixao GM, et al. Clinical course of 822 children with prenatally detected nephrouropathies. Clin J Am Soc Nephrol. 2012;7:444–51. Pubmed Central PMCID: 3302677, Epub 2012/01/24.eng.
70. Gonzalez Celedon C, Bitsori M, Tullus K. Progression of chronic renal failure in children with dysplastic kidneys. Pediatr Nephrol. 2007;22:1014–20.
71. Sanna-Cherchi S, Ravani P, Corbani V, Parodi S, Haupt R, Piaggio G, et al. Renal outcome in patients with congenital anomalies of the kidney and urinary tract. Kidney Int. 2009;76:528–33. Epub 2009/06/19.eng.
72. Wuhl E, van Stralen KJ, Verrina E, Bjerre A, Wanner C, Heaf JG, et al. Timing and outcome of renal replacement therapy in patients with congenital malformations of the kidney and urinary tract. Clin J Am Soc Nephrol. 2013;8:67–74. Pubmed Central PMCID: 3531653, Epub 2012/10/23.eng.

Chapter 2
Anatomy, Applied Embryology, and Pathogenesis of Congenital Anomalies of the Kidney and Urinary Tract

Amnah Al-Harbi and Paul Winyard

Abbreviations

CAKUT	Congenital anomalies of the kidney and urinary tract
CKD	Chronic kidney disease
MCDK	Multicystic dysplastic kidney
PKD	Polycystic kidney disease
RCAD	Renal cysts and diabetes syndrome
UPJ	Ureteropelvic junction
UVJ	Ureterovesical junction

Introduction

Congenital anomalies of the kidney and urinary tract (CAKUT spectrum) affect up to 3 % of human fetuses, accounting for one third of malformations detected antenatally [1, 2]. Thankfully, only a small proportion lead to chronic kidney disease (CKD) in childhood but they still present diagnostic and management challenges for fetal medicine and pediatric practitioners. It is critical to understand normal development

A. Al-Harbi
Nephrology Group, Developmental Biology and Cancer Programme (DBCP), Institute of Child Health (ICH), London WC1N 1EH, UK

P. Winyard, B.M., B.Ch., Ph.D. (✉)
Nephrology Section, Developmental Biology and Cancer Programme (DBCP), UCL Institute of Child Health (ICH), London, UK

Division of Pediatric Nephrology, Great Ormond Street Hospital for Children, Great Ormond Street, London, UK
e-mail: p.winyard@ucl.ac.uk

© Springer International Publishing Switzerland 2016
A.J. Barakat, H. Gil Rushton (eds.), *Congenital Anomalies of the Kidney and Urinary Tract*, DOI 10.1007/978-3-319-29219-9_2

of the kidney and urinary tract in order to frame the clinical implications of CAKUT. Many accounts focus predominantly on genetic causes of CAKUT, but it is also important to consider other contributors such as lower urinary tract obstruction, teratogens, and maternal diet. Ultimately, renal function in CAKUT is determined by the number of functioning nephrons formed during development in the first instance then the degree of ongoing disruption of this reduced nephron complement by factors such as obstruction or infections over the long term. Our role as physicians is to understand the former and take steps to correct or minimize the latter.

There are a wide spectrum of intrinsic kidney defects within CAKUT including aplasia, hypoplasia, dysplasia (with or without cysts), and multicystic dysplastic kidneys. Extrarenal parts of the spectrum encompass ureteric anomalies such as megaureter, ureteropelvic junction obstruction, ureterovesical junction (UVJ) obstruction or incompetence, and anomalies of the bladder and urethra [3]. Falling between these are conditions such as ectopic and horseshoe kidneys and duplex kidneys/ureters, where there are both renal and lower urinary tract issues. Around 50 % of the CAKUT cases associated with pediatric CKD5 have normal urinary tracts, whereas the rest have some degree of dysfunction ranging from significant flow impairment in boys with posterior urethral valves through varying degrees of vesicoureteric reflux [4]. It is important to detect the latter groups since further renal impairment can occur with undetected/suboptimally treated obstruction or urinary tract infections.

Anatomy and Embryology of Normal Renal Development

The human kidney develops from a few hundred cells at its inception into a mature organ with many hundreds of thousands of nephrons. Early reports estimated around one million nephrons per kidney, although definitive quantification was hampered by lack of material and differences in ascertainment techniques. More recent systematic studies demonstrate a normal range between 740,000 and 1,400,000 [5] with interesting links between renal size and a lower nephron complement, predisposing to hypertension and CKD in some populations [6, 7].

There are three phases of kidney development in humans with consecutive paired organs developing from intermediate mesoderm on the dorsal body wall (Fig. 2.1). The first two stages, the pronephros and mesonephros, degenerate during fetal life in mammals, whereas the metanephros develops into the mature kidney. This is a potential example of ontogeny recapitulating phylogeny because hagfish and some amphibians only have the pronephros for a kidney, while lampreys, other fishes, and amphibians stop at the mesonephros.

The pronephros develops around day 22–23 after fertilization; it starts as a small group of primitive epithelial structures called nephrotomes from the second through sixth somites in the neck/upper thorax, and then new tubules develop in subsequent somites. The pronephric duct is generated as the nephrotomes form at the level of the ninth somite, but it has nowhere to empty so none of these tubules are thought to be functional. The duct elongates rapidly in a caudal direction, reaching the cloaca by day 26, being rechristened the mesonephric, or Wolffian duct, as mesoneph-

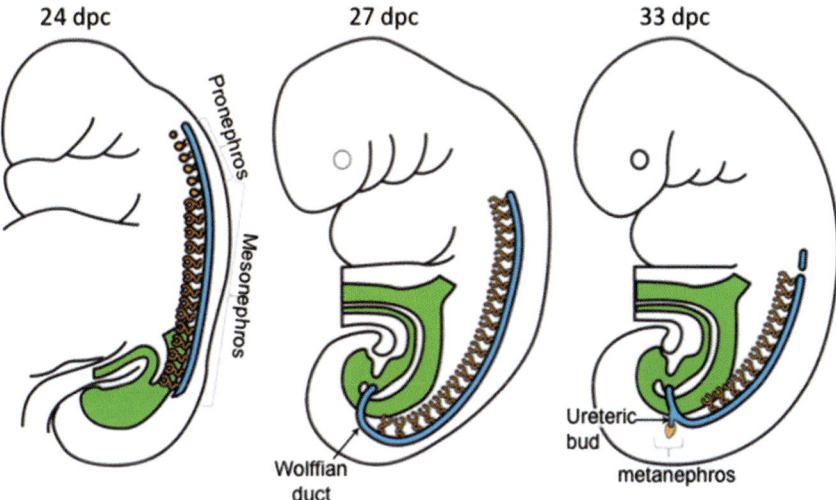

Fig. 2.1 Three phases of human kidney development between 24 and 33 days postconception (dpc). The pronephros, which develops in the upper thorax, consists of simple tubules connected to the pronephric duct which elongates caudally stimulating mesonephric glomeruli and tubules. This area is renamed the mesonephros and the duct becomes the mesonephric or Wolffian duct. Ongoing duct migration reaches the cloaca and the ureteric bud then branches from it into metanephric mesenchyme to form the metanephros. The latter will generate the definitive adult kidney, while more proximal pro- and mesonephric segments degenerate completely (aside from small contributions to the male urogenital system)

ric tubules develop alongside it. Caudal extension is accompanied by complete degeneration of nephrotomes and the pronephric part of the duct by day 25.

The mesonephros develops from around 24 days of gestation, comprising the craniocaudal duct and tubule-like structures. The mesonephric duct initially lacks a lumen, but this forms in a reverse caudocranial direction after fusion with the cloaca. Mesonephric tubules develop from intermediate mesoderm by 'mesenchymal to epithelial' transformation, a process which is subsequently reiterated in metanephric development. Approximately 40 mesonephric tubules are produced (several per somite), but synchronous cranial regression and caudal development means that there are never more than 30 pairs at any one time. The tubules contain segments analogous to those in the mature kidney including a vascularized glomerulus and proximal and distal tubules and are believed to produce small quantities of urine between weeks 6 and 10 (based on analogy with other large mammals). The mesonephros involutes during the third month of gestation, although caudal segments contribute to male urogenital structures including the epididymis, seminal vesicle, and ejaculatory duct.

The metanephros, the precursor to the mature human kidney, develops from around day 28. It consists of only two cell types at its inception: the epithelial cells of the ureteric bud and the mesenchyme cells of the metanephric mesenchyme. A series of reciprocal interactions between these tissues cause the ureteric bud to branch sequentially to form the ureter, renal pelvis, calyces, and collecting tubules, while mesenchymal cells either (1) undergo epithelial conversion to form the nephrons from glomerulus

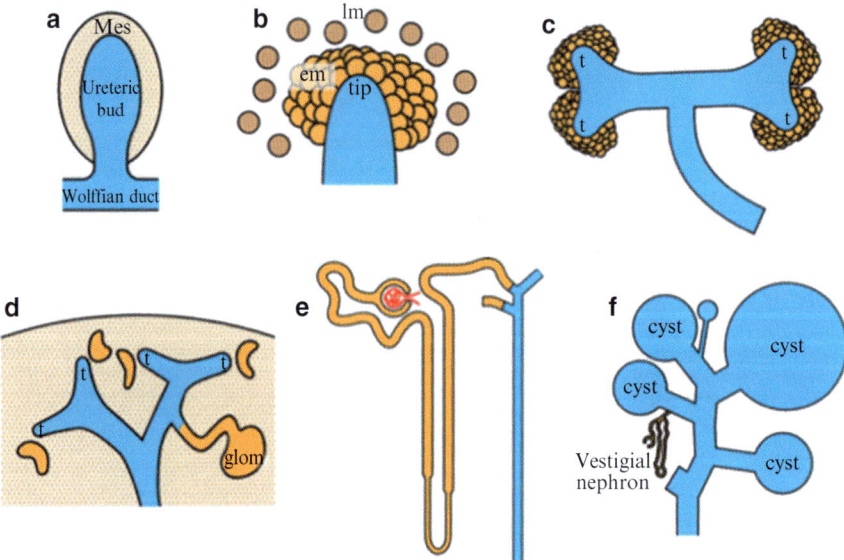

Fig. 2.2 Schematic of critical steps in metanephric development. (**a**) The first phase involves ingrowth of the epithelial ureteric bud (in *blue*) into the metanephric mesenchyme (in *white/orange*). (**b, c**) Mutual induction between the tip(s) of the ureteric bud and mesenchyme stimulates the bud to branch serially and the latter to delineate into two populations—the loose mesenchyme (lm) retains its phenotype and will form the stroma of the adult kidney, while cells adjacent to the bud tips compact and condense (cm) then undergo epithelial conversion. (**d, e**) These newly formed epithelia progress through vesicle, comma, and S-shaped stages as the nephron is formed. This includes glomerulus (glom) through distal tubule, which fuses with collecting ducts generated from repeated branching of the ureteric bud. (**f**) Dysplastic kidneys arise when induction fails or is incomplete; in the extreme case of multicystic dysplastic kidneys (MCDK), there are multiple cysts arising from ureteric structures and a few primitive, vestigial nephrons without any normal functioning renal tissue

to distal tubule or (2) give rise to interstitial cells (Fig. 2.2). Some mesenchymal cells also contribute to the renal vasculature.

The first phase of metanephric development occurs when the ureteric bud sprouts from the distal part of the mesonephric/Wolffian duct, and this penetrates the metanephric blastema, a specialized area of sacral intermediate mesenchyme (Fig. 2.2). The first glomeruli form by 8–9 weeks and nephrogenesis continues in the outer rim of the cortex until 34 weeks [8]. Nephrons elongate and continue to differentiate postnatally, but new nephrons are not formed. Similarly, nephrogenesis is completed before birth in most large mammals, but it must be noted that new nephrons are still formed for at least 7 days after birth in mice and rats which may confound some experimental analysis of kidney development.

Differentiation of the Ureteric Bud

The ureteric bud starts as a pseudostratified projection which grows into the metanephric blastema, becomes invested with mesenchyme, and begins to proliferate, extend, and branch, rapidly forming a polarized one-cell-thick epithelial tube. This process is contingent on mutual induction with the mesenchyme, and defects in either cell lineage can impair development. Branching occurs repeatedly, including exponential phases during nephrogenesis, hence generating a complex three-dimensional treelike collecting duct system. It is estimated that 18–20 rounds of branching occur in humans, but, in a similar fashion to pronephric and mesonephric structures, many of the early generations do not persist long term: it is difficult to be precise because of the scarcity of human fetal material, but Potter estimated that the first three to five generations are remodeled to form the renal pelvis while the next three to five give rise to the minor calyces and papillae [8].

Epithelial Differentiation of Parts of the Mesenchyme

Each nephron develops from the subpopulations of mesenchymal cells induced to condense around the ampullary tip of each ureteric bud branch. The mesenchyme is initially loosely arranged, but those cells destined to become nephrons condense around the bud tips and undergo phenotypic transformation into epithelial renal vesicles. Each vesicle elongates to form a comma shape which folds back on itself to become an S-shaped body. The proximal S-shape develops into the glomerulus, while distal parts generate the remaining nephron from proximal convoluted tubule to distal segments. These latter parts fuse with the collecting ducts thus generating the first part of the functional urinary tract.

Stromal Differentiation of the Mesenchyme

Much of the original work on nephrogenesis disregarded stromal cells, viewing them as unimportant supporting tissues. Recent mice studies have shown that stromal signaling is essential for normal ureteric bud and nephron formation as well as renal patterning; indeed one study linked aberrant stroma to both intrinsic dysplasia and fused horseshoe kidneys [9]. Stroma also contributes to the renal microvasculature which is increasingly highlighted in renal diseases [10].

The Spectrum of Maldevelopment in CAKUT

The wide spectrum of malformations within CAKUT is well covered in pathology textbooks [11], but we will highlight the most important ones here. As nephrologists, we tend to divide these into malformations with an intrinsic defect in the kidney such as agenesis, dysplasia, or polycystic kidney disease (PKD) versus extrarenal pathologies such as posterior urethral valves or vesicoureteric reflux. This simplifies understanding, but we must recognize that this is an artificial distinction since there is often combined maldevelopment of the kidney and urinary tract at the same time leading to a synergistic impairment of renal function [12].

Based on the renal embryology outlined above, there are several key phases that should be considered in CAKUT including:

1. Initial 'setup' of the renal field via pronephric and mesonephric stages.
2. Outgrowth of the ureteric bud into the correct area of prespecified metanephric mesenchyme.
3. Mutual induction between epithelial cells in the bud and mesenchyme that:

   • Cause the bud to branch repeatedly with each tip inducing new mesenchymal condensates
   • Induce mesenchyme to epithelial conversion which generates nephrons
   • Promote stromal patterning and microvasculature

Later stages include differentiation of segment specific cells and elongation and growth of tubules and the collecting systems. These may also be affected in CAKUT, but they are unlikely to have such a large impact on renal function in childhood because they affect nephron structure rather than nephron number.

Absent Kidneys: Agenesis or Aplasia

These result in the same thing, a missing kidney, but they have a different etiology—agenesis is a primary defect with aberrant initiation of the pronephros-mesonephros sequence and/or failure of ureteric bud outgrowth. In contrast, renal aplasia occurs when kidneys were initially induced but failed to progress through nephrogenesis and then involuted. Aplasia includes multicystic dysplastic kidneys (MCDK), since at least two thirds of these involute eventually; hence, there may be no trace of cysts if assessed after that point. Absence of both kidneys is rare at 1:7,000 to 1:10,000 births with a slight male bias. These babies usually die at birth with the Potter Sequence of anhydramnios-defective lung maturation-respiratory insufficiency, along with limb and face deformities. Lack of one kidney is commoner, affecting 1:1,000 individuals and affects both genders equally. Intriguingly, the left kidney is more often missing; no one knows why but there is slightly different timing of nephrogenesis on each side which may be important. Uncomplicated unilateral agenesis is increasingly detected on antenatal ultrasound; otherwise it may be silent because the other kidney can compensate if normal. Around half of cases have an associated urogenital anomaly when investigated. The commonest is vesicoureteric reflux (VUR), but others include contralateral renal dysplasia, absence of vas deference (perhaps indicating aberrant mesonephric develoment), absent adrenals, and pelvic renal ectopy. Bilateral or unilateral renal agenesis accompanies many syndromes such as the branchio-oto-renal syndrome, renal cysts and diabetes syndrome (RCAD) and the hypoparathyroidism, hypoparathyroidism, sensorineural deafness and renal disease syndrome (HDR), Fanconi's anemia, and Fraser, Kallmann, Di George, and Smith-Lemli-Opitz syndromes.

Dysplasia

Dysplastic kidneys fail to undergo normal differentiation; they usually accomplish phases 1 and 2 above, but there is disruption of the critical third phase (see genetics, obstructions, and teratogen section for causes). The dysplastic kidney can be either larger or smaller than normal and diffusely or partly cystic [2]. Diagnosis is routinely assigned on the basis of renal ultrasound although, in the strictest terms, it can only be made definitively by histology. Characteristic features include disrupted organization of normal nephrons, abundance of undifferentiated cells, thick vessels, metaplastic cartilage, and primitive, poorly branched ducts with smooth muscle collars. Cartilage is pathognomic but only present in around a third of cases. The extreme case is a multicystic dysplastic kidney (MCDK) where all of the renal parenchyma is replaced by cysts and poorly differentiated interstitial tissues, i.e., there is no functioning renal tissue. Such kidneys are often attached to an atretic ureter, raising the possibility of early pathology at the time of bud outgrowth and ureteric development. Dysplasia can occur as an isolated anomaly or in a multiorgan syndrome, such as RCAD.

Unilateral dysplasia is more common than bilateral, and coexisting abnormalities of the urinary tract occur in 50–75 % of patients, particularly renal ectopias such as horseshoe kidney, ureteral duplication, hydroureters, UPJ and UVJ obstruction, and vesicoureteric reflux. Prognosis is poor for bilateral dysplasias because they have an intrinsic nephron deficit, with severity ranging from the lethal Potter's sequence, through neonatal renal failure to later CKD. Conversely, children with unilateral dysplasia generally do well, with prognosis dependent on severity of coexisting anomalies. Historically, dysplastic kidneys were removed surgically because of case reports linking them to hypertension and Wilms' tumors. However, over 70 % of MCDK will eventually involute and disappear without intervention, as will a significant proportion of non-cystic dysplastic kidneys, and the systematic reviews conducted thus far do not substantiate these risks [13].

Hypoplasia

Hypoplastic kidneys are defined as (1) weighing less than 50 % of the normal mean for age and (2) lacking any primary histological abnormality—they may contain significantly fewer nephrons, but the formed nephrons appear normal and there are no undifferentiated tissues. In one variant, oligomeganephronia, both glomeruli and tubules are significantly enlarged [14]. Hypoplasia may be isolated or part of a wider malformation syndrome such as the renal coloboma syndrome. In theory, one should have detailed histologic examination of the kidney to exclude evidence of dysplasia before labeling as hypoplasia, but this is often not done if renal architecture looks normal (albeit in a small kidney) on ultrasound because of worries about the morbidity of biopsying a small kidney.

Table 2.1 Initial nephron number in CAKUT and renal diseases

Intrinsic renal conditions	Initial nephron number (100–0 %)	Range within extrarenal CAKUT spectrum			
• ADPKD					Vesicoureteric reflux
• ARPKD				Horseshoe kidneys	
• Nephronophthisis			Duplex kidneys		
• RCAD		Posterior urethral valves			
• Bardet-Biedl					
• (Cystic) dysplastic					
• MCDK					
• Agenesis					

Variants on hypoplasia include the small kidneys associated with low birth weight and prematurity, which are linked to low nephron number and increased risk of hypertension, proteinuria, and kidney disease in later life (Table 2.1) [15]. One component here may be the antenatal steroids given to stimulate lung development before premature birth—these are necessary to save the baby's life, but there is experimental animal evidence that high-dose corticosteroids halt or seriously retard nephrogenesis too. Bilateral small kidneys are occasionally seen in children with multiple congenital malformations, Down's syndrome, or long-standing disease or anomalies of the central nervous system. These may represent a failure of renal growth, rather than an intrinsic defect in early nephrogenesis.

Cystic Kidney Diseases and Ciliopathies

Renal cysts can develop at any stage of life, ranging from in utero through late adulthood. A key distinction between different conditions relating to CAKUT, however, is whether the cysts arise during kidney development or after the full nephron complement has been reached. Multicystic dysplastic kidneys clearly combine cysts and severe perturbation of early nephrogenesis (see panel f in Fig. 2.2). In contrast, most polycystic kidney disease (PKD) and the new group of diseases called ciliopathies (including Bardet-Biedl syndromes and nephronophthisis which have molecular defects in components of the primary cilium [16]) have relatively normal early development, then cysts develop later, i.e., there is a secondary, induced nephron defect so we will not consider them as CAKUT here.

Other CAKUT

There are many other parts of the spectrum including structural and functional lower urinary tract flow disruption (such as obstruction and reflux), ectopia, and renal fusion. To avoid repetition, these are considered in other parts of the book.

Intrinsic Nephron Number: A Key Concept in CAKUT

Functional renal mass is lost as all renal conditions progress through the CKD stages, but there is a fundamental difference at onset between CAKUT and diseases of the more mature kidney—the former start with the handicap of a reduced nephron number, particularly with intrinsic renal maldevelopment. Therefore, these children have less functional reserve and will show signs of CKD at earlier disease stages. The extreme examples are MCDK which have very low or zero functional nephrons versus conditions such as PKD and nephronophthisis where initial nephron count may be normal; nephrons are then lost as a secondary effect when cysts, inflammation, and fibrosis destroy normal functioning tissues.

The same principles apply to the extrarenal CAKUT spectrum, but these conditions tend to be more variable. The best example here is boys with posterior urethral valves where some have major disruption with very few functioning nephrons leading to renal failure form birth, while others have minimal initial perturbation. It is likely that all of these conditions have some deficit in nephron number, even when initial examination and blood tests are normal. Measurement of "functional" renal size may help predict how quickly CKD will progress [7], but it would be prudent to arrange lifelong renal follow-up in all of these cases.

Underlying Pathogenesis of CAKUT: Known Unknowns

There have been major advances in understanding the genetic and molecular pathogenesis of CAKUT over the last 20 years, with new causes being reported almost weekly [17]. It is striking that even with this increased knowledge, however, that less than a third of cases have been linked to gene mutations, which points to either inadequacies in current technologies or an (as yet) unfathomably complex interaction between genes, environment, and stochastic factors that we may never understand. We will briefly consider some of the most important molecular pathways identified thus far, along with the importance of obstruction and maternal dietary factors.

Important Genetic Factors in CAKUT

1. Regulating ureteric outgrowth and bud branching—The GDNF/RET system. Precise temporospatial control of ureteric bud outgrowth involves a large number of factors, but most function by regulating glial cell line-derived neurotrophic factor (GDNF) and its receptor Ret [18]. Both are expressed in the developing urogenital tract, genetic ablation abrogates metanephric development completely or causes severe dysplasia, and dysregulation can cause multiple ureters. One of the negative regulators is the SLIT2-ROBO pathway, and human mutations in this system have recently been implicated in cystic dysplastic kidneys, unilateral renal agenesis, and duplicated collecting system [19].

2. Mesenchymal-epithelial conversion—The PAX–EYA–SIX transcription cascade. PAX genes are well preserved from *Drosophila*, through zebrafish to human. Controlled expression of PAX2 is mandatory for normal kidney development and there is a direct correlation between expression and kidney phenotype [20]. PAX2 mutations cause the 'renal-coloboma' syndrome with optic nerve colobomas, renal anomalies, and vesicoureteric reflux [21], while polymorphisms with reduced PAX2 expression are associated with smaller kidneys inferred as having fewer nephrons [22]. PAX genes work in a functional cascade with SIX and EYA genes, and several of these have been linked to renal malformations including EYA1 in the branchio-oto-renal syndrome and SIX1 and SIX2 in familial CAKUT [23, 24].

3. Defective maturation and cysts—Hepatocyte nuclear factor (HNF) 1β. Mutations of the TCF2 gene, encoding the transcription factor hepatocyte nuclear factor 1β, cause the renal cysts and diabetes (RCAD) syndrome which is probably the major single cause of human congenital kidney malformations, accounting for up to a third of several antenatal presentations with 'bright' kidneys and 10 % of CAKUT overall [25]. Diverse renal malformations occur in RCAD, ranging from grossly cystic dysplastic kidneys, through hypoplasia with oligomeganephronia to apparent unilateral agenesis. Females may also have uterine abnormalities. An important issue is that cysts and diabetes can present at different times; hence, it is always worth asking at every appointment whether there have been any new diagnoses of diabetes since this may engender analysis for these mutations and gene deletions. We had one case of unexplained dysplasia where diabetes was not uncovered until the child was given steroids after renal transplantation.

Importance of Urinary Tract Obstruction in CAKUT

The second commonest cause of CKD5 in infancy is dysplasia brought on by urinary tract obstruction, particularly posterior urethral valves [4, 26]. Moreover, the most severely perturbed nephrogenesis seen in MCDK are classically reported to be connected to 'atretic' (i.e. obstructed) ureters. Experimental obstruction of the developing urinary tract has been known to generate typical morphology of renal malformations for over 40 years, and molecular analyses confirm similarities with human CAKUT [27].

Lower urinary tract issues are considered in detail elsewhere in this book, but it is worth noting that the pathology in human CAKUT contains a mixture of primary and secondary effects with a direct reduction in nephron number and later bladder dysfunction, which contributes to ongoing injury via ischemia and oxidative stress which promote proximal tubular cell death and interstitial fibrosis [28]. There are also conflicting data on whether correcting the obstruction is effective, with good results in large animals but poorer outcomes in mice and rats. The latter data are consistent with the generally poor results for in utero intervention to relieve obstruction in humans where shunting may improve perinatal survival but does not significantly improve the poor renal function [29].

Teratogens and Maternal Diet may Contribute to CAKUT

Many drugs and chemicals are teratogenic to the developing kidney [30]. They can be divided into two broad categories: exogenous factors such as drugs versus and endogenous factors which become teratogenic when present in abnormal quantities. An example of the former is the renin-angiotensin system: angiotensin-converting enzyme inhibitors and receptor blockers are prescribed to treat hypertension, but, when used during pregnancy, these can cause neonatal renal failure from a combination of hemodynamic compromise and renal tubular dysgenesis (along with skull malformations termed hypocalvaria). An example of the latter is retinoic acid, a natural metabolite of vitamin A, which perturbs nephrogenesis if depleted or in excess [31].

High glucose levels in diabetic mothers are associated with an increased incidence of kidney and lower urinary tract malformations, plus abnormalities in the nervous, cardiovascular, and skeletal systems [32]. This may not be a direct effect on the kidney, however, since diabetes is associated with caudal regression syndrome in the fetus which might clearly affect the lower urinary tract. It is also possible that some CAKUT cases ascribed to maternal diabetes had HNF1β mutations as reported in the RCAD syndrome above.

Maternal diet may have a more subtle effect on nephrogenesis, affecting nephron number without gross changes. This forms part of the 'Barker hypothesis' based on epidemiological data suggesting that fetal life programs the child for later diseases: individuals born to mothers with poor diets are much more likely to develop hypertension, cardiovascular disease, and diabetes in adulthood, and this has been ascribed to reduced nephron member [6, 33]. Clearly, dietary effects may be multiplied in CAKUT where there is already a nephron deficit.

References

1. Woolf AS, Price KL, Scambler PJ, Winyard PJ. Evolving concepts in human renal dysplasia. J Am Soc Nephrol. 2004;15:998–1007.
2. Winyard P, Chitty LS. Dysplastic kidneys. Semin Fetal Neonatal Med. 2008;13:142–51.
3. Renkema KY, Winyard PJ, Skovorodkin IN, Levtchenko E, Hindryckx A, Jeanpierre C, et al. Novel perspectives for investigating congenital anomalies of the kidney and urinary tract (CAKUT). Nephrol Dial Transplant. 2011;26:3843–51.
4. Pruthi R, O'Brien C, Casula A, Braddon F, Lewis M, Maxwell H, et al. UK Renal Registry 16th annual report: chapter 7 demography of the UK paediatric renal replacement therapy population in 2012. Nephron Clin Pract. 2013;125:127–38.
5. Puelles VG, Bertram JF. Counting glomeruli and podocytes: rationale and methodologies. Curr Opin Nephrol Hypertens. 2015;24:224–30.
6. Luyckx VA, Brenner BM. Birth weight, malnutrition and kidney-associated outcomes-a global concern. Nat Rev Nephrol. 2015;11:135–49.
7. Matsell DG, Cojocaru D, Matsell EW, Eddy AA. The impact of small kidneys. Pediatr Nephrol. 2015, 30:1501-9.
8. Potter EL. Normal and abnormal development of the kidney. Chicago, IL: Year Book Medical Publishers Inc.; 1972.
9. Hum S, Rymer C, Schaffer C, Bushnell D, Sims-Lucas S. Ablation of the renal stroma defines its critical role in nephron progenitor and vasculature patterning. PLoS One. 2014;9(2):e88400. doi:10.1371/journal.pone.0088400.eCollection2014.
10. Huang JL, Woolf AS, Kolatsi-Joannou M, Baluk P, Sandford RN, Peters DJ, et al. Vascular endothelial growth factor C for polycystic kidney diseases. J Am Soc Nephrol. 2015, pii: ASN.2014090856.
11. Jennette JC, Olson JL, Silva FG, D'agati VD. Heptinstall's pathology of the kidney. 7th Edition, 2015. Wolters Kluwer, Philadelpia, USA. ISBN 978-1-4511-4411-6.
12. Pope JC, Brock III JW, Adams MC, Stephens FD, Ichikawa I. How they begin and how they end: classic and new theories for the development and deterioration of congenital anomalies of the kidney and urinary tract, CAKUT. J Am Soc Nephrol. 1999;10:2018–28.
13. Narchi H. Risk of Wilms' tumour with multicystic kidney disease: a systematic review. Arch Dis Child. 2005;90:147–9.
14. Salomon R, Tellier AL, Attie-Bitach T, Amiel J, Vekemans M, Lyonnet S, et al. PAX2 mutations in oligomeganephronia. Kidney Int. 2001;59:457–62.
15. Luyckx VA, Bertram JF, Brenner BM, Fall C, Hoy WE, Ozanne SE, et al. Effect of fetal and child health on kidney development and long-term risk of hypertension and kidney disease. Lancet. 2013;382:273–83.
16. Arts HH, Knoers NV. Current insights into renal ciliopathies: what can genetics teach us? Pediatr Nephrol. 2013;28:863–74.
17. Hwang DY, Dworschak GC, Kohl S, Saiswat P, Vivante A, Hilger AC, et al. Mutations in 12 known dominant disease-causing genes clarify many congenital anomalies of the kidney and urinary tract. Kidney Int. 2014;85:1429–33.
18. Constantini F. GDNF/Ret signaling and renal branching morphogenesis: from mesenchymal signals to epithelial cell behaviors. Organogenesis. 2010;6:252–62.

19. Hwang DY, Kohl S, Fan X, Vivante A, Chan S, Dworschak GC, et al. Mutations of the SLIT2-ROBO2 pathway genes SLIT2 and SRGAP1 confer risk for congenital anomalies of the kidney and urinary tract. Hum Genet. 2015;134:905–16.
20. Harshman LA, Brophy PD. PAX2 in human kidney malformations and disease. Pediatr Nephrol. 2012;27:1265–75. doi:10.1007/s00467-011-2053-0. Epub 2011 Dec 3.
21. Sanyanusin P, Schimmentl LA, Mcnoe LA, Ward TA, Pierpoint MEM, Sullivan MJ, et al. Mutations of the PAX2 gene in a family with optic nerve colobomas, renal anomalies and vesicoureteral reflux. Nat Genet. 1995;9:358–64.
22. Quinlan J, Lemire M, Hudson T, Qu H, Benjamin A, Roy A, et al. A common variant of the PAX2 gene is associated with reduced newborn kidney size. J Am Soc Nephrol. 2007;18:1915–21.
23. Ruf RG, Xu PX, Silvius D, Otto EA, Beekmann F, Muerb UT, et al. SIX1 mutations cause branchio-oto-renal syndrome by disruption of EYA1-SIX1-DNA complexes. Proc Natl Acad Sci U S A. 2004;101:8090–5.
24. Weber S, Taylor JC, Winyard P, Baker KF, Sullivan-Brown J, Schild R, et al. SIX2 and BMP4 mutations associate with anomalous kidney development. J Am Soc Nephrol. 2008;19:891–903.
25. Raaijmakers A, Corveleyn A, Devriendt K, Van Tienoven TP, Allegaert K, Van Dyck M, et al. Criteria for HNF1B analysis in patients with congenital abnormalities of kidney and urinary tract. Nephrol Dial Transplant. 2015;30:835–42.
26. Penna FJ, Elder JS. CKD and bladder problems in children. Adv Chronic Kidney Dis. 2011;18:362–9.
27. Yang SP, Woolf AS, Quinn F, Winyard PJD. Deregulation of renal transforming growth factor-$\beta1$ after experimental short-term ureteric obstruction in fetal sheep. Am J Pathol. 2001;159:109–17.
28. Chevalier RL. Congenital urinary tract obstruction: the long view. Adv Chronic Kidney Dis. 2015;22:312–9.
29. Morris RK, Malin GL, Quinlan-Jones E, Middleton LJ, Hemmingh K, Burke D, et al. Percutaneous vesicoamniotic shunting versus conservative management for fetal lower urinary tract obstruction (PLUTO): a randomised trial. Lancet. 2013;382:1496–506.
30. Shepard TH. Catalog of teratogenic agents, Baltimore, MD: The Johns Hopkins University Press, 2010
31. Lee LM, Leung CY, Tang WW, Choi HL, Leung YC, McCaffery PJ, et al. A paradoxical teratogenic mechanism for retinoic acid. Proc Natl Acad Sci U S A. 2012;109:13668–73.
32. Woolf AS. Environmental influences on renal tract development: a focus on maternal diet and the glucocorticoid hypothesis. Klin Padiatr. 2011;223 Suppl 1:S10–7.
33. Fisher RE, Steele M, Karrow NA. Fetal programming of the neuroendocrine-immune system and metabolic disease. J Pregnancy. 2012;2012:792934. doi:10.1155/2012/792934.

Chapter 3
Congenital Anomalies of the Kidney: Number, Position, Rotation, and Vasculature

Paul H. Smith III and John H. Makari

Abbreviations

AVF	Arteriovenous fistula
CAKUT	Congenital anomalies of the kidney and urinary tract
CT	Computed tomography
DMSA	Dimercaptosuccinic acid
GDNF	Glial-derived neurotrophic factor
GFR	Glomerular filtration rate
IMA	Inferior mesenteric artery
MAG3	Mercaptoacetyltriglycine
MCDK	Multicystic dysplastic kidney
MR	Magnetic resonance
MRKH	Mayer-Rokitansky-Küster-Hauser syndrome
UPJ	Ureteropelvic junction
VCUG	Voiding cystourethrogram
VUR	Vesicoureteral reflux

A broad spectrum of developmental abnormalities of the genitourinary tract is known to occur within the pediatric population (Table 3.1). Given the complex

P.H. Smith III, M.D.
Division of Urology, University of Connecticut School of Medicine, Farmington, CT, USA

Division of Urology, Connecticut Children's Medical Center, Hartford, CT, USA

J.H. Makari, M.D., F.A.A.P., F.A.C.S. (✉)
Connecticut Children's Medical Center, Hartford, CT, USA

Departments of Urology and Pediatrics, University of Connecticut School of Medicine, Farmington, CT, USA
e-mail: jmakari@connecticutchildrens.org

© Springer International Publishing Switzerland 2016
A.J. Barakat, H. Gil Rushton (eds.), *Congenital Anomalies of the Kidney and Urinary Tract*, DOI 10.1007/978-3-319-29219-9_3

Table 3.1 Congenital
anomalies of the kidney

Congenital anomalies of the kidney
Anomalies of number
Renal agenesis
• Bilateral renal agenesis
• Unilateral renal agenesis
Functionally solitary kidney
• Multicystic dysplastic kidney
Supernumerary Kidney
Anomalies of position, fusion, rotation
• Malrotation
• Renal ectopia
Fusion anomalies
• Horseshoe kidney
• Crossed-fused ectopia
Anomalies of vasculature
• Multiple, accessory, and aberrant vessels
• Renal artery aneurysm
• Renal arteriovenous fistula

developmental process of the genitourinary system, it is not surprising that abnormalities of the genitourinary tract are among the most common congenital anomalies. Collectively, congenital anomalies of the kidney and urinary tract (CAKUT) occur in approximately 1 in 500 live births [1]. CAKUT represent a diverse group of anomalies with varying clinical implications; however, taken together, CAKUT are of great clinical significance as they encompass the most common causes of renal failure in children [1].

Anatomy and Embryology

Appreciation of normal genitourinary anatomy and embryology provides an essential framework to understanding conditions of anomalous renal development. The start of renal development is heralded by the formation of the nephric duct from the intermediate mesoderm on gestational day 22. Two transient primitive kidneys, the pronephros and mesonephros, develop sequentially in the mesoderm adjacent to the nephric duct. The pronephros is a vestigial structure, which provides no excretory renal function. The mesonephros, on the contrary, does provide transient renal function prior to its regression. Both pronephros and mesonephros regress and, ultimately, do not provide any structural contribution to the final renal system [1, 2].

During the fourth gestational week, the nephric duct gives rise to the ureteric bud, which invades the adjacent metanephric mesenchyme to initiate the development of the definitive, or metanephric, kidney. This process is orchestrated via highly regulated reciprocal interactions between the ureteric bud and metanephric mesenchyme. As the ureteric bud grows into the metanephric mesenchyme, it undergoes dichotomous branching to give rise to the ureter, pelvicalyceal system, and collecting ducts. The remaining stromal and epithelial components of the kidney are derived from the metanephric mesenchyme [1–3].

At the molecular level, branching of the ureteric bud is mediated by glial-derived neurotrophic factor (GDNF), which is secreted by the metanephric mesenchyme. GDNF interacts with RET receptor tyrosine kinase expressed on the ureteric bud to induce branching of the ureteric bud. The GDNF-RET pathway is influenced by multiple regulatory transcription and growth factors that augment local expression and activity of GDNF in the metanephric mesenchyme.

Development and propagation of a single ureteric bud is achieved through spatial restriction of GDNF expression to the caudal portion of the Wolffian duct and through modulation of Wolffian duct sensitivity to GDNF. GDNF expression in the metanephric mesenchyme is closely regulated through numerous molecular mediators including Eya1, Pax2, Six1, Six2, and Six4 [1]. Several molecular mechanisms prevent development and propagation of more than one ureteric buds. For example, SLIT2 and ROBO2 signaling pathways provide negative regulation of the GDNF-RET pathway by inhibiting GDNF expression outside of the caudal mesenchyme. Additionally, SPRY1 expression reduces the sensitivity of the Wolffian duct to GDNF, thereby preventing outgrowth of multiple ureteric buds [4, 5].

The epithelial components of the nephron are derived from the metanephric mesenchyme through the process of mesenchymal-epithelial transformation. This process is similarly mediated through interactions between the ureteric bud and metanephric mesenchyme. Key molecular mediators that orchestrate mesenchymal-epithelial transformation include the WNT proteins WNT9b and WNT4 and FGF8 [3].

The developing metanephric kidney originates within the pelvis. During the course of its development, the kidney ascends to its final location in the retroperitoneum at a vertebral level of approximately T12–L3. Renal ascent typically completed by the eighth week of gestation. During the process of ascent, the kidney rotates medially 90° [6]. The ascending kidney has a dynamic vascular supply during the course of its ascent, which drives from the adjacent common iliac or aortic segment. Progressively craniad aortic branches develop to supply the kidney at its current level, while more caudal branches regress [7]. The persistence of caudal arterial branches results in multiple renal vessels.

Anomalies of Number

Situations in which there is congenital absence of renal tissue, either unilateral or, less commonly, bilateral, represent the most common anomalies of renal number. In rare instances, an accessory, or supernumerary, kidney may be encountered. As discussed above, multiple molecular mechanisms are in place to ensure development and propagation of a single ureteric bud, which interacts with the ipsilateral metanephric mesenchyme to induce the formation of a single ipsilateral metanephric kidney. Abnormalities in any of these processes may result in absent, abortive, or abnormal renal development.

Renal Agenesis

Renal agenesis describes a condition in which the metanephric kidney fails to develop as a consequence of aberrations in the reciprocal interaction between the ureteric bud and the metanephric mesenchyme. Technically, renal agenesis should be distinguished from other causes of congenital absence of the kidney, such as the multicystic kidney that has undergone involution.

Renal agenesis may occur as an isolated finding or, commonly, in association with other anomalies or syndromic conditions. The spectrum of genetic aberrations leading to renal agenesis appears to be diverse and is still incompletely characterized. Because of the critical roles of GDNF and RET in the coordinated interaction between the ureteric bud and metanephric mesenchyme, genetic mutations impacting this pathway have been postulated to be important causes for renal agenesis. Indeed, mutations in RET are well described in human cases of non-syndromic unilateral renal agenesis; however, specific mutations in the GDNF gene do not appear to be a common cause of renal agenesis [8]. Myriad mutations in genes known to be involved in the renal development pathway, including WT1, HNF1β, PAX2, SALL1, SIX1, and EYA1, have been reported in association with syndromic renal agenesis [9].

Bilateral Renal Agenesis

Development of functional renal tissue plays an essential role in the fetal development of multiple organ systems. In particular, fetal urine production maintains appropriate amniotic fluid levels necessary to promote pulmonary development. Bilateral renal agenesis and other conditions in which functional renal tissue fails to develop are incompatible with life and often lead to fetal demise. Infants born with bilateral renal agenesis generally perish shortly after birth secondary to renal failure and pulmonary hypoplasia resulting from severe oligohydramnios. Bilateral renal agenesis occurs less commonly than unilateral renal agenesis, with an incidence of approximately 1 in 10,000 and is nearly twice as common in males [10]. Clinically, a diagnosis of bilateral renal agenesis is often made from prenatal sonographic findings of bilateral absence of renal tissue, severe oligohydramnios, and non-visualization of the bladder. It is believed that fetal urine production plays an important role in normal bladder development and, in its absence, the bladder fails to form. Additionally, other congenital anomalies are frequently seen in association with bilateral renal agenesis. Anomalies of nearly all major organ systems have been reported in patients with bilateral renal agenesis; however, the most consistently reported associated anomalies involve the genital tract, skeletal, cardiothoracic, and gastrointestinal systems. It is not surprising that mutations involving the GDNF-RET pathway are the most commonly identified genetic causes of bilateral renal agenesis [10].

Bilateral absence of functional renal tissue may also result from renal dysplasia, cystic dysplasia, and severe hypoplasia. Notably, it has been shown that combinations of these conditions may occur in an individual patient [10]. This suggests that discrete genetic mutations responsible for abnormal renal development do not necessarily result in a predictable phenotype.

Unilateral Renal Agenesis

Unilateral renal agenesis is thought to occur in approximately 1 in 1000–3000 live births [9]. There is a slight predilection for the left side and a nearly twofold higher incidence in males than in females [9]. Unless detected on prenatal ultrasonography, isolated unilateral renal agenesis may go undiagnosed early in life as patients are generally asymptomatic and physical exam findings may be absent or subtle. Historically, the diagnosis of unilateral renal agenesis is one that was often made as an incidental finding on imaging obtained as part of the diagnostic evaluation of other conditions. In the present era, the routine use of prenatal ultrasonography has allowed for better characterization of the natural history of unilateral renal agenesis and related conditions in utero. It is now apparent that a subset of patients previously presumed to have unilateral renal agenesis may actually have had a multicystic dysplastic kidney, which involuted prior to initial imaging [11].

Unilateral renal agenesis may occur in isolation or, commonly, in association with other congenital genitourinary and non-genitourinary anomalies. Anomalies of the contralateral kidney and collecting system have been reported to occur in 32–50 % of patients with unilateral renal agenesis. The most common abnormality affecting the contralateral kidney is vesicoureteral reflux, which occurs in approximately 24 % of patients with unilateral renal agenesis. Other less common associated urinary tract anomalies include ureteropelvic junction obstruction (6 %), megaureter (7 %), and duplicated collecting system (3 %) [9].

Ipsilateral genital duct anomalies are commonly seen in association with unilateral renal agenesis. Wolffian duct abnormalities, including congenital absence of the ipsilateral vas deferens, seminal vesicle, or epididymis, may occur in nearly 70 % of cases [12]. Conversely, the incidence of unilateral renal agenesis in males with congenital absence of the vas deferens is only approximately 11 % if bilateral and 26 % if unilateral [13]. Similarly, Müllerian duct anomalies are common in females with unilateral renal agenesis. During development of the female genital tract, the caudal portions of the Müllerian ducts fuse in the midline to give rise to the uterus and proximal two thirds of the vagina, while the more craniad portions remain unfused at the fallopian tubes. Anomalous Müllerian duct development may result in unicornuate, bicornuate, or didelphic uterus, duplication of the cervix or vagina, or complete uterine or proximal vaginal agenesis. Such Müllerian duct anomalies may occur in more than one third of females with unilateral renal agenesis [14]. Additionally, unilateral renal agenesis is often a component of the Mayer-Rokitansky-Küster-Hauser (MRKH) syndrome, a rare condition affecting approximately 1 in every 4–5000 females, which is characterized by a normal 46, XX karyotype and variable degrees of Müllerian duct agenesis. Renal anomalies, of which unilateral renal agenesis is the most common, are identified in 40–60 % of patients with MRKH [15].

Approximately one in three individuals with unilateral renal agenesis will have associated non-genitourinary anomalies. The most common associated non-genitourinary anomalies involve the gastrointestinal, cardiac, and musculoskeletal systems [9].

Compensatory Hypertrophy and Long-Term Renal Outcomes

Compensatory hypertrophy, defined as a renal length greater than two standard deviations above the mean, is a phenomenon commonly observed in patients with a congenitally solitary kidney. Although the mechanism driving compensatory hypertrophy is not well understood, it is hypothesized to occur as a response during fetal development to partially counter the globally decreased nephron endowment associated with an absent contralateral kidney [16].

Longitudinal series evaluating the long-term renal functional outcomes in patients with isolated unilateral renal agenesis are lacking. A recent meta-analysis of patients with unilateral renal agenesis demonstrated significant renal functional impairment as evidenced by a glomerular filtration rate (GFR) of <60 mL/min/1.73 m^2 in 10 % of patients [9]. The authors acknowledge that the majority of studies included in this meta-analysis evaluated pediatric patients and therefore may underestimate the incidence of renal injury in patients with unilateral renal agenesis as they enter adulthood. Another recent series identified renal injury in 37 % of 407 children with solitary functioning kidney. Renal injury was defined by the presence of hypertension, proteinuria, impaired GFR, and/or use of renoprotective medications. Of the 223 (55 %) patients with a congenital solitary functioning kidney, 99 patients carried a diagnosis of unilateral renal agenesis. The median time for development of renal injury was approximately 15 years. Furthermore, the authors note that evidence of renal injury was detected earlier among patients whose solitary functioning kidney did not achieve compensatory hypertrophy [17].

The hyperfiltration hypothesis was described by Brenner as an explanation for progressive renal injury resulting from a decreased overall number of nephrons [18]. According to this theory, individual glomeruli experience an increased filtration burden when the overall number of nephrons is decreased. The result is a cycle in which renal injury is induced by glomerular hypertension, which is further propagated as functional renal mass is reduced.

Taken together, the available data regarding the natural history of renal function in patients with congenital solitary functioning kidney would suggest that this condition is not universally benign. Thus, routine screening for hypertension and proteinuria, with intermittent assessment of renal function, into adulthood seems to be an advisable measure in this patient population. Serial sonographic follow-up of the solitary kidney to determine when or if compensatory hypertrophy is achieved may also serve as a valuable clinical metric in assessing an individual patient's risk for adverse long-term renal outcomes.

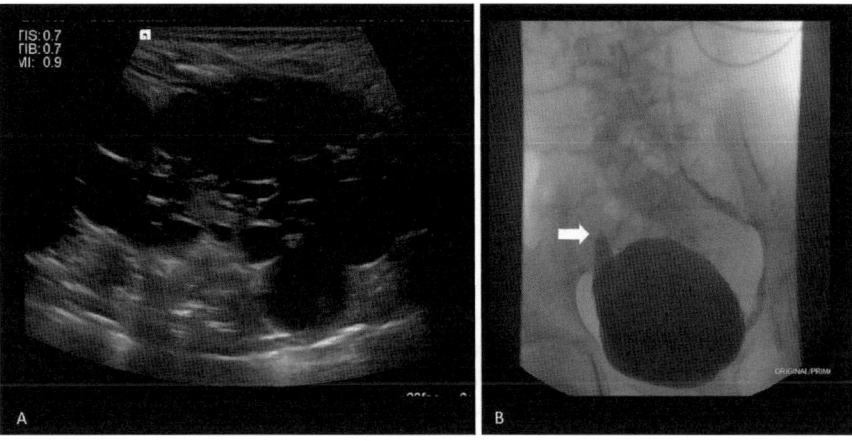

Fig. 3.1 Multicystic dysplastic kidney. (**A**) Renal sonogram demonstrating multiple cysts of variable sizes with no normal-appearing renal parenchyma. (**B**) Voiding cystourethrogram of a patient with right MCDK. Note that there is reflux into a blind-ending atretic right ureter (*arrow*) as well as reflux into the solitary left kidney

Multicystic Dysplastic Kidney

Multicystic dysplastic kidney (MCDK) is an anomaly of renal development, which is a common cause of congenital solitary functional kidney. It is estimated that MCDK occurs in approximately 1 in every 2400–4300 live births and occurs more frequently in males and on the left side [19]. The MCDK is composed of multiple noncommunicating cysts of various sizes and numbers, which replace all normal renal tissue (Fig. 3.1). By definition, no functional renal parenchyma is present, thereby making bilateral disease incompatible with life.

Grossly, the MCDK consists of multiple cysts separated by dysplastic stroma. The renal vessels are characteristically hypoplastic, and the ureter is atretic. A less common hydronephrotic variant has been described, in which a central cyst representing the renal pelvis is present [20].

MCDK is frequently cited as a common cause of abdominal mass in the newborn; however, in the present era of near-ubiquitous routine prenatal ultrasonography, the vast majority of MCDKs are detected in utero.

As with renal agenesis and other forms of renal dysplasia, aberrant interactions between the ureteric bud and the metanephric mesenchyme have been implicated in the pathogenesis of MCDK. Mutations in genes involved in ureteric bud-metanephric mesenchyme interaction, such as PAX2, EYA1, and SIX1, have been identified in various conditions of renal maldevelopment, including MCDK, and support the theory of aberrant bud-mesenchymal interactions as an etiology for MCDK [21]. Urinary obstruction secondary to ureteral atresia occurring in the early stages of renal development has also been proposed as a possible cause of MCDK [21].

A variety of associated urinary tract anomalies have been reported in conjunction with MCDK. The most common associated genitourinary anomaly is VUR into the contralateral kidney or the ipsilateral atretic ureter. VUR has been reported to occur in 15–28 % of patients with MCDK and is low grade in the majority of cases [22]. Ureteropelvic junction (UPJ) obstruction of the contralateral kidney has been reported in up to 15 % of patients with MCDK [21]. Many other urinary tract abnormalities have been reported in association with MCDK with lesser frequency including ureterocele, ureterovesical junction obstruction, and ureteral ectopia.

Risk of malignancy: Primary renal malignancies, typically Wilms' tumor and renal cell carcinoma, have been described to occur in the MCDK in rare instances. These anecdotal reports of malignant transformation in the MCDK have previously been used to rationalize nephrectomy in patients with MCDK. The risk of a Wilms' tumor developing in an MCDK has been estimated to be approximately 1 in 2000 based on a large series of 7500 Wilms' tumor samples collected by the National Wilms Tumor Study Pathology Center. All reported instances of Wilms' tumor developing in an MCDK have occurred before 4 years of age, and no cases of the tumor have been described to occur in the setting of an involuted MCDK [21]. Six cases of renal cell carcinoma developing in an MCDK have been described in the literature, which corresponds to a lower risk for renal cell carcinoma than in a normal kidney [22]. Therefore, the exceedingly low risk of malignant transformation of MCDK into Wilms' tumor or other primary renal malignancies argues against prophylactic extirpative management of the MCDK.

Involution: Involution of the MCDK is a well-described phenomenon. The timing and degree of involution are variable; however, the vast majority of MCDKs will involute to some degree over time. Variable rates of complete involution, ranging from 20 to 74 %, are reported in the literature. A large series reporting follow-up of patients with antenatally detected MCDK showed complete involution in 33 % at age 2 years, 47 % at age 5 years, and 59 % at age 10 years [23]. Additionally, complete in utero involution of MCDK is an increasingly recognized phenomenon.

Diagnosis: In the present era in which routine use of prenatal ultrasound has become the standard, the majority of congenital renal anomalies, including MCDK, are diagnosed prenatally. MCDK can typically be identified on prenatal ultrasonography after approximately 15 weeks gestation. The characteristic sonographic features include multiple noncommunicating cysts of variable sizes and numbers and absence of normal renal parenchyma or reniform shape. If MCDK is suspected on prenatal imaging, a confirmatory ultrasound should be obtained in the postnatal period.

Occasionally, a severely hydronephrotic kidney may masquerade as an MCDK. Distinguishing MCDK from an obstructed collecting system is of utmost importance as management of these two entities differs greatly. Traditionally, confirmatory nuclear renography (MAG3, DMSA) to demonstrate absence of ipsilateral function has been utilized to secure the diagnosis of the suspected MCDK. Recent reports have questioned the necessity of routine nuclear renography in all cases of suspected MCDK. In a recent series of 84 patients with a sonographic diagnosis of unilateral MCDK, a normal bladder, and no other major associated anomalies, nuclear renography confirmed absence of function in all patients [24]. The authors concluded that confirmatory nuclear renography is unnecessary in a healthy child with sonographically diagnosed unilateral MCDK and otherwise normal renal/bladder ultrasound.

VUR is the most common genitourinary abnormality associated with MCDK, with a reported incidence of 15–28 %. The ideal diagnostic and treatment approach for primary VUR remains an evolving and controversial topic. Due to the high incidence of VUR and potential for infection-induced scarring in a solitary kidney in patients with MCDK, VCUG is often recommended. The treatment of VUR in patients with MCDK is similar to that of primary VUR and is generally tailored according to the VUR grade and the presence or absence of breakthrough or recurrent urinary tract infection.

The vast majority of patients with MCDK are asymptomatic and may be safely managed conservatively. Similar to patients with unilateral renal agenesis, regular blood pressure monitoring and assessment for proteinuria are prudent for patients with MCDK. Renal sonography is a relatively inexpensive and noninvasive modality for surveillance of the MCDK. The rationale for obtaining serial imaging studies in patients with MCDK is to detect contralateral renal abnormalities and assess growth of the solitary kidney and involution of the MCDK. The ideal follow-up imaging protocol has not been established, but routine sonography after the first year is unnecessary in those MCDK demonstrating evidence of involution.

Supernumerary Kidney

Supernumerary kidney is a rare anomaly in which an extra or accessory kidney exists with independent vascular supply and collecting system (Fig. 3.2). Supernumerary kidney occurs more commonly on the left side and in males. The true incidence of supernumerary kidney is unknown; however, series indicating approximately 100 reported cases highlight the rarity of this condition [25]. The normal kidneys are typically in an orthotopic position with the supernumerary

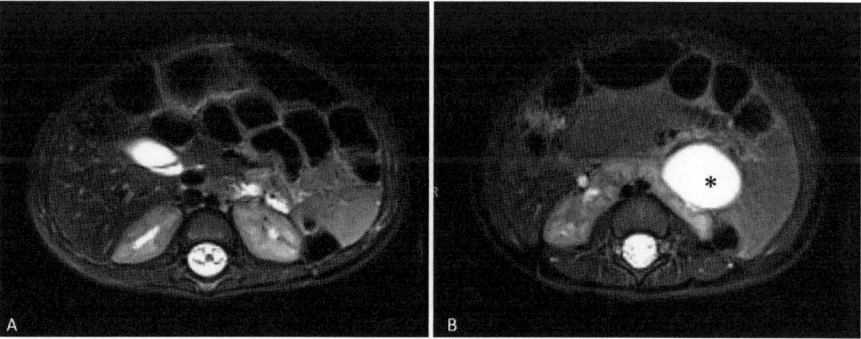

Fig. 3.2 MRI of patient with bilateral supernumerary kidneys. The normal kidneys are seen in an orthotopic position (**A**). The supernumerary kidneys are located caudal to the normal kidneys and are fused in a horseshoe configuration (**B**). The renal pelvis of left supernumerary kidney is dilated secondary to coexisting UPJ obstruction (*asterisk*)

kidney occupying a more caudal position. The supernumerary kidney often has a reniform morphology, but is frequently small.

Supernumerary kidney is generally diagnosed during the evaluation of flank pain, urinary tract infection, or hematuria. MR or CT excretory urography provides useful information in securing the diagnosis and clarifying the anatomy. Supernumerary kidneys are usually asymptomatic; thus, management is dictated by the presence of symptoms, function of the kidney, and associated anatomic abnormalities [26].

Abnormalities of Position, Rotation, and Fusion

Malrotation

Between the fourth and eighth weeks of gestation, the developing kidney ascends from the pelvis to its final retroperitoneal position adjacent to the second lumbar vertebra. The ascending kidney undergoes a 90° medial rotation along its longitudinal axis so that the final configuration of the normally positioned kidney is such that the renal pelvis is located in a medial position. Renal malrotation describes a situation in which the ascending kidney fails to undergo normal medial rotation. Autopsy series suggest that renal malrotation occurs in 1 in 939 individuals [27]. Often times, malrotation occurs as a component of anomalies of ascent and fusion, such as horseshoe kidney or pelvic kidney. Since rotation of the developing kidney occurs in an anteromedial direction, the most common configuration of the malrotated kidney is such that the renal pelvis is anteriorly located. Renal malrotation is often asymptomatic unless obstruction results from the abnormally configured collecting system. The diagnosis of renal malrotation may be confirmed on excretory or retrograde urography, which will demonstrate the calyces to project medial to the real pelvis.

Renal Ectopia

Renal ectopia refers to conditions in which the kidney is in an abnormal location and occurs with an incidence ranging between 1:500 and 1:1200. The possible sites of renal ectopia include pelvic, abdominal, and thoracic locations. Crossed ectopia discussed later in this chapter describes a kidney that crosses to the contralateral side of the body during its ascent. The most common variant of renal ectopia is the pelvic kidney (Fig. 3.3), which results from incomplete renal ascent. Morphologically, the pelvic kidney is frequently malrotated and may lack a reniform shape. As with horseshoe kidneys, the vascular supply to the pelvic kidney is generally abnormal and is derived from adjacent common iliac or aortic segments.

An increased incidence of other congenital anomalies, particularly those involving the urinary and genital systems, has been reported in individuals with ectopic kidney. The most common urinary tract abnormality associated with renal ectopia

Fig. 3.3 Pelvic kidney. The kidney is located adjacent to the bladder (*asterisk*)

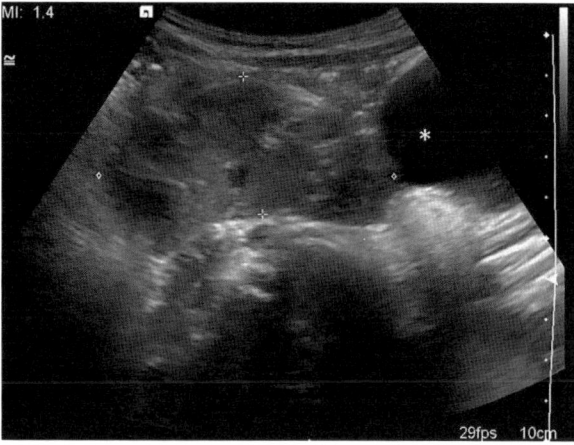

is VUR. In a report by Guarino et al. that evaluated associated urologic abnormalities in a large series of children with renal ectopia, VUR was identified in 26 % of patients with simple renal ectopia [28].

A variable incidence of UPJ obstruction in association with renal ectopia has been reported in the literature. Historic series have reported an incidence of UPJ obstruction as high as 33–52 % in symptomatic patients diagnosed with renal ectopia [29, 30]. The true incidence of UPJ obstruction in patients with renal ectopia may be lower than that reported in this select patient population, although it appears to be higher than that in the general population [28].

Presently, renal ectopia is most often detected on prenatal imaging studies or as an incidental finding on sonographic or cross-sectional imaging studies obtained for the evaluation of unrelated symptoms. Management of the patient with renal ectopia is generally directed according to symptoms and the presence of associated anomalies. Because of the increased incidence of VUR, evaluation with voiding cystourethrography may be considered for patients presenting with urinary tract infection or in infants and young children who were diagnosed on prenatal sonography. In patients presenting with nephrolithiasis associated with an ectopic kidney, formal metabolic evaluation is prudent as these patients are at risk for metabolic abnormalities that predispose to stone formation.

Renal Fusion Anomalies

Renal fusion anomalies refer to a subset of malformations in which the renal units are joined. The most common anomaly of renal fusion is horseshoe kidney, which occurs when kidneys are joined at poles by a common isthmus. This anomaly is identified in approximately 1 in 400–500 individuals and is nearly twice as common in males [31]. The embryogenesis of the horseshoe kidney is not completely understood. It is theorized that polar fusion of the left and right kidney occurs early during

Fig. 3.4 CT scan axial image showing a horseshoe kidney. The isthmus is located between the abdominal aorta (*large arrow*) and inferior mesenteric artery (*small arrow*). Both renal moieties are notably malrotated with anteriorly oriented renal pelves as is typical of the horseshoe kidney

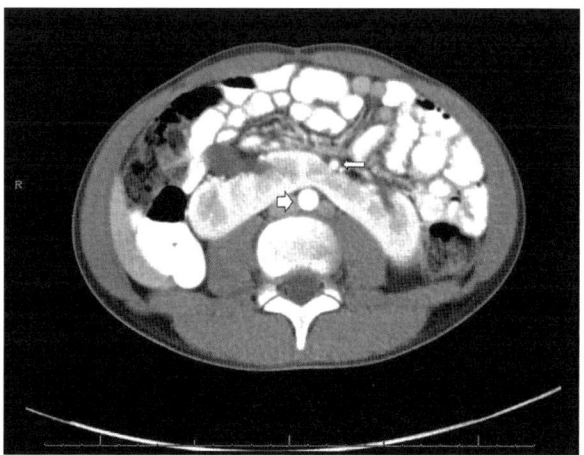

the development of the metanephric kidney. The left and right metanephric mesenchyme are in close proximity within the pelvis. If abutting, fusion of the poles may occur, thereby resulting in a horseshoe kidney.

Fusion occurs between the lower poles in 95 % of cases. The isthmus joining the two kidneys may be of variable compositions. In some instances, the isthmus is a relatively small fibrous structure, whereas in others it may be a more robust structure composed of functional renal parenchyma. During development, the isthmus of the ascending horseshoe kidney engages the inferior mesenteric artery at its junction with the abdominal aorta, thereby preventing normal ascent (Fig. 3.4). Therefore, horseshoe kidneys typically reside in an abnormal pelvic anatomic location with the isthmus situated at approximately the level of the 3rd to 5th lumbar vertebral body [31]. Additionally, fusion prohibits normal renal rotation during development, resulting in the renal pelves being anteriorly located in relation to the calyceal system. The proximal ureter typically courses over the anterior surface of the isthmus, which may result in UPJ obstruction. The renal vasculature of the horseshoe kidney is highly variable and is often complex. Arterial blood supply may originate from the abdominal aorta, inferior mesenteric artery, common iliac arteries, or combinations thereof. The isthmus commonly receives independent blood supply from the abdominal aorta. Additional accessory vessels may enter into the polar region of the kidney rather than the hilum [31, 32].

Etiology and Associated Congenital Anomalies/Syndromes

No specific genetic mutation has been identified as a cause for horseshoe kidney; however, horseshoe kidney is commonly seen in association with a variety of chromosomal and congenital anomalies. Associated congenital anomalies are present in approximately a third of patients, with skeletal, cardiovascular, neural tube, and anorectal anomalies being the most commonly associated findings. Horseshoe kidney is present in approximately 60 % of females with Turner's syndrome and 20 % of patients with trisomy 18.

Associated GU Anomalies

A variety of genitourinary anomalies have been described in association with horseshoe kidney. It has been suggested that more than half of patients with horseshoe kidney will have associated urinary tract anomalies with VUR occurring in up to 32 % of affected children [33–35].

The incidence of UPJ obstruction in the horseshoe kidney is estimated to be between 13 and 33 % [33, 36]. High insertion of the ureter on the renal pelvis is the most common cause of UPJ obstruction in the horseshoe kidney. Less commonly, obstruction may be due to the abnormal course of the ureter as it passes over the isthmus, congenital stricture, or as a complication of urolithiasis. UPJ obstruction of the horseshoe kidney is traditionally treated with dismembered pyeloplasty, sometimes in conjunction with isthmusectomy and nephropexy. Minimally invasive laparoscopic, robotic, and endoscopic treatments for UPJ obstruction of the horseshoe kidney are also described. Notably, division of the isthmus may not be necessary in all cases. Blanc et al. reported a series of 10 children who underwent successful laparoscopic pyeloplasty without division of the isthmus [37]. Preoperative imaging with CT or MR angiography provides valuable information regarding anomalous renal vasculature, which may be encountered during the procedure.

Individuals with horseshoe kidney are at particular risk for urolithiasis, which is reported in up to 60 % of patients [36]. Several factors contribute to stone formation in the horseshoe kidney, including infection, urinary stasis, or obstruction secondary to the abnormal anatomic configuration of the collecting system. Additionally, metabolic abnormalities that predispose to stone disease are present in most patients with horseshoe kidney and urolithiasis. Thus, metabolic evaluation is prudent in this subset of patients [36]. Surgical management of urolithiasis in the horseshoe kidney is similar to that in the anatomically normal kidney. The vast majority of stones may be successfully treated with minimally invasive techniques, including ureteroscopy, extracorporeal shockwave lithotripsy, percutaneous nephrolithotomy, or any combination thereof. Stone clearance following extracorporeal shockwave lithotripsy may be impaired by the abnormal anatomic configuration of the collecting system. Furthermore, targeting of stones for shockwave lithotripsy may prove challenging due to interference from the bony pelvis and vertebral column [36].

Risk of Malignancy

Development of primary renal malignancies in the horseshoe kidney is a phenomenon that has been well described in the literature. Renal cell carcinoma is the most commonly reported tumor of the horseshoe kidney; however, the incidence of renal cell carcinoma among patients with horseshoe kidney appears similar to that of the general population. Multiple series have indicated an increased risk of Wilms' tumor in the horseshoe kidney. Reports from the National Wilms Tumor Study Group suggest that there is approximately a two- to sevenfold increased risk for Wilms' tumor in the horseshoe kidney [38, 39]. In a review of 8617 patients enrolled in the National Wilms Tumor Study Group, 41 (0.48 %) patients had tumors arising in a horseshoe kidney [39]. Because of the slightly increased risk of Wilms' tumor, some advocate for use of sonographic screening for Wilms' tumor in children with horseshoe kidney once the diagnosis is made. Screening protocols utilize renal ultrasonography at 3–4-month intervals. Utilization of screening ultrasonography has shown to decrease stage of presentation when utilized in other high-risk patients, such as those with an aniridia or hemihypertrophy; however, a survival benefit has not clearly been shown [39]. Such a benefit has not been established in patients with a horseshoe kidney, and most pediatric urologists do not subscribe to long-term surveillance.

Diagnosis and Treatment

Horseshoe kidney is asymptomatic in the majority of cases and may be detected as an incidental finding on abdominal imaging studies obtained for other reasons. In children, the diagnosis is frequently made based on abnormalities detected on pre-natal ultrasonography. Among symptomatic patients, the most common complaints include urinary tract infection, abdominal pain, and gross hematuria. In young children newly diagnosed with horseshoe kidney or those with history of febrile urinary tract infection, a VCUG should be obtained due to the increased risk for VUR in this population. Females with horseshoe kidney and dysmorphic features consistent with Turner's syndrome should be evaluated with karyotype. Additional diagnostic measures should be tailored according to the patient's presenting symptoms and identification of associated anomalies. Diuretic renography is prudent in patients with clinical or radiographic features suggestive of UPJ obstruction. Patients presenting with urolithiasis should routinely be evaluated for metabolic abnormalities that may contribute to the development of urinary calculi.

Crossed-Fused Ectopia

Crossed-fused renal ectopia is the second most common anomaly of renal fusion. Crossed-fused ectopia describes a situation in which the kidney is localized on the opposite side of the body as that into which the ureter inserts into the bladder (Fig. 3.5). This anomaly is estimated to occur in approximately 1:1000–7500 with a male predominance of approximately 2–1. Left-to-right ectopia is the most common morphology. The crossed ectopic kidney is fused to the other kidney in approximately 90 % of cases. Although the exact embryologic mechanism leading to crossed-fused renal ectopia remains unclear, several theories have been proposed to

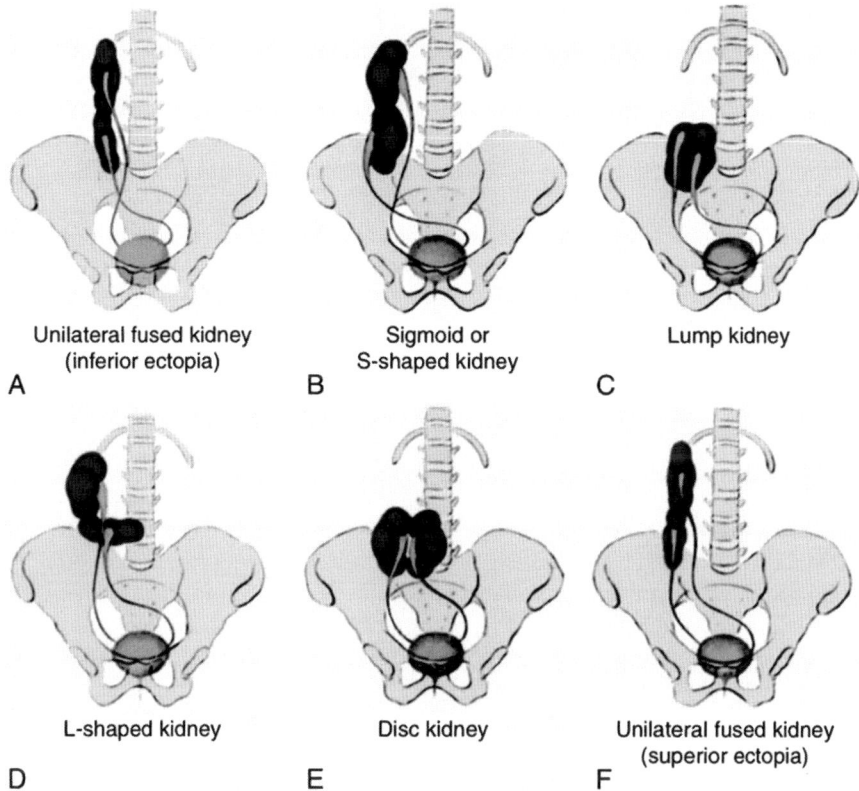

Unilateral fused kidney (inferior ectopia) **A**	Sigmoid or S-shaped kidney **B**	Lump kidney **C**
L-shaped kidney **D**	Disc kidney **E**	Unilateral fused kidney (superior ectopia) **F**

Fig. 3.5 Variants of crossed-fused renal ectopia. With permission from Wein AJ, Kavoussi LR, Novick AC, Partin AW, Peters CA, eds. Campbell-Walsh Urology. Philadelphia, PA: Saunders; 2012:3141. © Elsevier. [51]

explain this finding. One theory offers that crossed ectopia is the result of an abnormally oriented ureteric bud, which interacts with the contralateral metanephric mesenchyme to induce renal development. It has also been proposed that crossed ectopia may result from displacement of the developing kidney to the contralateral side by an abnormal umbilical or common iliac artery or other pelvic structures.

A diagnosis of crossed-fused renal ectopia may be suggested by sonographic findings or on cross-sectional abdominal imaging. Excretory urography or retrograde pyelography remains the gold standard for securing the diagnosis of crossed-fused ectopia as these modalities will demonstrate a renal collecting system of the ectopic moiety, which is subtended by a ureter that crosses the midline. Notably, the trigonal position of the ureteral orifice is orthotopic in the majority of cases; however, the incidence of VUR is approximately 20 % in patients with crossed-fused ectopia (Fig. 3.6) [28]. As with horseshoe kidney, the vascular supply to the crossed-fused ectopic kidney is often abnormal and variable. Thus, preoperative assessment

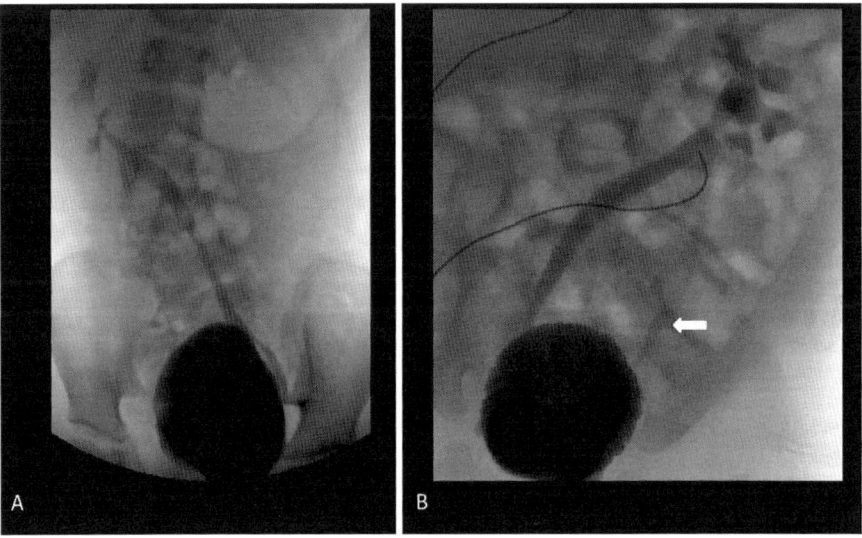

Fig. 3.6 Voiding cystourethrogram demonstrating vesicoureteral reflux associated with crossed-fused renal ectopia. (**A**) Left to right crossed-fused renal ectopia represents the most common variant of crossed-fused ectopia. (**B**) Right-to-left crossed-fused renal ectopia associated with vesicoureteral reflux into both the ectopic kidney and the normally positioned left kidney (*arrow*)

of the renal vasculature with MR or CT angiography is prudent when planning renal surgery.

Isolated crossed-fused renal is generally asymptomatic; however, it is notable that up to half of patients will have associated anomalies, which may involve the genitourinary, gastrointestinal, or skeletal systems [32]. In addition to the increased incidence of VUR, an incidence of UPJ obstruction has been reported to be between 5 and 33 % [40]. Life expectancy and long-term outcome for patients with crossed-fused renal ectopia are normal, unless impacted by associated anomalies. Similarly, management for patients with crossed-fused ectopia is dictated by the presence of symptoms or associated anomalies.

Anomalies of Renal Vasculature

During the course of its ascent, the developing kidney is revascularized by successively more craniad branches from the common iliac arteries and aorta. Classically, the kidney receives its vascular supply via a single arterial branch from the aorta at approximately vertebral level L2. Failure of more caudal branches to regress during the ascent of the kidney may result in an anatomic variation in which there are multiple renal arteries. A renal artery is described as *aberrant* if it is derived from a vessel other than the aorta or common iliac artery. The vascular supply to the kidney is via end arteries. Thus, compromise to a renal artery will generally result in ischemia to the corresponding renal parenchyma. Occasionally, multiple arteries may supply a common segment of renal parenchyma. In this situation, the additional vessel is described as an *accessory renal artery*.

The presence of multiple renal arteries is a common finding. Series reviewing CT scan data suggest an approximately 28 % incidence of multiple renal arteries [41]. Thus, consideration should be given to the possibility of multiple renal arteries any time renal surgery is planned. Not surprisingly, there is a high incidence of multiple and abnormal renal vascular supply to abnormally positioned kidneys, such as the horseshoe, ectopic, or crossed-fused kidneys. In such patients, CT or MR angiography can provide valuable information when planning renal surgery.

The presence of multiple renal arteries does not generally cause symptoms or have adverse effects on renal health. A notable exception is the situation in which a caudal renal artery impinges on the ureter resulting in UPJ obstruction. The phenomenon of a lower pole-crossing vessel causing UPJ obstruction is, in fact, a common etiology of UPJ obstruction. Treatment involves transposition of the ureter anterior to the crossing vessel. The artery is preserved to avoid ischemic injury to the renal parenchyma it supplies.

Renal artery aneurysms are uncommon, particularly in children, with an overall incidence of 0.1–1 % [42]. Several renal artery aneurysm morphologies have been described, including saccular, fusiform, dissecting, and arteriovenous variants [27]. Of these, the saccular variant is the most common. In pediatric patients, renal artery aneurysm may be related to infection, trauma, connective tissue disease, arteritides, fibromuscular dysplasia, or idiopathic causes [43, 44]. Hypertension is the most common presenting symptom of renal artery aneurysm in children, and it is not uncommon for patients to be asymptomatic. Other presenting symptoms may include hematuria, pain, or rarely ureteral obstruction from a large aneurysm [42, 45].

On exam, patients may have an abdominal bruit or pulsatile mass. The diagnosis of renal artery aneurysm was previously made with renal angiography; however, in the present era, formal angiography has recently given way to CT and MR angiography, which are now the most commonly utilized studies to assess for aneurysmal disease [46].

Treatment of renal artery aneurysms is intended to correct associated hypertension, limit ongoing thrombotic/ischemic renal injury, and prevent aneurysm rupture. Rupture of a renal artery aneurysm is a rare but devastating complication. The size criteria at which intervention should be recommended are controversial; however, most studies support surgical intervention for aneurysms >2 cm, regardless of symptoms. Additionally, repair is recommended for any female of childbearing age as this patient population is at increased risk for rupture and associated mortality from rupture during pregnancy [46]. Surgical repair of renal artery aneurysms traditionally involves open vascular reconstruction of the renal artery with vascular grafting. Additionally, there is increasing experience with endovascular coiling and stenting techniques, which may ultimately translate to greater utilization of these less invasive techniques in select patients [46].

Arteriovenous fistula (AVF) of the renal vasculature is a rare anomaly, particularly in children, in which there is direct communication between the renal arterial and venous system through enlarged, tortuous vascular spaces. Renal AVF may be acquired or congenital, with the former representing the majority of cases. Percutaneous renal biopsy is the most common cause of acquired renal AVF. Additional etiologies include blunt or penetrating trauma, percutaneous endoscopic procedures, or partial nephrectomy. Approximately 25 % of renal AVFs are congenital [47]. A *cirsoid* AFV is an unusual congenital anomaly, which is characterized by the presence of multiple vascular communications [48, 49].

Treatment of renal AVF is directed by the size of the lesion and presence of associated signs and symptoms. Small lesions secondary to a traumatic etiology may often be managed nonoperatively as they are often asymptomatic and resolve spontaneously. Hematuria is a common, although nonspecific, symptom of AVF. Large lesions may result in diastolic hypertension, renovascular hypertension, and high-output heart failure, which are often reversed with treatment of the AVF. Endovascular treatment with selective embolization is safe and effective for most lesions; however, surgical resection with total or partial nephrectomy may be required for larger, complex, or recurrent lesions [50].

References

1. Song R, Yosypiv IV. Genetics of congenital anomalies of the kidney and urinary tract. Pediatr Nephrol. 2011;26:353–64.
2. Glassberg KI. Normal and abnormal development of the kidney: a clinician's interpretation of current knowledge. J Urol. 2002;167:2339–50. discussion 50–1.
3. Fanos V, Loddo C, Puddu M, Gerosa C, Fanni D, Ottonello G, et al. From ureteric bud to the first glomeruli: genes, mediators, kidney alterations. Int Urol Nephrol. 2015;47:109–16.
4. Nagalakshmi VK, Yu J. The ureteric bud epithelium: morphogenesis and roles in metanephric kidney patterning. Mol Reprod Dev. 2015;82:151–66.
5. Shapiro E. Clinical implications of genitourinary embryology. Curr Opin Urol. 2009; 19:427–33.
6. Sadler TW, Langman J. Urogenital System. Langman's medical embryology. 9th ed. Philadelphia, Pa.: Lippincott Williams & Wilkins; 2004. p. 321-62.
7. Cocheteux B, Mounier-Vehier C, Gaxotte V, McFadden EP, Francke JP, Beregi JP. Rare variations in renal anatomy and blood supply: CT appearances and embryological background. A pictorial essay. Eur Radiol. 2001;11:779–86.
8. Skinner MA, Safford SD, Reeves JG, Jackson ME, Freemerman AJ. Renal aplasia in humans is associated with RET mutations. Am J Hum Genet. 2008;82:344–51.
9. Westland R, Schreuder MF, Ket JC, van Wijk JA. Unilateral renal agenesis: a systematic review on associated anomalies and renal injury. Nephrol Dial Transplant. 2013;28:1844–55.
10. Harewood L, Liu M, Keeling J, Howatson A, Whiteford M, Branney P, et al. Bilateral renal agenesis/hypoplasia/dysplasia (BRAHD): postmortem analysis of 45 cases with breakpoint mapping of two de novo translocations. PLoS One. 2010;5:e12375.
11. Mesrobian HG, Rushton HG, Bulas D. Unilateral renal agenesis may result from in utero regression of multicystic renal dysplasia. J Urol. 1993;150:793–4.
12. Robson WL, Leung AK, Rogers RC. Unilateral renal agenesis. Adv Pediatr. 1995;42: 575–92.

13. Schlegel PN, Shin D, Goldstein M. Urogenital anomalies in men with congenital absence of the vas deferens. J Urol. 1996;155:1644–8.
14. Heinonen PK. Gestational hypertension and preeclampsia associated with unilateral renal agenesis in women with uterine malformations. Eur J Obstet Gynecol Reprod Biol. 2004;114:39–43.
15. Guerrier D, Mouchel T, Pasquier L, Pellerin I. The Mayer-Rokitansky-Kuster-Hauser syndrome (congenital absence of uterus and vagina)--phenotypic manifestations and genetic approaches. J Negat Results Biomed. 2006;5:1.
16. Lankadeva YR, Singh RR, Tare M, Moritz KM, Denton KM. Loss of a kidney during fetal life: long-term consequences and lessons learned. Am J Physiol Renal Physiol. 2014;306:F791–800.
17. Westland R, Kurvers RA, van Wijk JA, Schreuder MF. Risk factors for renal injury in children with a solitary functioning kidney. Pediatrics. 2013;131:e478–85.
18. Hostetter TH, Olson JL, Rennke HG, Venkatachalam MA, Brenner BM. Hyperfiltration in remnant nephrons: a potentially adverse response to renal ablation. Am J Physiol. 1981;241:F85–93.
19. Kuwertz-Broeking E, Brinkmann OA, Von Lengerke HJ, Sciuk J, Fruend S, Bulla M, et al. Unilateral multicystic dysplastic kidney: experience in children. BJU Int. 2004;93:388–92.
20. Thomsen HS, Levine E, Meilstrup JW, Van Slyke MA, Edgar KA, Barth JC, et al. Renal cystic diseases. Eur Radiol. 1997;7:1267–75.
21. Hains DS, Bates CM, Ingraham S, Schwaderer AL. Management and etiology of the unilateral multicystic dysplastic kidney: a review. Pediatr Nephrol. 2009;24:233–41.
22. Cambio AJ, Evans CP, Kurzrock EA. Non-surgical management of multicystic dysplastic kidney. BJU Int. 2008;101:804–8.
23. Aslam M, Watson AR. Unilateral multicystic dysplastic kidney: long term outcomes. Arch Dis Child. 2006;91:820–3.
24. Whittam BM, Calaway A, Szymanski KM, Carroll AE, Misseri R, Kaefer M, et al. Ultrasound diagnosis of multicystic dysplastic kidney: is a confirmatory nuclear medicine scan necessary? J Pediatr Urol. 2014;10:1059–62.
25. Oto A, Kerimoglu U, Eskicorapci S, Hazirolan T, Tekgul S. Bilateral supernumerary kidney: imaging findings. JBR-BTR. 2002;85:300–3.
26. Sureka B, Mittal MK, Mittal A, Sinha M, Thukral BB. Supernumerary kidneys--a rare anatomic variant. Surg Radiol Anat. 2014;36:199–202.
27. Bauer SB. Anomalies of the Upper Urinary Tract. In: Campbell MF, Wein AJ, Kavoussi LR, editors. Campbell-Walsh urology/editor-in-chief, Alan J Wein ; editors, Louis R Kavoussi [et al]. 9th ed. Philadelphia: W.B. Saunders; 2007. p. 3291..
28. Guarino N, Tadini B, Camardi P, Silvestro L, Lace R, Bianchi M. The incidence of associated urological abnormalities in children with renal ectopia. J Urol. 2004;172:1757–9. discussion 9.
29. Gleason PE, Kelalis PP, Husmann DA, Kramer SA. Hydronephrosis in renal ectopia: incidence, etiology and significance. J Urol. 1994;151:1660–1.
30. Kramer SA, Kelalis PP. Ureteropelvic junction obstruction in children with renal ectopy. J Urol (Paris). 1984;90:331–6.
31. Natsis K, Piagkou M, Skotsimara A, Protogerou V, Tsitouridis I, Skandalakis P. Horseshoe kidney: a review of anatomy and pathology. Surg Radiol Anat. 2014;36:517–26.
32. Glodny B, Petersen J, Hofmann KJ, Schenk C, Herwig R, Trieb T, et al. Kidney fusion anomalies revisited: clinical and radiological analysis of 209 cases of crossed fused ectopia and horseshoe kidney. BJU Int. 2009;103:224–35.
33. Cascio S, Sweeney B, Granata C, Piaggio G, Jasonni V, Puri P. Vesicoureteral reflux and ureteropelvic junction obstruction in children with horseshoe kidney: treatment and outcome. J Urol. 2002;167:2566–8.
34. Pitts Jr WR, Muecke EC. Horseshoe kidneys: a 40-year experience. J Urol. 1975;113:743–6.
35. Segura JW, Kelalis PP, Burke EC. Horseshoe kidney in children. J Urol. 1972;108:333–6.
36. Yohannes P, Smith AD. The endourological management of complications associated with horseshoe kidney. J Urol. 2002;168:5–8.

37. Blanc T, Koulouris E, Botto N, Paye-Jaouen A, El-Ghoneimi A. Laparoscopic pyeloplasty in children with horseshoe kidney. J Urol. 2014;191:1097–103.
38. Mesrobian HG, Kelalis PP, Hrabovsky E, Othersen Jr HB, deLorimier A, Nesmith B. Wilms tumor in horseshoe kidneys: a report from the National Wilms Tumor Study. J Urol. 1985;133:1002–3.
39. Neville H, Ritchey ML, Shamberger RC, Haase G, Perlman S, Yoshioka T. The occurrence of Wilms tumor in horseshoe kidneys: a report from the National Wilms Tumor Study Group (NWTSG). J Pediatr Surg. 2002;37:1134–7.
40. Arena F, Arena S, Paolata A, Campenni A, Zuccarello B, Romeo G. Is a complete urological evaluation necessary in all newborns with asymptomatic renal ectopia? Int J Urol. 2007;14:491–5.
41. Bouali O, Labarre D, Molinier F, Lopez R, Benouaich V, Lauwers F, et al. Anatomic variations of the renal vessels: focus on the precaval right renal artery. Surg Radiol Anat. 2012;34:441–6.
42. Mercier C, Piquet P, Piligian F, Ferdani M. Aneurysms of the renal artery and its branches. Ann Vasc Surg. 1986;1:321–7.
43. Callicutt CS, Rush B, Eubanks T, Abul-Khoudoud OR. Idiopathic renal artery and infrarenal aortic aneurysms in a 6-year-old child: case report and literature review. J Vasc Surg. 2005;41:893–6.
44. Robitaille P, Lord H, Dubois J, Rypens F, Oligny LL. A large unilateral renal artery aneurysm in a young child. Pediatr Radiol. 2004;34:253–5.
45. Netsch C, Gross AJ, Bruning R. Symptomatic hydronephrosis from renal artery aneurysm associated with fibromuscular dysplasia: management with transarterial embolization. J Endourol. 2011;25:569–72.
46. Klausner JQ, Lawrence PF, Harlander-Locke MP, Coleman DM, Stanley JC, Fujimura N. The contemporary management of renal artery aneurysms. J Vasc Surg. 2015;61:978–84. e1.
47. van der Zee JA, van den Hoek J, Weerts JG. Traumatic renal arteriovenous fistula in a 3-year-old girl, successfully treated by percutaneous transluminal embolization. J Pediatr Surg. 1995;30:1513–4.
48. Maldonado JE, Sheps SG, Bernatz PE, Deweerd JH, Harrison Jr EG. Renal arteriovenous fistula. A reversible cause of hypertension and heart failure. Am J Med. 1964;37:499–513.
49. Kopchick JH, Bourne NK, Fine SW, Jacobsohn HA, Jacobs SC, Lawson RK. Congenital renal arteriovenous malformations. Urology. 1981;17:13–7.
50. Takebayashi S, Hosaka M, Kubota Y, Ishizuka E, Iwasaki A, Matsubara S. Transarterial embolization and ablation of renal arteriovenous malformations: efficacy and damages in 30 patients with long-term followup. J Urol. 1998;159:696–701.
51. Wein AJ, Kavoussi LR, Novick AC, Partin AW, Peters CA, editors. Campbell-Walsh Urology. Saunders: Philadelphia PA; 2012. p. 3141.

Chapter 4
Renal Dysplasia and Congenital Cystic Diseases of the Kidney

Matthew D. Mason and John C. Pope IV

Abbreviations

ADPKD	Autosomal dominant polycystic kidney disease
AML	Angiomyolipoma
ARPKD	Autosomal recessive polycystic kidney disease
CT	Computed tomography
ESRD	End-stage renal disease
JNPH	Juvenile nephronophthisis
MCDK	Multicystic dysplastic kidney
MCKD	Medullary cystic kidney disease
MLCN	Multilocular cystic nephroma
MRI	Magnetic resonance imaging
TSC	Tuberous sclerosis complex
UTI	Urinary tract infection
VCUG	Voiding cystourethrography
VHL	Von Hippel-Lindau disease
VUR	Vesicoureteral reflux

M.D. Mason, M.D.
Division of Pediatric Urology, Upstate Medical University,
725 Irving Ave, Suite 406, Syracuse, NY 13210, USA
e-mail: masonm@upstate.edu

J.C. Pope IV, M.D. (✉)
Division of Pediatric Urologic Surgery, Vanderbilt University Medical Center,
4102 Doctor's Office Tower, 200 Children's Way, Nashville, TN 37232-9820, USA
e-mail: john.pope@vanderbilt.edu

© Springer International Publishing Switzerland 2016
A.J. Barakat, H. Gil Rushton (eds.), *Congenital Anomalies of the Kidney and Urinary Tract*, DOI 10.1007/978-3-319-29219-9_4

Introduction

Renal dysplasia and congenital cystic diseases of the kidney together encompass a wide spectrum of entities with varied presentations and clinical significance. These conditions can range from those with incidental discovery of a radiographically abnormal kidney with minimal consequence to those associated with stage 5 chronic kidney disease (end-stage renal disease (ESRD)) or even neonatal demise. Some of these conditions have well-established genetic and developmental mechanisms and inheritance patterns, whereas others are poorly understood. These conditions are often associated with other syndromes or abnormalities, making evaluation and treatment of renal abnormalities just one element of the care for such patients.

Renal Dysplasia and Hypoplasia

Abnormal development of the kidney has been described using many different terms in the past, which can cause some confusion. In this chapter, we will utilize terminology as established by the Committee on Terminology, Nomenclature and Classification of the American Academy of Pediatrics (AAP) Section on Urology [1]. Renal dysgenesis is a broad term, defined as abnormal renal development that affects the size, shape, or structure of the kidney. This includes the entities of renal dysplasia and hypoplasia, which will be discussed individually in this chapter. Renal agenesis will be discussed elsewhere in this textbook (see Chapter 15).

Renal Dysplasia

Definition: Renal dysplasia refers to abnormal renal tissue, and, as such, this is a histological diagnosis seen in a variety of clinical conditions, rather than a clinical condition in and of itself. The diagnosis is made by identifying kidney tissue containing primitive renal elements in the setting of immature mesenchyme [2].

Clinical features: Renal dysplasia is one of the most common causes of pediatric ESRD. It is often seen in the setting of other congenital abnormalities of the urinary tract, such as vesicoureteral reflux (VUR), congenital urinary obstruction, or ureteral ectopia. Renal dysplasia is also associated with a number of syndromes, such as Fraser, branchio-oto-renal, Kallmann, renal-coloboma, Simpson-Golabi-Behmel, Smith-Lemli-Opitz, and other syndromes. Varying amounts of dysplastic tissue can be present within the affected kidneys, with the extent of associated renal insufficiency dependent upon whether one or both kidneys are affected and the number of preserved mature functioning nephrons. Given the heterogeneity of this group of patients, the clinical course of patients with renal dysplasia is also highly variable [2].

Pathogenesis: The etiology of renal dysplasia is not clearly understood, but is considered to be the result of either disrupted renal development secondary to urinary outflow obstruction or a primary defect in the embryological activity of the ureteric bud and metanephric differentiation. A number of candidate genes have been implicated in a number of studies, but no clear pattern of inheritance has been established [2].

Presentation: Renal dysplasia is seen in a wide variety of conditions. As such, it is usually discovered in the evaluation and treatment of patients with other associated conditions such as the above named syndromes or anatomic abnormalities of the urinary tract (which may be detected by antenatal imaging or postnatal evaluation of urinary tract infection (UTI) or urological symptoms).

Evaluation: On ultrasound examination, the parenchyma of renal dysplasia is hyperechoic compared to the liver or spleen. A kidney composed entirely of dysplastic parenchyma will typically appear small with no discernable corticomedullary differentiation. There can be variable amounts of renal cysts present, from no visible cysts to a dysplastic kidney apparently composed entirely of cysts (see multicystic dysplastic kidney, later in this chapter). An example of renal dysplasia seen on ultrasonography is shown in Fig. 4.1. On nuclear renography, areas of renal dysplasia may appear as photopenic renal cortical abnormalities. It is important to note that radiographic findings are not diagnostic of renal dysplasia, as the ultimate diagnosis can only be made histologically [3]. Overall renal function is assessed by serum laboratory testing. Urinalysis may reveal proteinuria earlier in the course of renal insufficiency.

Histology: Renal dysplasia is hallmarked by the presence of primitive renal tissue in the setting of immature mesenchyme. Primitive ducts lined by columnar epithelium are seen scattered throughout, surrounded by concentric rings of fibromuscular cells. Immature glomerular structures and nests of cartilage can be seen. As with imaging, cysts may or may not be present (Figs. 4.2 and 4.3).

Fig. 4.1 Ultrasound appearance of a kidney with renal dysplasia in a newborn. The kidney is small with echogenic parenchyma and contains cysts

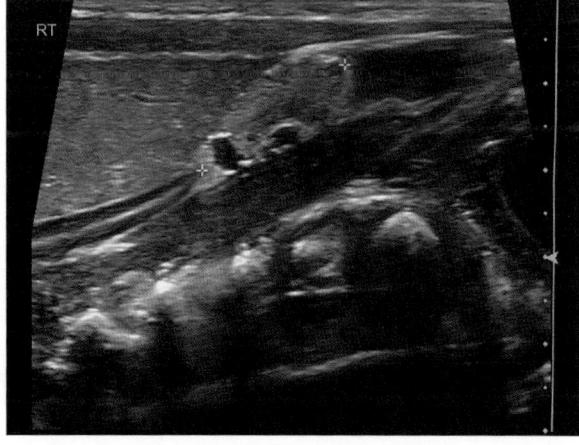

Fig. 4.2 Gross appearance
of a kidney (and ureter)
with renal dysplasia.
Courtesy of Raina
R. Flores, M.D.

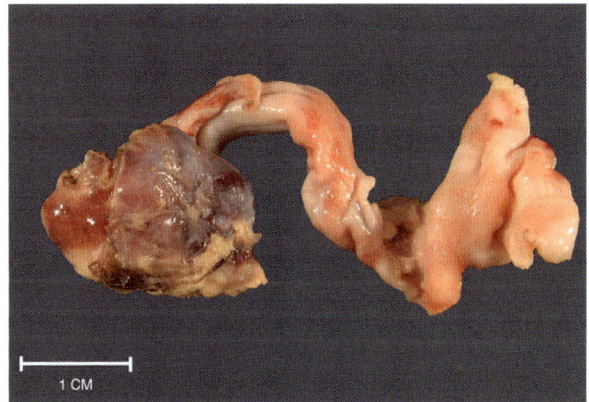

Fig. 4.3 Histologic
appearance of a kidney
with renal dysplasia.
Courtesy of Raina
R. Flores, M.D.

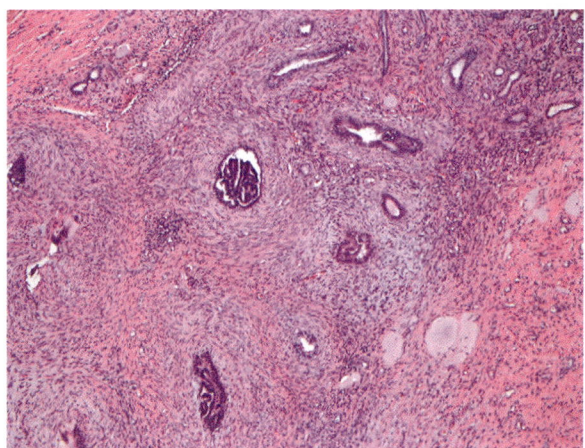

Treatment: Treatment of patients with renal dysplasia is usually dictated by the other associated syndromes or conditions and the degree of renal dysfunction. Medical treatment of hypertension and chronic renal disease may be necessary. Surgical treatment may be indicated for the other associated urinary tract conditions in these patients to preserve existing renal function, but is not a primary treatment of renal dysplasia itself.

Renal Hypoplasia

Definition: Renal hypoplasia describes a small kidney with decreased renal mass, due to decreased number of nephrons or smaller nephrons, but with normal renal architecture without dysplasia.

Clinical features: Like renal dysplasia, the clinical features of renal hypoplasia are highly variable, with renal insufficiency dependent upon the number of functioning nephrons. Renal hypoplasia can be unilateral or bilateral, and can be associated with other urological conditions, such as VUR. In the setting of unilateral hypoplasia, the contralateral kidney can demonstrate compensatory hypertrophy [4].

Pathogenesis: The etiology of isolated renal hypoplasia is unclear, but its association with other conditions such as VUR may indicate abnormal renal development secondary to abnormal urine outflow. Alternatively, hypoplasia and associated conditions may stem from a common genetic or developmental abnormality.

Presentation: Less severe renal hypoplasia without impact on overall renal function may only be discovered incidentally on imaging of the kidneys for another reason. Bilateral hypoplasia, if significant, may present with failure to thrive, anorexia, vomiting, delayed growth, proteinuria, or polyuria /polydipsia, indicative of renal insufficiency [2].

Evaluation: Ultrasonography of the kidneys will reveal smaller renal size, usually with normal-appearing echotexture (unlike the increased echogenicity seen in kidneys with dysplasia). In cases of unilateral hypoplasia, contralateral hypertrophy may be present. Nuclear renography may be useful in evaluating the relative renal function of the hypoplastic kidney. Typically this will demonstrate good and uniform uptake of the radioisotope in a smaller kidney. Consequently, when unilateral, relative differential renal function will be reduced compared to the normal contralateral kidney. Urinalysis may reveal proteinuria indicative of renal dysfunction prior to serum laboratory abnormalities. In more severe cases of bilateral hypoplasia, renal failure will be evident on laboratory testing [2, 5].

Histology: Hypoplastic kidneys exhibit decreased renal mass, but the nephrons themselves appear histologically normal.

Treatment: Similar to renal dysplasia, treatment of patients with renal hypoplasia is usually dictated by other associated conditions and the degree of renal dysfunction. Patients with isolated unilateral renal hypoplasia may not require intervention. In patients with bilateral renal hypoplasia who develop renal dysfunction, medical treatment of hypertension, anemia, acidosis, and fluid and electrolyte imbalance may be necessary, with eventual dialysis and renal transplant for patients who develop ESRD. Surgical treatment of associated urological conditions such as VUR may be indicated to prevent further deterioration in renal function but will not treat existing hypoplasia.

Oligomeganephronia

Definition: Oligomeganephronia is a severe variant of renal hypoplasia with small kidneys containing reduced overall nephron number, with hypertrophy of the individual nephrons.

Clinical features: Oligomeganephronia typically affects both kidneys and has a more predictable course than other types of hypoplasia, progressing to chronic kidney disease.

Oligomeganephronia is seen in a number of syndromes, such as branchio-otorenal and acrorenal syndromes. Due to significantly reduced nephron number, hyperfiltration injury will result in progressive nephron loss with eventual ESRD, typically in the second decade of life.

Pathogenesis: Oligomeganephronia appears to result from halted development of the metanephric blastema early in nephrogenesis (at 14–20 weeks gestation). In these kidneys, there is no continued increase in nephron number as in normal nephrogenesis, but the existing nephrons become hypertrophic. The disease does not appear to be familial.

Presentation: Oligomeganephronia presents similarly to other cases of significant renal insufficiency in children, with failure to thrive, anorexia, vomiting, delayed growth, proteinuria, polyuria, and polydipsia. Patients typically present in the first 1–2 years of life, but may present as early as the neonatal period with spontaneous pneumothorax [2, 5].

Evaluation: Renal ultrasound of patients with oligomeganephronia reveals small, normally shaped kidneys, which may or may not be hyperechoic. Urinalysis typically shows proteinuria and a specific gravity no greater than 1.012. Renal failure will be evident on laboratory testing, with reduced creatinine clearance in the range of 10–50 ml/min/1.73 m^2. Neonates with suspected oligomeganephronia should be evaluated for other associated syndromes mentioned above [2, 5].

Histology: A diagnosis of oligomeganephronia can only truly be made histologically, with kidneys exhibiting decreased nephron number and individual nephrons being widened and elongated. Enlarged glomeruli and tubules are seen. In later stages of this disease, glomeruli exhibit hyalinosis and segmental sclerosis, and renal tubules become atrophic with interstitial fibrosis [2, 5].

Treatment: Oligomeganephronia is typically treated medically, with treatment of hypertension, anemia, acidosis, and fluid and electrolyte imbalance. Patients may benefit from restriction of dietary protein and initiation of angiotensin-converting enzyme inhibitor. Upon development of ESRD, patients will need dialysis and renal transplantation.

Segmental Renal Hypoplasia (Ask-Upmark Kidney)

Definition: This form of segmental renal hypoplasia was first described by Ask-Upmark in 1929, being found primarily in adolescent females with severe hypertension. This is a rare disease, but is potentially a surgically treatable form of severe hypertension [2, 6].

Clinical features: Cases of Ask-Upmark kidney have typically been reported in adolescents with severe hypertension. The majority of these patients have a history of UTI or VUR. Patients may exhibit headaches, hypertensive encephalopathy, or retinopathy. The disease may be unilateral or bilateral [2, 6].

Pathogenesis: Ask-Upmark kidney was originally considered a congenital anomaly, but now many feel this is an acquired lesion, possibly due to chronic atrophic pyelonephritis associated with VUR. These segmental lesions may cause abnormal renin secretion with subsequent secondary hypertension, although not all patients have elevated plasma renin activity upon testing. Studies have reported normalization of blood pressure following nephrectomy or segmental resection of the lesion [6].

Presentation: Patients with Ask-Upmark kidney may present with hypertension in 35 %, UTI in 41 %, or impaired renal function in 24 %. Females are affected twice as often as males [6].

Evaluation: Patients with bilateral disease may reveal proteinuria, and serum laboratory testing may reveal renal insufficiency. Ultrasonography, computed tomography (CT), or magnetic resonance imaging (MRI) classically reveal a small kidney with one or multiple deep, narrow, segmental "slit scars" [2, 6].

Histology: Affected kidneys are small with one or more deep grooves in the lateral convexity. These grooves mark the sites of underlying abnormal, elongated renal calyces with only a thin associated band of parenchyma and no renal pyramid, sharply demarcated from the surrounding renal tissue. The overlying renal cortex contains atrophic tubules without glomeruli and can exhibit hyperplastic vessels or arteriosclerosis and epithelial-lined cysts [2, 6].

Treatment: Nephrectomy or partial nephrectomy of the lesion has been shown to correct hypertension in affected patients, regardless of plasma renin activity. Persistent hypertension after resection of the lesion may represent another unrecognized lesion or arteriosclerosis of the remaining renal tissue. Cases of bilateral disease are typically managed medically. Surgical treatment of VUR may be indicated to prevent further renal deterioration but will likely not improve existing hypertension.

Congenital Renal Cystic Diseases

Renal cysts are fluid-filled cavities lined with dedifferentiated epithelial cells, containing urine-like fluid or semisolid material, which may form for a variety of reasons and have varying shapes or sizes. Congenital renal cystic diseases encompass a broad spectrum of conditions that may be inheritable or sporadic. These conditions may exist solely with abnormalities of the kidney or may be a part of a syndrome with numerous extrarenal manifestations. There are different conditions with multiple renal cysts, and nomenclature can be confusing. The term polycystic refers to genetically determined renal cysts as a result of either autosomal dominant or autosomal recessive polycystic kidney disease. The term multicystic refers to multiple cystic lesions within a kidney, usually sporadic and typically within a dysplastic kidney. The term pluricystic has been used to refer to kidneys with multiple renal cysts in the setting of a syndrome with extrarenal findings [7]. Congenital renal cystic diseases can be classified into those that are noninheritable and inheritable. Table 4.1 summarizes the modes of inheritance and features of various congenital renal cystic diseases.

Multicystic Dysplastic Kidney

Definition: Multicystic dysplastic kidney (MCDK) is a form of renal dysplasia in which the kidney is composed of dysplastic parenchyma containing many renal cysts of varying sizes.

Clinical features: MCDK is considered a noninheritable sporadic type of congenital renal cystic disease. It is the most common type of congenital renal cystic disease and the second most common cause of a newborn abdominal mass, after hydronephrosis with an incidence of 1 in 1000–4000 live births. These kidneys can vary widely in size from a tiny "nubbin" of tissue to those that encompass a large portion of the abdominal cavity and subsequently can cause respiratory or digestive difficulty. MCDK is a benign entity, and the lesions within MCDK are not progressive. However, MCDKs are non functional, and bilateral MCDK is a fatal condition due to anhydramnios and pulmonary hypoplasia. Patients with unilateral MCDK may have contralateral renal hypertrophy and often have normal overall renal function and longevity. However, the contralateral kidney is frequently associated with other urological abnormalities, including VUR in up to 18–43 % of cases and ureteropelvic junction obstruction in as many as 3–12%. MCDKs do not have a significant association with increased risk of hypertension or neoplasm and typically involute over time in about 40 % of cases [2].

Pathogenesis: MCDK is caused by abnormal metanephric differentiation. It is postulated to arise from a primary abnormality of the metanephric blastema, abnormal induction of the metanephric blastema, or severe urinary outflow obstruction early in renal development [2]. It is typically associated with ureteral atresia which may be segmental.

Presentation: MCDK is frequently discovered prenatally on routine ultrasonography. In the absence of prenatal imaging, larger MCDKs may present as a palpable abdominal mass, potentially with respiratory insufficiency or interference with digestive function in the newborn due to mass effect.

Evaluation: MCDK is typically discovered by routine prenatal ultrasound, but can be difficult to discern from severe hydronephrosis. MCDK typically appears as a lesion within the renal fossa containing multiple cysts of varying sizes without

Table 4.1 Congenital renal cystic diseases

Disease	Inheritance pattern	Typical renal manifestations	Typical extrarenal manifestations
Multicystic dysplastic kidney	Noninheritable	Nonfunctioning kidney composed of dysplastic tissue and many cysts of varying sizes	None
Multilocular cystic nephroma	Noninheritable	Multiloculated cystic neoplasm within an otherwise normal kidney	None
Simple cysts	Noninheritable	Single asymptomatic cyst within a normal kidney	None
Autosomal dominant polycystic kidney disease	Inheritable (autosomal dominant)	Large cystic kidneys Renal failure (variable in timing but typically in adult life)	Other organ cysts (liver, pancreas, spleen, lung, seminal vesicle) Mitral valve prolapse Aortic aneurysms Colonic diverticula Circle of Willis aneurysms Subarachnoid hemorrhage
Autosomal recessive polycystic kidney disease	Inheritable (autosomal recessive)	Large echogenic kidneys in the newborn Renal failure (variable in timing but more frequent in early life)	Congenital hepatic fibrosis
Juvenile nephronophthisis	Inheritable (autosomal recessive)	Cysts of the corticomedullary junction Renal failure in children	Tapetoretinal degeneration in Senior-Loken syndrome Hepatic fibrosis Skeletal anomalies Bardet-Biedl syndrome Neurologic defects
Medullary cystic disease	Inheritable (autosomal dominant)	Cysts of the corticomedullary junction Renal failure in early adult life	None
Tuberous sclerosis	Inheritable (autosomal dominant)	Renal cysts Renal angiomyolipomas (40–80 % of cases) Renal cell carcinoma (3 % of cases)	Cranial tumors Mental retardation Epilepsy Adenoma sebaceum
Von Hippel-Lindau	Inheritable (autosomal dominant)	Renal cysts (75 % of cases) Clear cell renal cell carcinoma (35 % of cases) Renal adenomas	Cerebellar hemangioblastomas Retinal angiomas Pheochromocytomas Pancreatic cysts Epididymal cystadenoma
Glomerulocystic kidney disease	Inheritable (autosomal dominant)	Numerous minute cysts in the renal cortex Renal failure (of varying severity and timing)	Dependent on presence of other syndromes

Fig. 4.4 Ultrasound appearance of a multicystic dysplastic kidney in a neonate. The kidney is large and composed of numerous cysts of varying sizes with intervening echogenic parenchyma

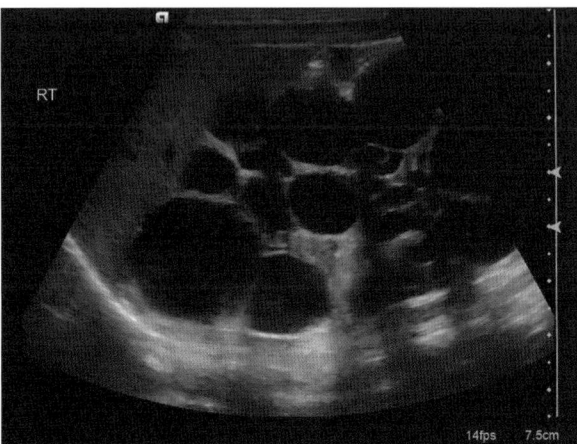

apparent communication between cysts (Fig. 4.4). There is typically no large central fluid collection which would suggest a hydronephrotic kidney. The kidney can be of varying sizes, from much smaller to much larger than the contralateral kidney. At times the renal shape can be so distorted that it becomes difficult to tell if this lesion is the kidney. Ultrasound imaging should be repeated postnatally for clearer evaluation of the lesion and to evaluate the contralateral kidney. In cases where it is difficult to discern MCDK from hydronephrosis, nuclear renography will usually demonstrate radionuclide update in a hydronephrotic kidney but not in MCDK. Recent studies suggest that routine voiding cystourethrography (VCUG) may not be indicated in cases of MCDK with a normal-appearing contralateral kidney and bladder, given the low rate of clinically significant VUR. Patients should be monitored for signs and symptoms of UTI with implementation of VCUG when clinically indicated. Although MCDK does not have a significant association with hypertension or neoplasm, patients should be evaluated periodically by their primary care physician for hypertension or abdominal mass [2, 8, 9].

Histology: MCDKs are grossly composed of numerous cysts of varying sizes and may resemble a "bunch of grapes" (Fig. 4.5). These cysts are lined by cuboidal epithelium and contain proteinaceous or sanguineous fluid. There can be varying amounts of intervening solid stromal tissue containing primitive renal ducts, immature cartilage, and dysplastic elements as seen in other kidneys with renal dysplasia (Fig. 4.6). The kidney often does not have a reniform shape, and the renal vessels, ureter, or renal pelvis may be absent [2, 7].

Treatment: In the rare cases where MCDK is so large during the neonatal period as to cause respiratory or digestive difficulty, a nephrectomy may be necessary. In most cases, the MCDK will spontaneously involute. Nephrectomy may also be necessary for rare cases of hypertension or cyst rupture causing hemorrhage or pain. There is no clear evidence to show that surveillance ultrasonography is beneficial for these patients.

Fig. 4.5 Gross appearance of a multicystic dysplastic kidney. Courtesy of Raina R. Flores, M.D.

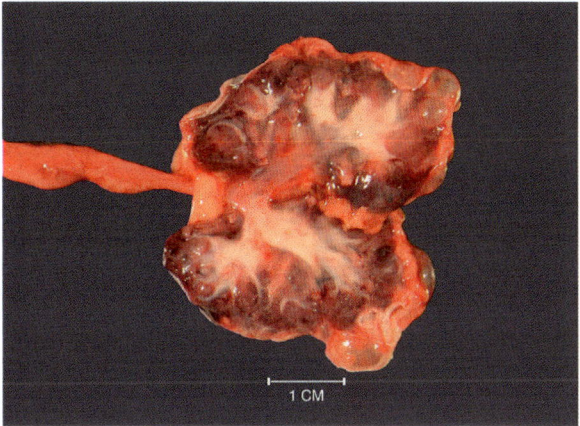

Fig. 4.6 Histologic appearance of a multicystic dysplastic kidney. Courtesy of Raina R. Flores, M.D.

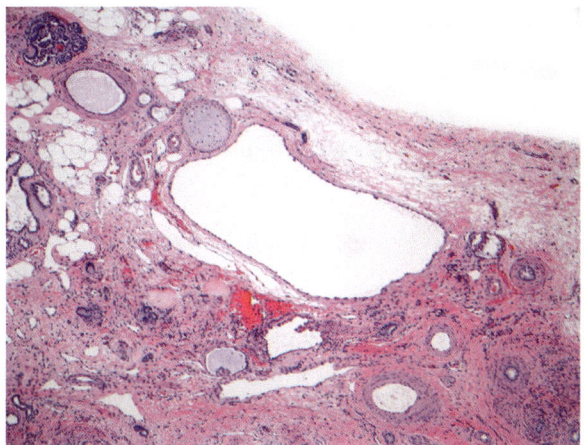

Simple Renal Cysts

Definition: A simple renal cyst is a round, fluid-filled structure, usually asymptomatic and of no clinical consequence, within an otherwise normal kidney.

Clinical features: Simple cysts are the most common cystic lesion encountered in the adult kidney (estimated at 33 % of patients over 60 years of age), but are rare in infants and children. In the pediatric population, they are typically solitary and unilateral. They can be detected prenatally as early as 14 weeks of gestation, but many of these cysts resolve before birth. Typically, they are discovered incidentally, occur within a non-diseased kidney, and have no symptoms or clinical impact. Rarely are cysts large enough to cause symptoms from mass effect. There have been reports of initially small simple cysts in children growing in size over time with eventual mass effect requiring surgical intervention, suggesting a possible role for follow-up imaging to monitor the size and character of these lesions [7, 10].

Pathogenesis: Simple renal cysts are thought to arise from the distal convoluted tubule or collecting duct of the nephron. They likely represent a portion of a nephron with some degeneration and abnormal fluid handling with resultant cyst formation [7].

Presentation: The majority of simple renal cysts present incidentally on imaging of the kidney for other reasons. They typically are not associated with symptoms or laboratory abnormalities, but rarely can cause pain or hematuria with rupture or an abdominal mass in the setting of a very large cyst [2].

Evaluation: Ultrasound evaluation of a simple cyst will show a spherical- or oval-shaped collection of anechoic fluid with a thin smooth margin within a normal kidney, usually located in the renal cortex. A simple cyst will not have solid components, internal echoes, septations, or calcifications, which if present would require further evaluation with contrast-enhanced CT or MRI using the Bosniak classification system [2, 11].

Histology: Simple cysts are typically found in the renal cortex, containing clear serous fluid within a fibrous wall lined by a single layer of flattened epithelial cells. They can vary widely in size from under one centimeter to over 15 cm in diameter [2, 7].

Treatment: Intervention for asymptomatic simple renal cysts is not indicated. In the setting of a large renal cyst causing pain or mass effect, intervention may be warranted in the form of surgical unroofing of the cyst or percutaneous aspiration, with or without injection of a sclerosing agent [2, 10].

Multilocular Cystic Nephroma

Definition: Multilocular cystic nephroma (MLCN), also known as benign multilocular cyst, is a neoplastic but not dysplastic process that occurs focally within a usually otherwise normal kidney. It is considered to be part of a spectrum of diseases including Wilms' tumor, with MLCN representing the most benign form of this spectrum.

Clinical features: MLCN is one of four disease processes composing a spectrum from most benign to most malignant, including MLCN, multilocular cystic partially differentiated Wilms' tumor, multilocular cyst with nodules of Wilms' tumor, and cystic Wilms' tumor. MLCN is considered to be a neoplastic process rather than a form of renal dysplasia or MCDK. There are two general forms of this disease, a pediatric form and an adult form. The pediatric form typically presents in children under age 2 years and is twice as common in males. The adult form typically presents in women over age 30 years. The cysts of MLCN can have mass effect upon the renal pelvis causing urinary obstruction and pain, or even prolapse through the transitional epithelium, presenting with hematuria caused by bleeding into the renal collecting system. These lesions can have progression in size at variable rates, from slow enlargement over years to rapid growth of many centimeters over months [2, 7, 12, 13].

Pathogenesis: The pathogenesis of MLCN is somewhat debated, but it is thought to be a neoplastic process. Supporting this idea are reports of MLCN arising in patients with previously normal kidneys and the progressive growth seen in MLCN. Additionally, there have been rare reports of local recurrence after resection or metastasis [2, 13].

Presentation: The most common presentation of MLCN in children is an asymptomatic flank mass. Adults with MLCN may present with some combination of flank mass, abdominal pain, and/or hematuria [2, 13].

Evaluation: Physical examination should rule out hemihypertrophy or aniridia, which may be associated with Wilms' tumor but have not been reported in association with MLCN. Ultrasound evaluation reveals a complex intrarenal mass, sometimes with extension into the renal pelvis or extrarenal space. The mass typically contains highly echogenic septations separating the lesion into multiple anechoic locules; however, there may be debris within locules creating internal echoes. In some lesions, the locules may be so small as to give the appearance of numerous internal echoes without distinct locules. CT or MRI will typically show the intrarenal mass to have a well-defined capsule and septa that typically enhance with intravenous contrast medium. Ultrasound, CT, or MRI will help to characterize this lesion and differentiate it from other cystic diseases of the kidney, such as MCDK, but cannot differentiate these lesions from other neoplastic processes. Surgical excision and histopathologic examination is required to clearly discern MLCN from malignant neoplasm [2, 13].

Histology: These lesions are of varying sizes but are typically a bulky lesion circumscribed by a thick capsule with compression of the adjacent renal parenchyma. There may be extension of the lesion into the adjacent perinephric space or the renal pelvis. Multiple noncommunicating cysts separated by thin fibrous septa are seen of varying sizes, from a few millimeters to a few centimeters, containing fluid that is clear to yellow in color. Microscopically, the septa are fibrous and may contain well-differentiated renal tubules. The cysts are lined by either flattened or "hobnail" epithelium, so-called because of eosinophilic cuboidal cells which project into the cyst lumen [2, 7, 13].

Treatment: Suspected MLCN should be treated with surgical excision, as these lesions can have progressive growth. Additionally, histopathologic examination of the lesion is required to evaluate for malignancy, such as nodules of Wilms' tumor. Surgical excision is usually achieved by nephrectomy, but partial nephrectomy may be feasible if the location and extent of the lesion is amenable. There have been rare reports of recurrence after excision of MLCN, which likely represent inadequate excision of the original lesion. Surveillance with periodic abdominal imaging can evaluate for local recurrence. Patients found to have malignancy will need management according to tumor staging and treatment protocols [2, 7, 13].

Autosomal Recessive Polycystic Kidney Disease (ARPKD)

Definition: ARPKD is an inheritable genetic disease that causes varying, often severe, congenital renal insufficiency and hepatic impairment due to diffuse bilateral renal cystic disease and hepatic fibrosis. It has previously been referred to as "infantile" polycystic kidney disease, although it can present at varying ages.

Clinical features: ARPKD has an incidence of 1 in 10,000–50,000 live births, with 30–50 % of affected newborns dying shortly after birth. Renal impairment is highly variable, with potential ESRD in infancy to those with some preservation of renal function into adulthood. Generally, the earlier the disease presents, the more severe the phenotype. Congenital hepatic fibrosis is present in all patients regardless of the severity of renal disease and becomes more prevalent as patients age. For infants surviving the neonatal period, survival is approximately 50 % at 10 years. Most ARPKD is diagnosed on prenatal ultrasound and appear as bilateral enlarged hyperechoic kidneys. There may be oligohydramnios due to insufficient fetal urine production, with subsequent pulmonary hypoplasia. Severe oligohydramnios may result in respiratory failure and facial and limb deformities. Kidneys may be so enlarged as to cause difficulty with labor and delivery or occupy so much of the infant's abdominal volume as to cause respiratory or digestive difficulty after birth. Beyond the neonatal period, patients have progressive renal insufficiency and hypertension, with 20–45 % progressing to ESRD by age 15. Patients with less severe renal disease still have progressive hepatic fibrosis, and liver disease becomes the dominant clinical complication as these patients age (2, 7).

Pathogenesis: The gene responsible for ARPKD has been identified as PKHD1 on the short arm of chromosome 6 (6p12). This gene encodes fibrocystin (also known as polyductin), a protein highly expressed in the kidney and liver. This protein is localized to the primary cilia, a mechanosensing structure involved in regulation of cellular arrangement and proliferation. Dysfunction of the polyductin protein results in dysfunction of the primary cilia with subsequent cyst formation [2, 7, 14].

Presentation: Approximately half of patients with ARPKD are diagnosed prenatally, with discovery of renal abnormality and possible oligohydramnios on ultrasonography. Infants present with large palpable abdominal masses and variable respiratory distress. Hypertension typically occurs early in life and can be severe. A minority of patients with ARPKD may present later in childhood or even adulthood, typically with symptoms caused by congenital hepatic fibrosis and hepatomegaly [2, 15].

Evaluation: Ultrasound examination of the kidneys prenatally or in infancy reveals bilaterally enlarged kidneys. The cysts present within the kidney are often too small to be individually resolved on ultrasound in infancy, creating numerous acoustic interfaces resulting in a very echogenic kidney (Fig. 4.7). Macroscopic cysts are not typically seen in infants with ARPKD and are suggestive of autosomal dominant polycystic kidney disease (ADPKD). Later in life, macroscopic renal cysts, hepatosplenomegaly, and increased echogenicity of the liver may

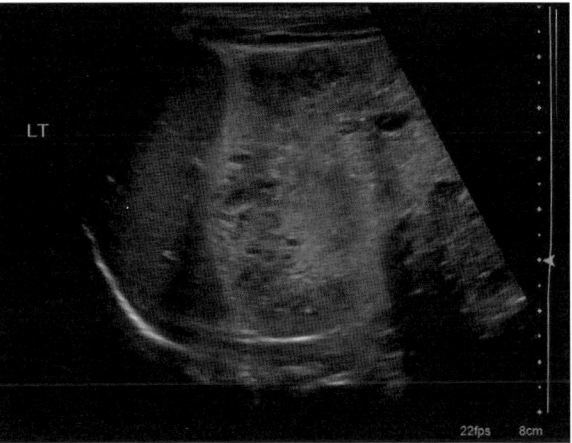

Fig. 4.7 Ultrasound appearance of a kidney in a 6-month-old patient with autosomal recessive polycystic kidney disease (ARPKD). The kidney is enlarged and echogenic (as compared to the spleen seen superiorly), and the cysts that are visible are small. This patient also had intrahepatic biliary duct dilation typical of ARPKD on ultrasound

become apparent. Physical examination reveals bilateral firm abdominal masses that do not transilluminate. In most cases, serum laboratory evaluation will reveal renal insufficiency, evidenced by rising blood urea nitrogen and creatinine shortly after birth. Diagnosis of ARPKD can typically be made by imaging as well as one or more of the following: no renal cysts seen in either parent, a sibling affected by ARPKD, consanguineous parents, or evidence of hepatic fibrosis. ARPKD and ADPKD can both present in infancy in a similar manner, so a careful family history to evaluate for cystic kidney disease with an autosomal dominant or autosomal recessive pattern is important. Genetic testing is possible but may not detect mutations in PKHD1 in up to 40 % of patients. A liver or renal biopsy can be done if the diagnosis is unclear [2, 15].

Histology: Kidneys are enlarged bilaterally, up to 20 times the normal size, but maintain a normal reniform shape. The cut surface of the kidney shows fusiform collecting duct cysts arranged in a radiating pattern from the renal pyramids to the cortex (Fig. 4.8). More severe cases have nearly 100 % of collecting ducts affected. There are numerous minute cysts throughout the renal cortex (Fig. 4.9). The liver exhibits periportal fibrosis and enlargement in all patients, regardless of the current severity of liver disease [2, 7].

Treatment: There is no cure or disease-specific treatment for ARPKD. In the neonatal period, management should focus on respiratory support when needed as well as management of hypertension and fluid/electrolyte imbalance. In infants with respiratory or digestive difficulty due to compression from enlarged kidneys, unilateral or bilateral nephrectomy may be beneficial. Affected families should be referred for genetic counseling, as siblings will have a 25 % chance of being affected by this disease and a 50 % chance of being a carrier. Patients will need ongoing medical management of hypertension, chronic kidney disease, and hepatic failure. Surgical treatment for complications of portal hypertension may be required. As ESRD develops, patients will require dialysis and possible renal transplantation.

Fig. 4.8 Gross appearance of the cut surface of a kidney from a patient with autosomal recessive polycystic kidney disease. Courtesy of Raina R. Flores, M.D.

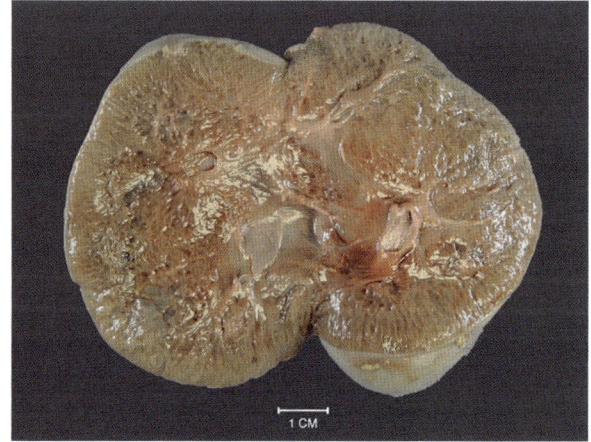

Fig. 4.9 Histologic appearance of a kidney from a patient with autosomal recessive polycystic kidney disease. Courtesy of Raina R. Flores, M.D.

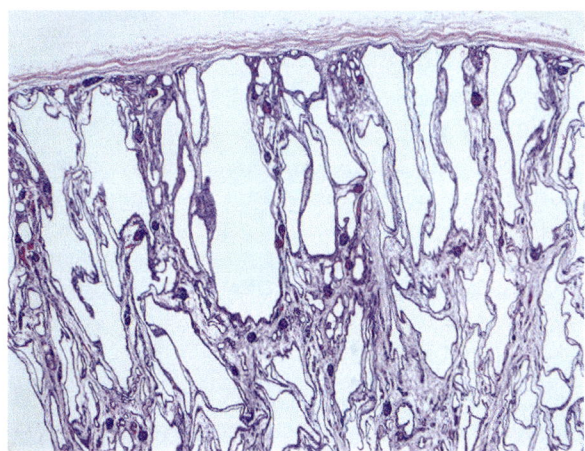

Autosomal Dominant Polycystic Kidney Disease (ADPKD)

Definition: ADPKD is an inheritable genetic disease that causes multiple cysts within the kidneys bilaterally and renal failure leading to ESRD. ADPKD has previously been referred to as "adult" polycystic kidney disease, although this is a misnomer as patients can present as early as infancy.

Clinical features: ADPKD is the most common inheritable type of renal cystic disease, with an incidence estimated at 1–2 per 1000 live births. Approximately 10 % of patients receiving hemodialysis in the United States have ADPKD. The majority of cases present between 30 and 40 years of age, with 96 % of patients manifesting the disease by 90 years of age. This disease also can present in neonates, which indicates a more severe disease process and can even result in fetal demise or neonatal death. Similarly, renal dysfunction is highly variable, ranging from renal failure in infancy to preserved renal function into old age. Hypertension is common in this population, occurring in half of patients aged 20–35 (despite normal renal function) and nearly all patients with ESRD. ADPKD cysts have been associated with pain due to mass effect, hemorrhage, UTI, or nephrolithiasis. Patients have extrarenal manifestations of ADPKD in the form of cysts of the liver, pancreas, spleen, and lungs, as well as aortic aneurysms, mitral valve prolapse, colonic diverticula, and "berry aneurysms" of the circle of Willis. The consequences of these extrarenal manifestations are quite variable. Approximately 10–30 % of patients have berry aneurysms, and 9 % of these patients die due to subarachnoid hemorrhage [2, 7].

Pathogenesis: ADPKD is caused by mutations in PKD1 (located on the short arm of chromosome 16) or PKD2 (located on the long arm of chromosome 4), genes that encode for the proteins polycystin-1 and polycystin-2, respectively. These proteins together form a complex responsible for regulating calcium transport that is localized to the primary cilia of renal epithelial cells (similar to the polyductin protein implicated in ARPKD). Dysfunction of this protein complex causes dysregulation of cellular arrangement and proliferation and subsequently results in cyst formation. ADPKD is transmitted in an autosomal dominant fashion, with an inherited mutation in one allele of either PKD1 or PKD2 in all cells. The Knudson two-hit hypothesis suggests that a somatic mutation in the remaining functional allele then causes loss of functional protein, accounting for why only 1–2 % of nephrons undergo cystic change when all cells contain the inherited mutation. Studies have suggested that regardless of whether the inherited mutation was on PKD1 or PKD2, a second mutation in either PKD1 or PKD2 is sufficient to disrupt the entire protein complex and cause cyst formation (Fig. 4.10). Ten percent of cases of ADPKD have no family history of the disease and are thought to be new mutations in either PKD1 or PKD2. PKD1 mutations account for 85 % of

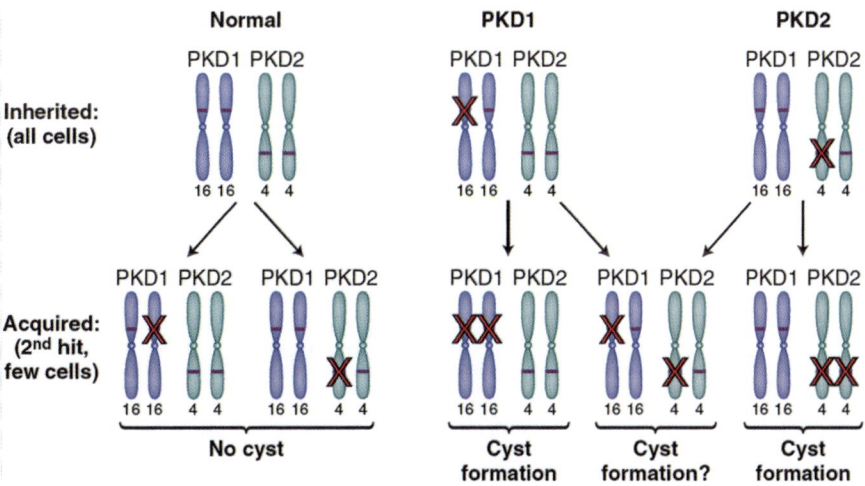

Fig. 4.10 Schematic of "two-hit" hypothesis for genetic basis of cystogenesis in autosomal dominant polycystic kidney disease

cases of ADPKD and usually create a more rapidly progressive phenotype, with over half of patients showing cysts by 10 years of age and ESRD occurring in the sixth decade of life. ADPKD can be seen in conjunction with tuberous sclerosis, as the PKD1 gene is adjacent to the TSC2 gene of tuberous sclerosis on chromosome 16, so large deletions of chromosome 16 can cause both diseases simultaneously. A suspected third gene, PKD3, has not yet been identified [2, 7, 15, 16].

Presentation: Given the variable nature of ADPKD, the disease can present anytime from in utero to late in adult life. Infants may present with abnormal renal appearance detected on prenatal ultrasonography or with palpable abdominal masses after birth. The typical case of ADPKD presents with signs or symptoms between age 30 and 50 years. Patients most frequently present with abdominal or flank pain as mentioned above. Patients can also present with hematuria, hypertension, or gastrointestinal symptoms possibly due to mass effect upon the gastrointestinal tract or the associated colonic diverticulosis. Screening of family members may detect the disease in others once a case has been identified [2, 15].

Evaluation: ADPKD is most commonly diagnosed by ultrasonography, showing the presence of macroscopic renal cysts (Figs. 4.11, 4.12, and 4.13). Ninety percent of patients will have a positive family history consistent with an autosomal dominant pattern of inheritance. Ultrasonographic diagnostic criteria for individuals with a genetic risk for ADPKD are shown in Table 4.2. Given the rarity of simple renal cysts in children, a single renal cyst in a child with a genetic risk for ADPKD is concerning for a diagnosis of the disease. The disease may manifest in children before it does in the parents, especially when parents are young, and further family history and ultrasound examination of the kidneys of grandparents may be helpful in certain cases. Evaluating asymptomatic children of affected individuals with annual blood pressure measurement and urinalysis is appropriate. Screening by ultrasound exam is somewhat controversial, as there is currently no disease-specific treatment. CT or MRI may be utilized in patients

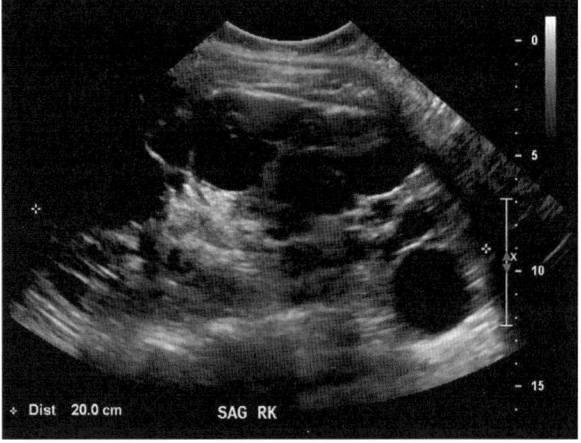

Fig. 4.11 Ultrasound appearance of a kidney in a 40-year-old patient with autosomal dominant polycystic kidney disease. The kidney is enlarged and contains numerous large cysts

Fig. 4.12 Ultrasound appearance of a kidney in a 12-year-old patient with autosomal dominant polycystic kidney disease. Several renal cysts are seen in the kidney. On subsequent imaging over the next several years, the patient developed many more cysts within both kidneys

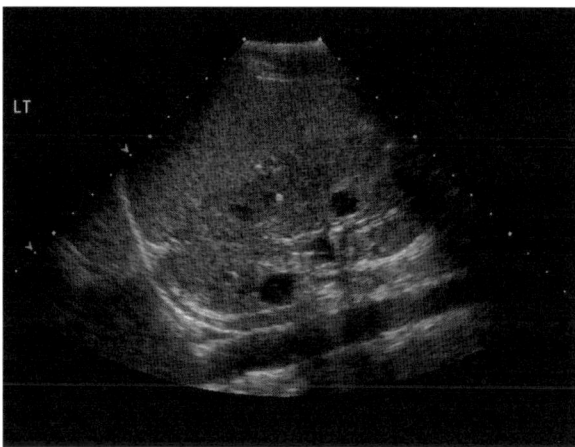

Fig. 4.13 Ultrasound appearance of a kidney in a newborn with bilaterally enlarged kidneys palpable on abdominal exam and family history positive for autosomal dominant polycystic kidney disease. The renal parenchyma is echogenic and contains numerous macroscopic cysts

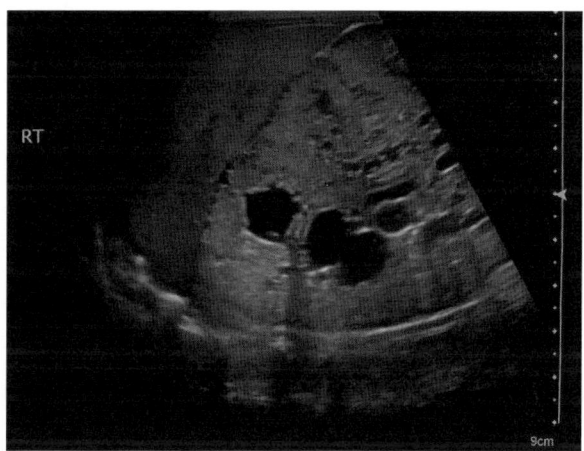

Table 4.2 Ultrasound criteria for the diagnosis of ADPKD in individuals with genetic risk

Age of patient	Minimum ultrasound criteria for diagnosis
Younger than 30 years	Two renal cysts (unilateral or bilateral)
30–59 years	Two cysts in each kidney
60 years or older	Four cysts in each kidney

with ADPKD to evaluate for cysts in other organs when the diagnosis is in question or in evaluating for hemorrhage into cysts. Genetic testing for mutations of PKD1 and PKD2 is commercially available and may be useful in the setting of unclear diagnoses or in potential family members who wish to be donors for renal transplantation [2, 7, 15].

Fig. 4.14 Gross appearance of the exterior surface of a kidney from a patient with autosomal dominant polycystic kidney disease. Courtesy of Raina R. Flores, M.D

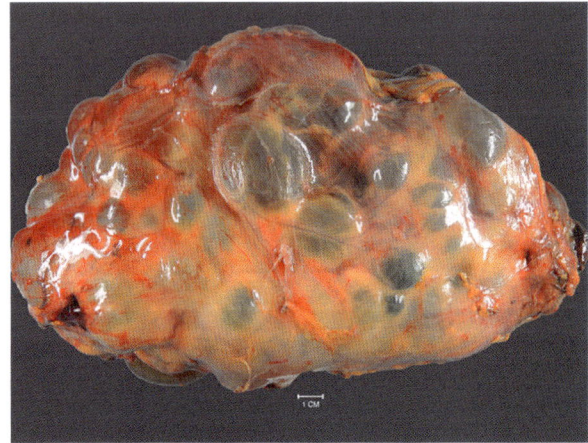

Fig. 4.15 Gross appearance of the cut surface of a kidney from a patient with autosomal dominant polycystic kidney disease. Courtesy of Raina R. Flores, M.D

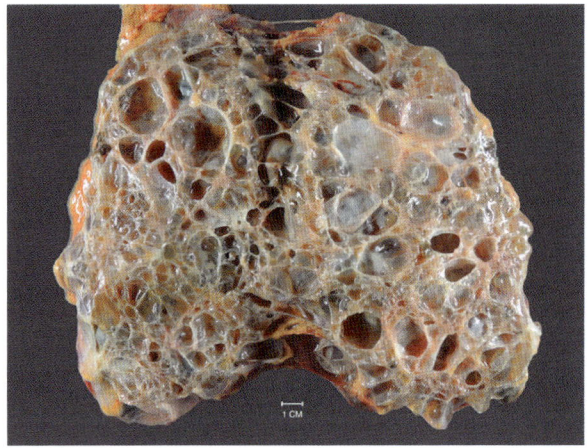

Histology: ADPKD kidneys have variable sizes, from relatively normal size to severely enlarged kidneys as the disease progresses. The kidneys retain their reniform shape, with numerous cysts evenly distributed throughout the renal cortex and medulla, ranging in diameter from 0.1 to several centimeters (Figs. 4.14 and 4.15). Microscopically, cysts can be seen in early stages as focal outpouchings of the renal tubules, eventually becoming detached and no longer communicating with the nephron (Fig. 4.16) [2, 7].

Treatment: There is no cure or disease-specific treatment for ADPKD at this time, although studies are ongoing. Management of patients presenting with severe disease in the newborn period can be taken with a similar approach to infants with ARPKD, with management of respiratory failure, renal insufficiency, hypertension, and rarely surgical removal of one or both kidneys. Families should be referred for genetic counseling if they have not already, given the autosomal dominant mode of

Fig. 4.16 Histologic appearance of a kidney from a patient with autosomal dominant polycystic kidney disease. Courtesy of Raina R. Flores, M.D.

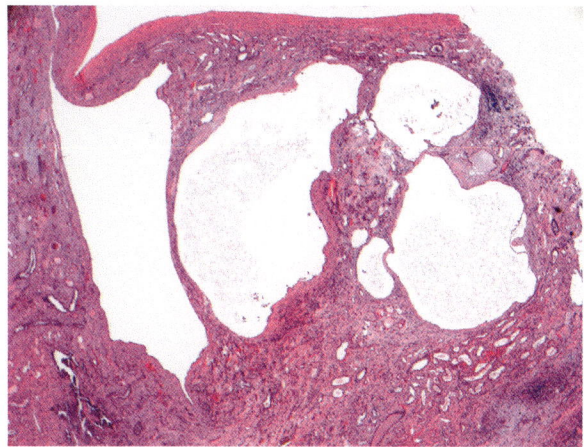

inheritance of this disease. Long term, patients will need medical management of renal insufficiency and hypertension. Adequate management of hypertension is especially critical in this population, in order to slow renal deterioration and minimize risk of intracranial hemorrhage. In ADPKD patients with flank or abdominal pain, evaluation for infection, urinary stone, or tumor should be performed and treated accordingly. Aspiration for diagnostic and therapeutic purposes can be performed when cyst infection is suspected. In the setting of a large cyst causing pain or mass effect, intervention may be warranted in the form of surgical unroofing of the cyst or percutaneous aspiration, with or without injection of a sclerosing agent. Nephrectomy can be performed for symptomatic patients if they have already progressed to ESRD. Patients with ESRD will require dialysis and potential renal transplantation. Family members of affected individuals that wish to be renal donors need to first be evaluated for presence of the disease [2, 15, 17].

Juvenile Nephronophthisis and Medullary Cystic Kidney Disease

Definition: Juvenile nephronophthisis (JNPH) and medullary cystic kidney disease (MCKD) are two distinct inheritable renal cystic diseases with similar features and similar histology of interstitial nephritis and corticomedullary junction cysts [2].

Clinical features: JNPH accounts for 10–20 % of chronic kidney disease in children, leading to ESRD at a mean age of 13 years. It is estimated that 1–5 % of all patients with ESRD have JNPH. MCKD typically manifests in early adult life, progressing to ESRD usually by 40 years of age. Both conditions are associated with a urinary concentrating defect, leading to salt wasting with subsequent polyuria and polydipsia in 80 % of cases. Ten percent to 20 % of cases of JNPH are associated with extrarenal malformation, such as tapetoretinal degeneration in Senior-Loken syndrome (also known as "renal-retinal syndrome"), hepatic fibrosis, skeletal anomalies, Bardet-Biedl syndrome, or neurologic defects. In contrast, MCKD appears to be free of extrarenal manifestations [2, 7].

Pathogenesis: JNPH is typically inherited as autosomal recessive and MCKD as autosomal dominant, although either can appear sporadically in about 15 % of cases. Six different genes have been identified in JNPH, namely, NPHP1, NPHP2/INVS, NPHP3, NPHP4, NPHP5/IQCB1, and NPHP6/CEP290. MCKD is caused by mutations in the MCKD1 or MCKD2 gene. The cysts in JNPH and MCKD appear to arise from the distal convoluted and collecting tubules, accounting for the cysts seen at the corticomedullary junction and deeper within the renal medulla [2, 7].

Presentation: JNPH can present with polyuria and polydipsia in infancy or growth retardation in childhood. MCKD typically presents in adulthood during the third or fourth decade, again with polyuria and polydipsia. Both diseases have fairly non-specific symptoms.

Evaluation: Ultrasound examination may reveal small or relatively normal-sized kidneys. Cysts may or may not be seen on imaging, especially early on in the disease, as they may be too small to discern. In patients with significant tubulointerstitial fibrosis, the kidney may appear echogenic. Contrast-enhanced CT and MRI are more sensitive imaging modalities for detecting small cysts in the medulla and corticomedullary junction.

Histology: The histological appearances of JNPH and MCKD are very similar. Kidneys are small to normal in size. Both diseases show interstitial nephritis and fibrosis, numerous small cysts at the corticomedullary junction and deeper in the medulla, and irregular thickening and disintegration of the tubular basement membrane.

Treatment: There is no cure or disease-specific treatment for JNPH or MCKD. Treatment of the salt-wasting urine concentrating defect consists of sodium replacement and avoidance of diuretics. Patients will eventually progress to ESRD and need dialysis and possible renal transplantation. Family members wishing to donate a kidney for transplantation must be evaluated for this disease given the autosomal recessive or dominant inheritance.

Tuberous Sclerosis Complex (TSC)

Definition: Tuberous sclerosis complex (TSC) is a multiple malformation syndrome which manifests with hamartomas throughout the body, renal cysts, and other renal abnormalities.

Clinical features: TSC is considered an autosomal dominant inherited disorder, affecting up to 1 in 6000 individuals. TSC classically manifests with a triad of mental retardation, epilepsy, and adenoma sebaceum. Adenoma sebaceum is red/brown telangiectatic papule typically in the nasolabial folds and on the chin and cheeks. The 2012 International Tuberous Sclerosis Complex Consensus Conference established updated criteria for a diagnosis of TSC, involving demonstration of a number of major and minor clinical features. The predominant organ system impacted by TSC is the central nervous system, but the second most common organ is the kidney. Approximately 20 % of patients with TSC will develop renal cysts, usually before age 3 years, and as such renal cysts may be one of the earlier manifestations of TSC in some patients. Angiomyolipomas (AML) are much more common in TSC, affecting 40–80 % of these patients, but do not typically present until after 6 years of age. AMLs can grow progressively and have increasing risk for hemorrhage with increasing size. AMLs can cause a palpable flank mass and have been associated with renal insufficiency and hypertension [2, 7, 18].

Pathogenesis: TSC is considered to be an autosomal dominant inheritable condition, although this seems to be in only 25–40 % of cases, due to either sporadic mutations or variable penetrance. There are two genes implicated in this disease. TSC1 is located on the short arm of chromosome 9 and encodes the protein hamartin. TSC2 is located on the short arm of chromosome 16 and encodes the protein tuberin. Hamartin and tuberin inhibit the mTOR pathway. Loss of function of either protein leads to diffuse hamartoma formation. The TSC2 gene is located in close proximity to the PKD1 gene of ADPKD, and large deletions in the short arm of chromosome 16 can cause both diseases concurrently.

Presentation: Patients are diagnosed with TSC at a wide range of ages, from birth to over 70 years of age. However, average age at diagnosis is 7.5 years and the vast majority of patients are diagnosed before age 10. The most common signs and symptoms leading to a diagnosis of TSC are not related to the kidney and typically involve seizure activity, family history of TSC, and cardiac or dermatologic abnormalities [19].

Evaluation: Renal cysts in TSC appearing on ultrasound examination as other renal cysts do, with a spherical or ovoid anechoic collection within the kidney. AMLs appear to have a white, "fluffy" appearance due to numerous acoustic interfaces within the lesion and the presence of fat. On CT imaging, AMLs classically contain areas less dense than water, indicative of macroscopic fat. In patients with TSC that have renal cysts and no AMLs, the kidneys can mimic the appearance of ADPKD [2].

Histology: Cysts in patients with TSC are classically lined by granular eosinophilic cells containing large nuclei, with some areas forming papillary tufts. There may be associated metanephric hamartomata within the kidney. AMLs are composed of proliferative vessels, smooth muscle, and adipose tissue [2, 7].

Treatment: Renal cysts in TSC are typically asymptomatic and do not require treatment. Patients with TSC do develop hypertension and renal failure and must be managed accordingly. AMLs are typically asymptomatic; however, current recommendations are to embolize or excise AMLs that enlarge to a diameter greater than 4 cm due to an increase risk of spontaneous hemorrhage. As such, patients with AMLs are followed annually by ultrasound or CT to monitor the size of their lesions. Patients with AMLs who are considering pregnancy or estrogen administration should be warned about potential hemorrhage [2].

Von Hippel-Lindau Disease

Definition: Von Hippel-Lindau disease (VHL) is an autosomal dominant inherited multiple malformation syndrome which has renal cysts as one of its many manifestations, with hemangioblastomas, cysts, and tumors in various other organs.

Clinical features: VHL has an incidence of 1 in 30,000 to 1 in 50,000. It is inherited in an autosomal dominant fashion, with 95 % penetrance of the disease by 65 years of age.

Approximately 20 % of patients have no family history of the disease and are thought to be new mutations. Patients may develop hemangioblastomas of the cerebellum and retina; cysts of the kidney, pancreas, and epididymis; epididymal cystadenoma; pheochromocytoma; and clear cell renal cell carcinoma. Mean age at presentation is 35–40 years of age. Renal cysts are the most common lesions in patients with VHL (present in approximately 75 % of patients) and are frequently the earliest manifestation of the disease. Cysts are often bilateral and multifocal. Renal cell carcinoma occurs in about half of patients with VHL and often occurs in kidneys with renal cysts. Both the cysts and tumors are typically asymptomatic unless large enough to cause mass effect or hemorrhage. The renal lesions of VHL do not typically cause renal failure, but renal cell carcinoma has been reported as the leading cause of death in this population [2, 20, 21].

Pathogenesis: The disease VHL is caused by an inherited mutation in one allele of the VHL gene, a tumor suppressor gene located on the short arm of chromosome 3 (3p25). A somatic mutation in the remaining functioning VHL allele causes loss of function of the resultant protein, pVHL. pVHL is part of a complex of proteins responsible for degradation of HIF1α, a transcription factor with many target genes encoding growth factors. With loss of pVHL function, HIF1α levels increase causing vasculogenesis and tumorigenesis [2].

Presentation: Patients typically present between age 35 and 40 years, although the disease can become apparent in infancy. Common presenting symptoms are altered neurological function or hematuria, and the most common initial lesions in VHL are retinal angiomas, cerebellar hemangiomas, and renal cell carcinoma. Patients with genetic risk for VHL may be detected based on screening [2, 20].

Evaluation: Genetic testing for VHL mutations is commercially available and can be utilized to determine if family members of VHL patients have genetic risk for the disease. Patients with an established genetic risk for VHL can be given a diagnosis of VHL themselves if they develop a single retinal or cerebellar hemangioblastoma, pheochromocytoma, or renal cell carcinoma. For patients without a family history, two or more of these lesions can lead to diagnosis. Ophthalmoscopic examination can diagnose retinal angiomas and should be performed annually for patients with VHL or those with genetic risk for the disease. These patients should also be evaluated annually with physical exam and 24-h urine collection for catecholamine metabolites and with imaging of the brain and abdomen every 3 years. Renal cysts on ultrasound have the typical ovoid or spherical hypoechoic collection within the kidney, with absence of internal echoes or septations. Renal tumors will typically have a more complex appearance, with internal echoes or heterogeneity suggestive of solid components. Contrast-enhanced CT or MRI is useful in discerning renal cell carcinoma from renal cyst in cases where diagnosis is in question [2].

Histology: Once the disease has manifested, renal cysts and tumors are found in multiple locations in bilateral kidneys. The cysts in VHL appear similar to simple renal cysts, although some cysts may be lined by hyperplastic cells that could indicate a precancerous lesion [2].

Treatment: Treatment of VHL is a multidisciplinary approach, given the various organ systems involved in this disease. The goal of renal management in VHL is to control renal cancer while preserving renal parenchyma as long as feasible, in order to delay renal insufficiency and ESRD. Current approaches to renal cell carcinomas in VHL employ frequent surveillance of the kidneys, with nephron-sparing surgery when tumors become large. Renal cysts in VHL do not require specific treatment [2].

Glomerulocystic Kidney Disease

Definition: *Glomerulocystic kidney disease* refers to a disease of bilateral kidneys containing diffuse cysts of Bowman's space and the adjacent proximal convoluted tubule. This is in contrast to *glomerulocystic kidney*, which refers to kidneys containing glomerular cysts in the setting of other pathology, usually within a multiple malformation syndrome [2, 7, 12].

Clinical features: Glomerulocystic kidney disease can present in infancy or may not present until adulthood. The disease is usually inherited in an autosomal dominant pattern, although it can present sporadically. Sporadic cases of the disease are thought to represent new mutations. The disease causes progressive renal failure with a wide range in severity, from patients who are asymptomatic into adulthood to those who die in the neonatal period. The different presentations in children and adulthood may represent different subtypes of this disease [2, 7, 12].

Pathogenesis: The etiology and pathogenesis of glomerulocystic kidney disease is unclear. The inheritance pattern is autosomal dominant, although a responsible gene has not been identified [2, 7, 12].

Presentation: Patients who present in infancy or childhood are typically discovered on the basis of imaging findings or symptoms of renal failure. Patients who present in adulthood, similarly, may present with hypertension, hematuria, proteinuria, renal insufficiency, or incidental discovery of cystic renal lesions on imaging [2, 7, 12].

Evaluation: Ultrasound examination shows bilateral kidneys with numerous minute cysts in the renal cortex without cysts in the renal medulla. Urinalysis and serum laboratory evaluation may reveal proteinuria, hematuria, and renal insufficiency. A renal biopsy may be necessary to make the definitive diagnosis [2, 7, 12].

Histology: Numerous renal cysts are seen throughout the renal cortex, from the subcapsular zone to the inner cortex, and are all less than 1 cm in diameter. There are cystic dilations of Bowman's space and the adjacent proximal convoluted tubule as well as glomerular degeneration [7].

Treatment: Treatment of this disease is based on the degree of renal failure, with medical treatment of hypertension and electrolyte imbalance when indicated. Patients who progress to ESRD will need dialysis and possible transplantation.

References

1. Glassberg KI, Stephens FD, Lebowitz RL, et al. Renal dysgenesis and cystic disease of the kidney: a report of the Committee on Terminology, Nomenclature and Classification, Section on Urology, American Academy of Pediatrics. J Urol. 1987;138:1085–92.
2. Pope IV JC. Renal dysgenesis and cystic disease of the kidney. In: Wein AJ, Kavoussi LR, Partin AW, Peters CA, Novick AC, editors. Campbell-Walsh Urology. 10th ed. Philadelphia: Elsevier Saunders; 2012. Chapter 118.
3. Peters C, Rushton HG. Vesicoureteral reflux associated renal damage: congenital reflux nephropathy and acquired renal scarring. J Urol. 2010;184:265–73.
4. Schaefer F, Bakkaloglu SA. Diseases of the kidney and urinary tract in children. In: Taal MW, Chertow GM, Marsden PA, Skorecki K, Yu ASL, Brenner BM, editors. Brenner and Rector's the Kidney, 9th Edition. Philadelphia: Elsevier Saunders, 2012. Chapter 75, p. 2622–79.
5. Lane PH. Oligomeganephronia. In: Drugs and Diseases. Medscape. 2014. http://emedicine. medscape.com/article/983074-overview. Accessed 28 Jan 2015.
6. Arant Jr BS, Sotelo-Avila C, Bernstein J. Segmental "hypoplasia" of the kidney. J Pediatr. 1979;95:931–9.
7. Bisceglia M, Galliani CA, Senger C, Stallone C, Sessa A. Renal cystic diseases: a review. Adv Anat Pathol. 2006;13:26–56.
8. Angtuaco TL, Miller SF, Ferris EJ. Congenital urinary tract abnormalities: prenatal and neonatal diagnosis. Curr Probl Diagn Radiol. 1990;19:165–98.
9. Calaway AC, Whittam B, Szymanski KM, Misseri R, Kaefer M, Rink RC, et al. Multicystic dysplastic kidney: is an initial voiding cystourethrogram necessary? Can J Urol. 2014;21:7510–4.
10. Bayram MT, Alaygut D, Soylu A, Serdaroglu E, Cakmakci H, Kavukcu S. Clinical and radiological course of simple renal cysts in children. Urology. 2014;3:433–7.
11. Israel GM, Bosniak MA. An update of the Bosniak renal cyst classification system. Urology. 2005;66:484–8. doi:10.1016/j.urology.2005.04.003.
12. Obata Y, Furusu A, Miyazaki M, Nishino T, Kawazu T, Kanamoto Y, et al. Glomerulocystic kidney disease in an adult with enlarged kidneys: a case report and review of the literature. Clin Nephrol. 2011;75:158–64.
13. Madewell JE, Goldman SM, Davis Jr CJ, Hartman DS, Feigin DS, Lichtenstein JE. Multilocular cystic nephroma: a radiographic-pathologic correlation of 58 patients. Radiology. 1983;146:309–21.
14. Menezes LF, Cai Y, Nagasawa Y, Silva AM, Watkins ML, Da Silva AM, et al. Polyductin, the PKHD1 gene product, comprises isoforms expressed in plasma membrane, primary cilium, and cytoplasm. Kidney Int. 2004;66:1345–55.
15. Dell KM. The spectrum of polycystic kidney disease in children. Adv Chronic Kidney Dis. 2011;18:339–47. doi:10.1053/j.ackd.2011.05.001.
16. Koptides M, Mean R, Demetriou K, Pierides A, Deltas CC. Genetic evidence for a transheterozygous model for cystogenesis in autosomal dominant polycystic kidney disease. Hum Mol Genet. 2000;9:447–52.

17. Wuthrich RP, Mei C. Pharmacological management of polycystic kidney disease. Expert Opin Pharmacother. 2014;15:1085–95. doi:10.1517/14656566.2014.903923.
18. Northrup H, Krueger DA. Tuberous sclerosis complex diagnostic criteria update: recommendations of the 2012 International Tuberous Sclerosis Complex Consensus Conference. Pediatr Neurol. 2013;49:243–54. doi:10.1016/j.pediatrneurol.2013.08.001.
19. Staley BA, Vail EA, Thiele EA. Tuberous sclerosis complex: diagnostic challenges, presenting symptoms, and commonly missed signs. Pediatrics. 2011;127:e117–25. doi:10.1542/peds.2010-0192. Epub 2010 Dec 20.
20. O' Brien FJ, Danapal M, Jairam S, Lalani AK, Cunningham J, Morrin M, et al. Manifestations of Von Hippel Lindau syndrome: a retrospective national review. Q J Med. 2014;107:291–6. doi:10.1093/qjmed/hct249.
21. Maher ER, Yates JR, Harries R, Benjamin C, Harris R, Moore AT, et al. Clinical features and natural history of von Hippel-Lindau disease. Q J Med. 1990;77:1151–63.

Chapter 5
Congenital Hydronephrosis

Ardalan E. Ahmad and Barry A. Kogan

Abbreviations

APD	Anteroposterior diameter
GA	Gestational age
SFU	Society for Fetal Urology
UPJ	Ureteropelvic junction
UTI	Urinary tract infection
UVJ	Ureterovesical junction
VCUG	Voiding cystourethrogram

Introduction

Congenital anomalies of the genitourinary system are common. Some involve the genitalia, but many involve the kidneys. Though originally thought to be uncommon, with the advent of prenatal ultrasound, these anomalies are now being discovered with increasing frequency. Of these, hydronephrosis is the most common.

Prior to routine use of antenatal ultrasonography, the majority of the children with hydronephrosis came to medical attention due to an abdominal mass or symptoms (e.g., urinary tract infection (UTI), stones, hematuria). This turns out to be quite rare. The advent of ultrasound technology changed this. It became readily

A.E. Ahmad, M.D.
Division of Urology, University of Toronto, Toronto, ON, Canada

B.A. Kogan, M.D. (✉)
Division of Urology, Department of Surgery and Pediatrics, Albany Medical College,
23 Hackett Blvd, Albany, NY 12208-3436, USA
e-mail: bkogan@communitycare.com

© Springer International Publishing Switzerland 2016
A.J. Barakat, H. Gil Rushton (eds.), *Congenital Anomalies of the Kidney and Urinary Tract*, DOI 10.1007/978-3-319-29219-9_5

77

apparent that ultrasound was both safe and beneficial for monitoring the fetus. As fluid collections are easily seen on ultrasound, fetal hydronephrosis was readily diagnosed. The quality of ultrasound has steadily improved and, increasingly, prenatal ultrasound has become routine. Hence, the finding of some form of fetal hydronephrosis has become common. This has created an interesting medical dilemma. Since hydronephrosis is now most often diagnosed before birth in asymptomatic infants, should it be treated aggressively to prevent future complications, or does that lead to overdiagnosis and overtreatment of conditions that would never need treatment? This chapter will review the epidemiology, grading, and etiology of congenital hydronephrosis with a focus on evaluation and treatment.

Embryology

During embryogenesis, humans develop three sets of kidneys: pronephros, mesonephros, and metanephros. Although the pronephros and mesonephros regress in utero, the metanephros develops to become the permanent kidney. Around the fourth week of gestation, the caudal end of the mesonephric duct forms the ureteric bud which will converge with and induce the metanephric blastema to form the future kidney. The metanephric mesenchyme continues to develop into glomerulus, proximal convoluted tubules, loop of Henle, and distal convoluted tubules, while the collecting ducts, calyces, renal pelvis, and ureter are derived from the ureteric bud. The mesonephric ducts connect to the urogenital sinus to form the future bladder trigone. The apical and pelvic portions of the urogenital sinus become the bladder and the urethra to the level of the urogenital diaphragm, while the phallic portion becomes the penile urethra in males and the lower third of vagina and vestibule in females [1].

Epidemiology

With the routine use of prenatal ultrasonography, there has been a dramatic increase in the rate of detection of fetal anomalies. Hydronephrosis is the most common anomaly identified on prenatal ultrasound, affecting 1–5 % of all pregnancies [2]. Although there is a high incidence of hydronephrosis, the clinical significance of this finding is uncertain, as the overwhelming majority of these infants will ultimately not have significant urological abnormalities [3].

Classification/Grading

Hydronephrosis is defined as abnormal increased intrarenal fluid associated with accumulation of urine in the renal collecting system (dilation of the renal pelvis and calyces). Classifying and grading the hydronephrosis is key as the severity of the hydronephrosis and its effect on the renal parenchyma are important factors in determining prognosis and treatment.

Renal Parenchyma

As a simple general rule, ultrasound can determine not only the degree of hydronephrosis but the health of the renal parenchyma. An ultrasound should ascertain the thickness of the renal parenchyma and its volume (usually in three dimensions). This has been shown to correlate well with the degree of function. In addition, ultrasound should be used to determine whether there is corticomedullary differentiation (a good sign for renal function), the parenchymal echogenicity (if more than the liver echogenicity this is a poor prognostic sign), and whether there are cortical cysts (a sign of renal dysplasia). Though not a functional test, considerable functional information can be obtained from the ultrasound (Fig. 5.1).

Degree of Hydronephrosis

Different classification systems have been used to describe the degree of hydronephrosis. Although the goal of these classifications has been to develop a uniform, objective, and reproducible method to grade hydronephrosis, the systems used remain somewhat subjective and have not been uniformly accepted.

The most common method that has been utilized for classification of prenatal hydronephrosis is measurement of the anteroposterior diameter (APD) in a transverse plane (Table 5.1, Fig. 5.2). This is thought to be reasonably objective and reproducible, but even with this one simple measurement, there is variability (e.g., depending

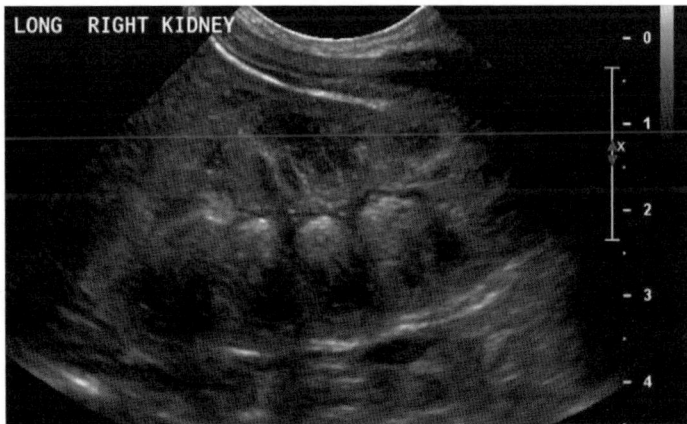

Fig. 5.1 Longitudinal ultrasound of the right kidney. The kidney is normal in size; there is good parenchymal thickness and excellent corticomedullary differentiation. Though ultrasound is not a functional test, it is highly likely this kidney has excellent function

Table 5.1 SFU proposed classification of prenatal urinary tract dilation by AP diameter

Degree of CHN	Second trimester (mm)	Third trimester (mm)
Mild	4 to <7	7 to <9
Moderate	7–10	9–15
Severe	>10	>15

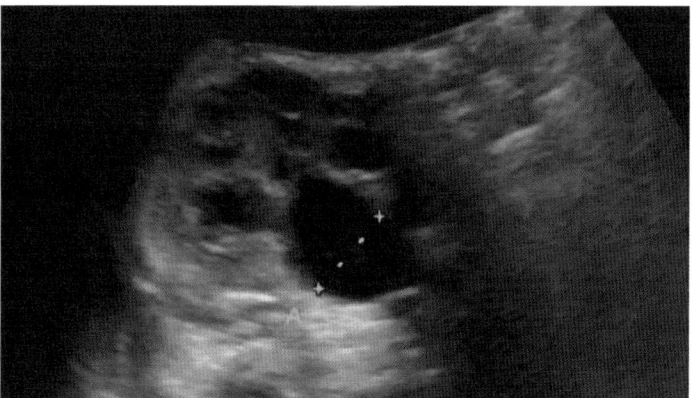

Fig. 5.2 Transverse ultrasound of the kidney, demonstrating an AP diameter of 16 mm

on the position of the fetus at the time of the measurement). Nonetheless, an APD of <4 mm at <28 weeks' gestation, a <7 mm at 28 weeks, is almost always predictive of no need for future intervention (and hence no need for postnatal workup). On the other end of the spectrum, one study showed that an AP diameter of ≥4 mm before 33 weeks' gestation or ≥7 mm after 33 weeks of gestation was 100 % sensitive in identifying patients with abnormal renal function or those who required subsequent intervention postnatally [4]. Since the "need" for surgery is not well defined, in our opinion, a clear cutoff value for defining obstruction requiring surgical intervention has not been determined.

Measurement of APD has also been used postnatally by many centers. However, in 1993, the Society for Fetal Urology (SFU) proposed a classification based not on the size of the renal pelvis (APD), but on the appearance of the intrarenal collecting system [1, 4]. The SFU grading system is a spectrum, with Grade 1 demonstrating normal parenchymal thickness and only renal pelvis splitting and Grade 4 revealing distention of the renal pelvis and calyces in addition to parenchymal thinning (Table 5.2, Fig. 5.3). This likely has been the most commonly used system of classification until recently. Indeed, many studies of outcome of patients with hydronephrosis are based on the SFU classification. In 2014, a revision of the SFU classification was published that proposed a common nomenclature for both pre- and postnatal grading of urinary tract dilation. This system should provide more standardized and reproducible description of hydronephrosis and is described in more detail later in this chapter [5, 6].

Table 5.2 SFU grading of infant hydronephrosis

SFU grade	Pattern of renal sinus splitting
Grade 0	No splitting
Grade 1	Urine in pelvis barely splits sinus
Grade 2	Dilation of major calyces
Grade 3	Uniform dilation of major and minor calyces, no parenchymal thinning
Grade 4	SFU Grade 3 and parenchymal thinning

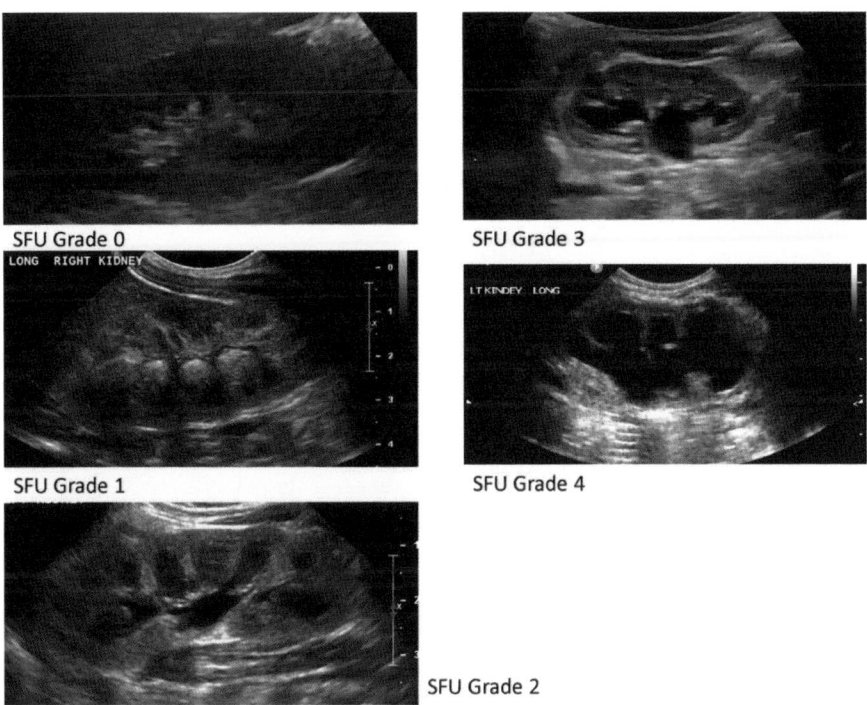

SFU Grade 0

SFU Grade 3

SFU Grade 1

SFU Grade 4

SFU Grade 2

Fig. 5.3 Ultrasound views of representative SFU Grades 0 to 4

Prenatal Evaluation/Management

There are no accepted guidelines for the evaluation and management of urinary tract dilation prenatally, but a general scheme is outlined (Fig. 5.4). Suffice it to say that the need for prenatal intervention of any kind is extremely rare. If the hydronephrosis is unilateral and the dilation is limited to the upper urinary tract, very limited prenatal follow-up of any type is needed for the hydronephrosis. Routine obstetrical care should be advised, and a postnatal evaluation beginning with a renal/bladder ultrasound should be performed, optimally 7–10 days after birth. The delay is thought to be valuable in low-risk patients as early postnatal ultrasound has been

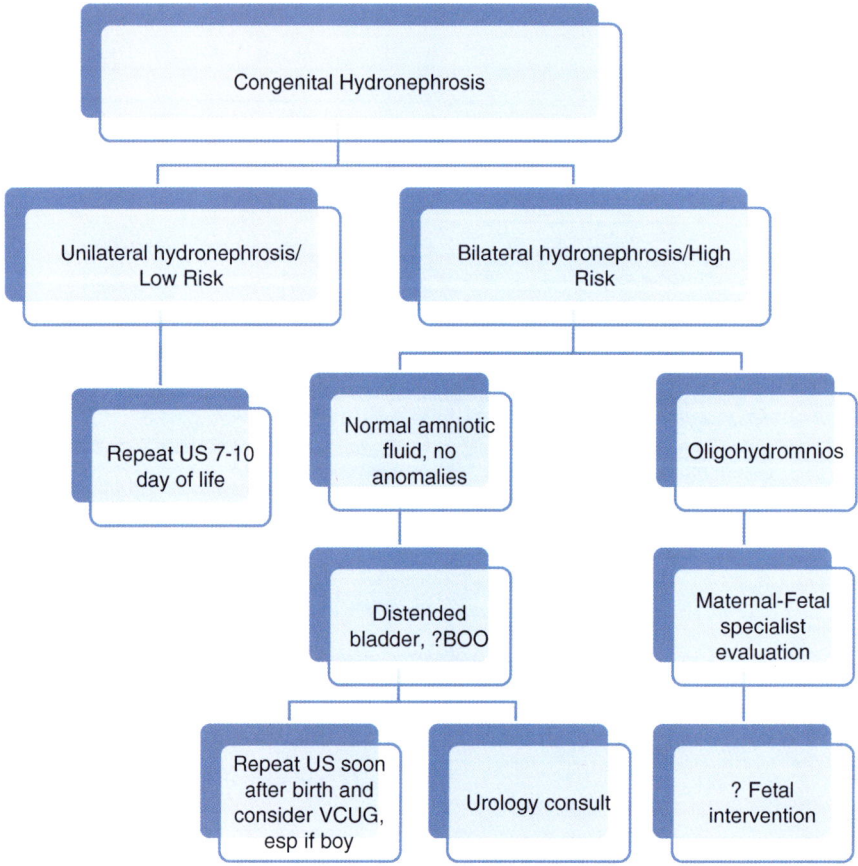

Fig. 5.4 Prenatal management of hydronephrosis. *BOO* bladder outlet obstruction, *US* ultrasound

associated with a significant false-negative rate (i.e., the early ultrasound significantly underestimates the degree of hydronephrosis, presumably due to low urine out of the neonate), providing a false sense of security. A neonatal circumcision in boys need not be withheld and may well reduce the rate of urinary tract infections in the first few months of life. The use of prophylactic antibiotics (generally amoxicillin or cephalexin 10 mg/kg/day) is controversial and is probably unnecessary unless there is significant ureteral dilation.

In the more unusual fetal cases in which there is bladder dilation as well, it is important to look for other anomalies in the fetus and to monitor amniotic fluid volumes. In the absence of other anomalies and when there are normal amniotic fluid volumes, interventions of any kind should be rare. If there is significant bladder dilation (or a "key hole sign") suggestive of posterior urethral valves (Fig. 5.5), the only concensus recommendation is to plan for delivery of the infant in a center where

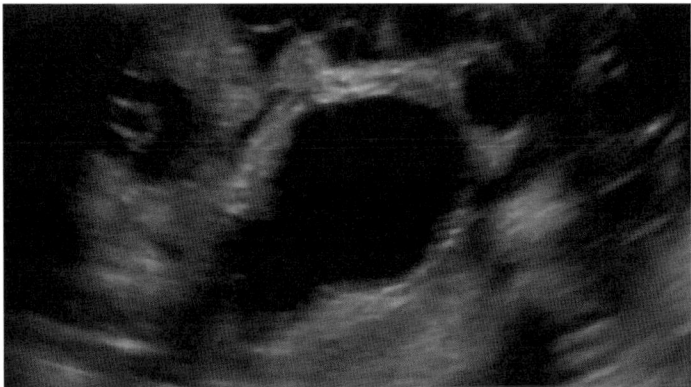

Fig. 5.5 Prenatal US demonstrating thick wall, dilated bladder "key hole sign" suggestive of bladder outlet obstruction. *BL* bladder, *PU* prostatic urethra

pediatric urology care is available. In the event of oligohydramnios, an evaluation by a high-risk maternal/fetal medicine specialist is warranted. These findings suggest neonatal demise and potentially could lead to the very rare circumstance in which prenatal intervention might be warranted. Even in expert hands however, there are limited data demonstrating improvement in long-term renal function. There has been some efficacy demonstrated for benefit in survival and in neonatal pulmonary function. Even so, significant specialized counseling is required as this brings up a major ethical dilemma. These rare neonates likely would have succumbed to pulmonary hypoplasia; with prenatal intervention, they might survive but be afflicted with neonatal renal failure, all the while putting the mother at considerable risk.

Postnatal Evaluation

The evaluation after birth depends again on whether the lower tract appears to be involved (Fig. 5.6). In boys, if the bladder is distended and/or if there is hydroureteronephrosis on both sides, a voiding cystourethrogram (VCUG) should be performed soon after birth to rule out posterior urethral valves. In girls, a VCUG is probably also warranted to rule out significant reflux, but not as urgently. In these cases, neonatal prophylactic antibiotics are usually recommended. Management is determined by the results of the VCUG and the severity of the abnormality on ultrasound.

If the hydronephrosis does not involve the bladder, then consideration is given to two main factors: (a) if the ureters are involved and (b) whether both kidneys are involved. The rate of urinary tract infection is higher in those with ureteral dilation, and hence if there is a suggestion of ureteral dilation on the ultrasound, prophylactic antibiotics are generally recommended. If there is ureteral dilation,

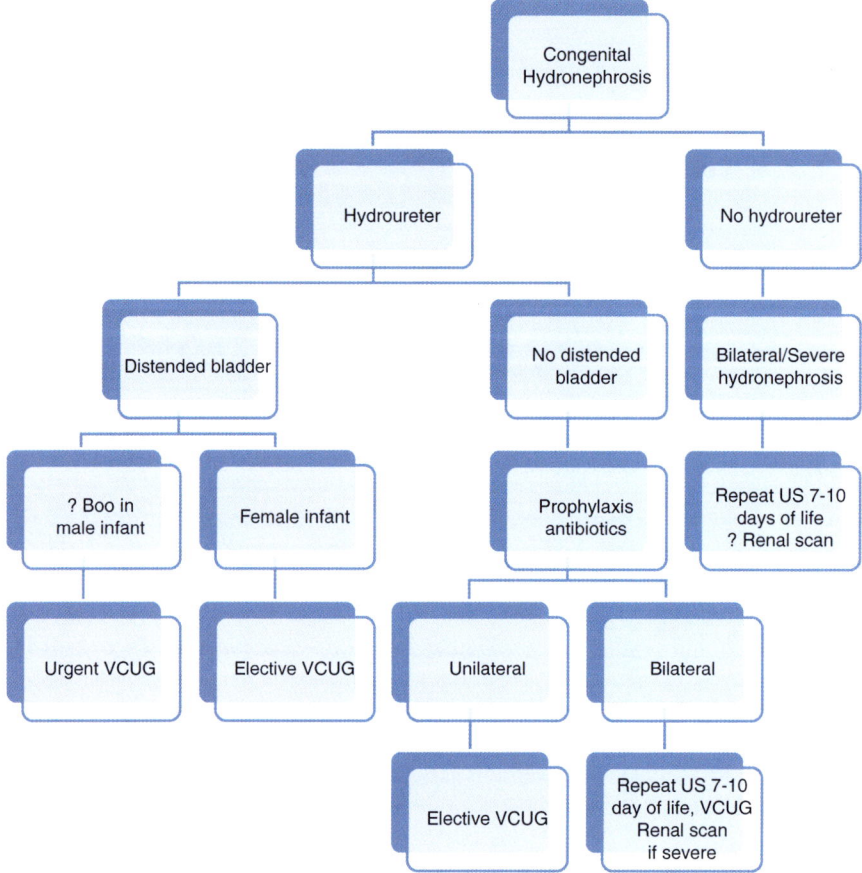

Fig. 5.6 Postnatal management of prenatal hydronephrosis. *BOO* bladder outlet obstruction, *US* ultrasound

the causes include either a functionally obstructed megaureter or VUR (or both). Alternatively, the infant may have nonobstructive, non-refluxing hydroureteronephrosis which resolves spontaneously over time. Evaluation consists of a postnatal ultrasound at about 7–10 days and a VCUG. In severe cases, a renal scan (MAG-3 diuretic renogram to determine function and drainage) may be valuable. The timing of these tests is not urgent if the condition is unilateral.

In the absence of ureteral dilation, then the urgency of the evaluation depends on whether the problem is bilateral. If so, then workup would be more urgent (depending also on the severity). In the past, workup would have included an ultrasound and VCUG, but currently in the absence of ureteral dilation, a VCUG is generally not recommended. A Mag-3 renal scan may become necessary, but that depends on the severity of the hydronephrosis.

Postnatal Management: Hydronephrosis (Without Ureteral Dilation)

Neonatal urinary tract dilation should not be confused with obstruction. Hydronephrosis is diagnosed by visualizing dilation of the collecting system, and obstruction is one cause of hydronephrosis, but there are many others (Tables 5.3 and 5.4) [6, 7]. For example, hydronephrosis can be the result of resolved obstruction. During embryogenesis, the ureter goes through a period when it is solid and does not have an open lumen; later, it will recanalize. If this is delayed, hydronephrosis may result, but as the lumen fully opens, there will be no residual obstruction. As another example, high urine flow may cause hydronephrosis. This is often true later in life in patients with diabetes insipidus. This also is likely a cause of prenatal hydronephrosis as renal tubular reabsorption has not fully developed and urine output on a per kg basis is high. Similarly, it is well known that maternal progesterone relaxes the maternal bladder and

Table 5.3 Differential diagnosis of congenital hydronephrosis [6]

Etiology	Incidence (%)
Transient hydronephrosis	50–70
Ureteropelvic junction obstruction (UPJO)	10–30
Vesicoureteral reflux (VUR)	10–20
Ureterovesical junction obstruction (UVJO)	5–15
Multicystic dysplastic kidney (MCDK)	2–6
Posterior urethral valves (PUVs)	1–2
Ureterocele/duplex system/ ectopic ureter	5–7
Other	<1

Table 5.4 Risk of uropathology based on degree of congenital hydronephrosis [7]

Estimated degree of hydronephrosis		
Pathology	Mild (percent 95 % CI)	Moderate (percent 95 % CI)	Severe (percent 95 % CI)
---	---	---	---
Any	11.9 (4.5–28.0)	45.1 (25.3–66.6)	88.3 (53.7–97.0)
UPJO	4.9 (2.0–11.9)	17.0 (7.6–33.9)	54.3 (21.7–83.6)
VUR	4.4 (1.5–12.1)	14.0 (7.1–25.9)	8.5 (4.7–15.0)
PUV	0.2 (0.0–1.4)	0.9 (0.2–2.9)	5.3 (1.2–21.0)
Ureteral obstruction	1.2 (0.2–8.0)	9.8 (6.3–14.9)	5.3 (1.4–18.2)
Other[a]	1.2 (0.3–4.0)	3.4 (0.5–19.4)	14.9 (3.6–44.9)

UPJO ureteropelvic junction obstruction, *VUR* vesicoureteral reflux, *PUV* posterior urethral valve
[a]Prune belly syndrome, VATER syndrome, solitary kidney, renal mass, and unclassified

ureteral musculature, and it has been shown that progesterone has the same effect in the fetus, resulting in prenatal hydronephrosis. Finally, another main cause of hydronephrosis in the neonate is VUR (discussed in Chap. 6). All these causes of hydronephrosis are nonobstructing. They are nearly all self-limiting and require no surgical treatment. In contrast, there are some cases of neonatal hydronephrosis that are the result of obstruction. In these cases, the most common location of the obstruction is at the junction of the ureter and pelvis, and this is generally referred to as ureteropelvic junction (UPJ) obstruction. It should be noted that nearly all of these cases are partial obstructions, and in many instances these partial obstructions do not need treatment. Even marked dilation has been shown to resolve nonoperatively in some cases [8].

One of the main challenges for the clinician is to determine when postnatal hydronephrosis is the result of significant obstruction, that is, not only obstruction but obstruction that is severe enough to result in renal damage. In addition to the standard history and physical exam, attention should be focused in several areas. Occasionally, as in the case of a boy with a posterior urethral valve, a very weak voiding stream will have been noted, or there may be a positive family history of VUR. However, as mentioned above, nearly all these infants are asymptomatic. Physical examination should include the lower abdomen (looking especially for a distended bladder), the genitalia (looking for penile abnormalities that may affect urine flow), and the spine to rule out a neurogenic bladder as a cause of hydronephrosis. Unless the hydronephrosis is bilateral and severe, no laboratory studies are needed. Ultrasound is the mainstay of the immediate workup. Since most research has been focused on the previous SFU grading system, this should be used as a reference when reviewing the literature. For most Grade 1 and 2 hydronephrosis, little workup is needed, and repeat ultrasounds to look for progression should be limited. Repeat ultrasound is more warranted in Grade 3 hydronephrosis, mostly to determine if there is progression to Grade 4.

Grade 4 hydronephrosis (hydronephrosis with associated parenchymal thinning) is the main cause for concern. Again, the mainstay of evaluation is serial ultrasound examinations. Progression of dilation and continued thinning of parenchyma are generally signs of significant obstruction warranting intervention (as they appear to be causing renal injury). However, it is important to be somewhat cautious when interpreting the ultrasound as a full bladder, increased hydration, and even supine vs. prone positioning may all make the hydronephrosis appear worse, so they must be comparable on each study. Some clinicians use AP diameter as the best judge of the need for surgery (<2 cm, very unlikely to need surgery; 2–5 cm, questionable; and >5 cm will almost always need surgery) [9]. Because there is a large "gray zone," this is not as helpful as clinicians would like. Although it was at one time mandatory, a VCUG is generally not performed unless there is ureteral dilation noted.

Most clinicians will obtain a diuretic renogram for Grade 3 and 4 hydronephrosis (Fig. 5.7). The purpose of this test is to determine the relative renal function of the hydronephrotic kidney, and the washout after the diuretic is

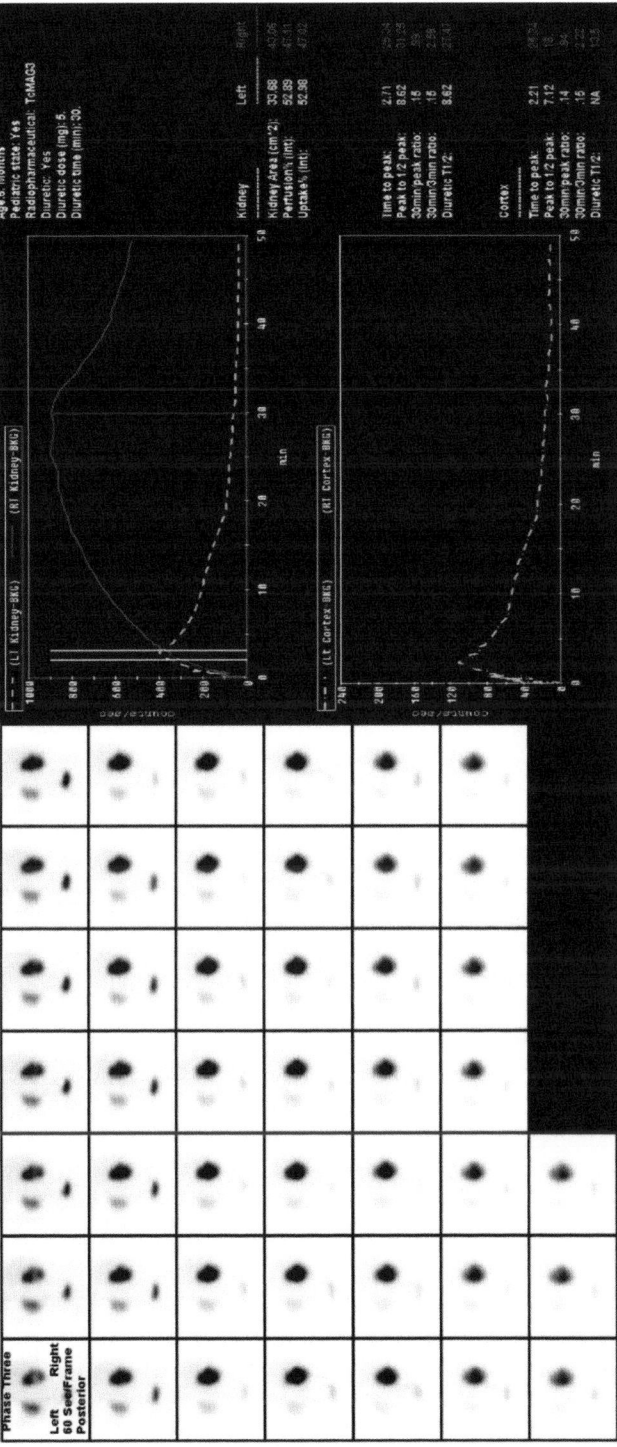

Fig. 5.7 Diuretic renogram in patients with SFU Grade 4 hydronephrosis. The relative function of the right and left kidneys is almost equal. The left kidney starts draining within a couple of minutes. The right kidney demonstrates no drainage until furosemide is given and then only moderate drainage

given. Indeed, some clinicians place great importance on the relative function. If >40 %, they generally do not recommend intervention, whereas if <40 % there is thought to be less margin for error, and if there is any suggestion of obstruction, surgery is recommended. Again, there are many caveats. In large hydronephrotic kidneys, the background subtraction can be tricky, and the measurements may overestimate the function of the hydronephrotic kidney, especially when it is on the right [10]. Also, the amount of washout is dependent not only on the degree of obstruction but also on the size and compliance of the collecting system as well as the degree of response to the diuretic. In general, <40 % relative function of the affected kidney (or a drop of 10 % from a previous study) and progression of hydronephrosis on ultrasound are the main indications for operative intervention in infants. Progressive deterioration in drainage on Lasix MAG-3 renography is another indication for intervention. In two small but randomized and controlled studies of patients with Grade 4 hydronephrosis, about 25 % of those observed ultimately were felt to need operative intervention [11, 12].

In older children, there are some significant differences. Whereas most infants with significant hydronephrosis and UPJ obstruction are boys, the ratio of girls to boys increases and indeed reverses [13]. Further, the majority of older children are symptomatic from the obstruction. The major symptoms are usually intermittent pain and often emesis. Hematuria may also be present and rarely the children will develop stones in the hydronephrotic kidney. Surgical correction of UPJ obstruction is generally straightforward. The findings in neonates are almost always a kink and fibrosis around the UPJ and are thought to represent an "intrinsic obstruction." The great majority of cases are treated with a dismembered pyeloplasty [14]. The obstructing segment is removed and the healthy ureter below is sewn to the healthy renal pelvis above. In some cases, a stent is left indwelling to help insure proper healing, but this usually requires a second procedure later (albeit minor) to remove it. In older children with symptomatic intermittent obstruction, the obstruction is more likely to be "extrinsic," in many cases from a crossing vessel. This should be looked for carefully at the time of operation and preserved. In most cases again, a dismembered pyeloplasty is performed, doing the anastomosis on the anterior side of the vessel, but there are some techniques that "hitch" the vessel cephalad to the ureteropelvic junction.

The biggest controversy currently is over the approach. The procedure can be done with the traditional open approach or using a laparoscopic approach. In some centers, infant pyeloplasty is performed with a robot-assisted laparoscopic technique, but this is challenging due to the size of the robot and the robotic equipment [15]. Most patients are discharged the next day, so the principal advantages of the laparoscopic approaches are cosmetic (with multiple small incisions vs. one larger one). At one time, there was enthusiasm for endopyelotomy (incising the UPJ internally and leaving a stent for the ureter to heal over), but the results are not good enough for use in primary cases. The technique may be helpful in cases of restenosis. Fortunately in children, this is rarely needed with initial pyeloplasty success rates of >95 % reported routinely. Success is usually defined as less hydronephrosis and thicker parenchyma on ultrasound, but in questionable cases a diuretic renogram may be helpful which typically demonstrates stable or improved differential renal function and improved drainage.

Postnatal Management: Hydroureteronephrosis

When the ureter is dilated, the level of the problem is at the ureterovesical junction (UVJ). There are a variety of etiologies that can cause this condition, most prominently VUR, UVJ obstruction, or both. As noted above, a VCUG is usually performed to determine whether there is reflux present and a Mag-3 renal Lasix scan to rule out distal obstruction as a cause of the problem. Also, because ureteral dilation is associated with a higher rate of urinary tract infections, prophylactic antibiotics are generally recommended.

UVJ obstruction in infants is a fascinating condition. Rather than an actual stenosis, the pathophysiology is thought to be a segment of ureter just outside the bladder that has only circular and no longitudinal muscle [16]. This then causes the ureter to close as it contracts, inhibiting peristalsis. On older fluoroscopic studies, peristalsis is noted starting in the renal calyces and continuing down the ureter to the aperistaltic segment. At this point, the ureter closes on itself and the peristalsis reverses, heading back up to the kidney and ending again in the calyces. This leads to the classic radiographic picture of calyces dilated out of proportion to the proximal ureter and the distal ureter being very dilated to a normal caliber segment just outside the bladder (Fig. 5.8).

For reasons that are unclear (maybe the longitudinal muscle grows into the abnormal segment of ureter), the natural history of the condition is one of spontaneous improvement. Hence, observation is the treatment of choice. At least 50 % will improve spontaneously and another 30–40 % will remain stable.

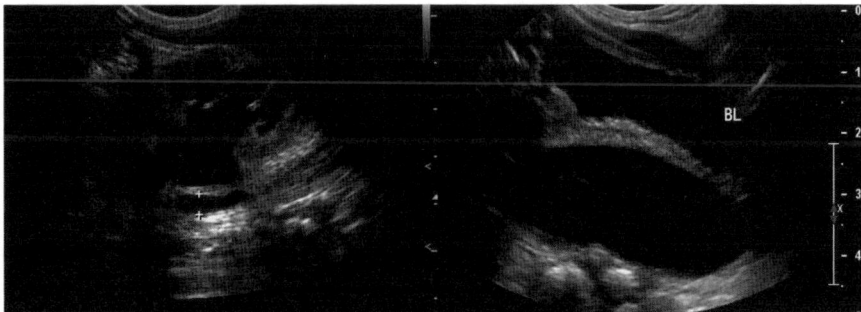

Fig. 5.8 Renal and bladder ultrasound in a patient with UVJ obstruction. The calyces (*white arrows*) are dilated out of proportion to the proximal ureter (*left* picture), and in the *right* picture, the distal ureter (DU) is very dilated up to a normal caliber segment just outside the bladder. *U* proximal ureter, *BL* bladder, *DU* distal ureter Labels missing and the figures need more contrast to see the urine (black) and the tissues around them (grey)

Although a number of ingenious surgical repairs have been devised, operative intervention is reserved for those rare cases of progression of hydronephrosis on ultrasound, worsening drainage and/or poor renal function on renal scan or recurrent UTI that cannot be prevented by prophylactic antibiotics. When surgery is performed, the ureter above the aperistaltic segment is tailored to a smaller diameter and reimplanted into the bladder.

Modern Classification of Hydronephrosis

The SFU has recently convened a multidisciplinary panel and proposed a new standardized system for describing and measuring hydronephrosis [6]. It is hoped that future clinical care and research in this field will take advantage of this standardization. The new SFU classification system utilizes the APD, calyceal dilation, parenchymal thickness, and appearance as well the appearance of ureter and bladder to classify patients (Table 5.5). In contrast to the previous SFU classification system, the new classification is meant to be used both prenatally and postnatally to risk stratify patients and to determine the appropriate follow-up schedule (also discussed in Chap. 13).

Prenatally, the new SFU system stratifies fetuses with hydronephrosis (based on gestational age (GA)) to a low-risk or an increased-risk group for postnatal uropathy (Fig. 5.9). A fetus is considered to be at increased risk of postnatal uropathy if APD is ≥ 7 mm at <28 weeks or ≥ 10 mm at ≥ 28 weeks or if there are any one of the following findings: dilation of peripheral calyces, abnormal parenchymal thickness,

Table 5.5 SFU proposed ultrasound parameters included in the classification of urinary tract dilation [6]

US parameters	Measurement/findings (mm)	Note
Anteroposterior renal pelvic diameter (APRPD)		Measured on transverse image at the maximal diameter of intrarenal pelvis
Calyceal dilation Central (major calyces) Peripheral (minor calyces)	Yes/no Yes/no	
Parenchymal thickness	Normal/abnormal	Subjective assessment
Parenchymal appearance	Normal/abnormal	Evaluate echogenicity, corticomedullary differentiation, and for cortical cysts
Ureter	Normal/abnormal	Dilation of ureter is considered abnormal; however, transient visualization of the ureter is considered normal postnatally
Bladder	Normal/abnormal	Evaluate wall thickness, for the presence of ureterocele and for a dilated posterior urethra

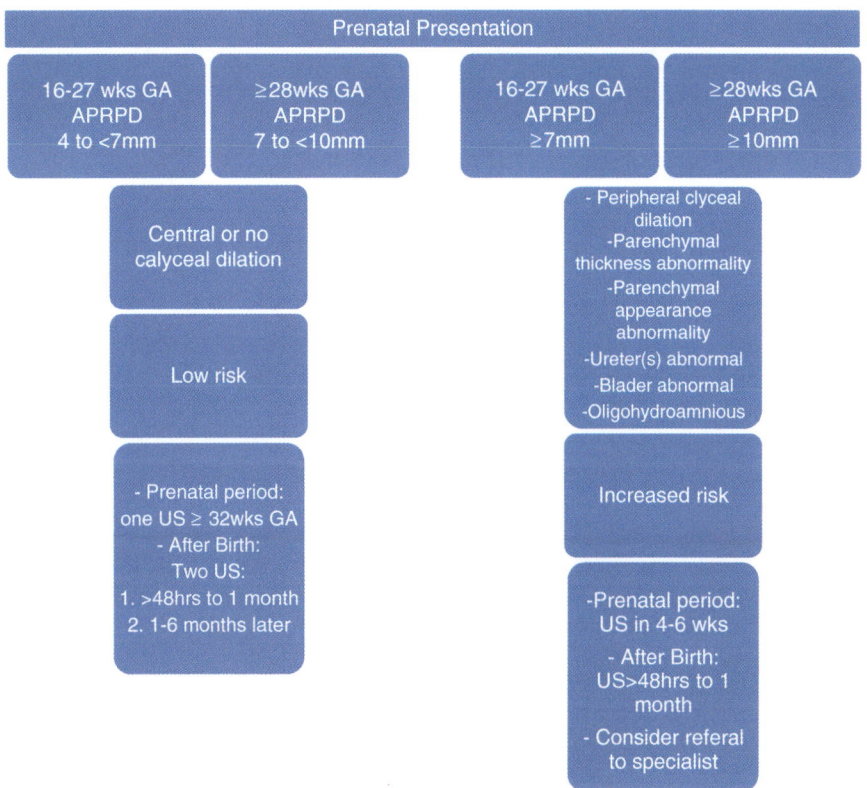

Fig. 5.9 SFU proposed risk stratification and management schema for prenatal urinary tract dilation

appearance of visibly dilated ureter, an abnormal bladder, or the presence of oligo-hydramnios suspected to be related to the urinary tract [6]. Management then is based on this risk assessment. For example, in a fetus categorized as low risk based on ultrasound prior to 32 weeks' GA, only one further repeat ultrasound at ≥32 weeks' GA is recommended. On the other hand, fetuses with persistent or worsening hydronephrosis are followed with a postnatal ultrasound at >48 h of life. Patients with increased risk of postnatal uropathy are routinely reevaluated with an ultrasound in 4–6 weeks, with certain conditions requiring a more stringent follow-up (e.g., posterior urethral valves, bilateral severe hydronephrosis, solitary kidney) (Fig. 5.9) [6].

Similarly, the ultrasound findings after 48 h of life are used to categorize patients to three groups for postnatal risk assessment (Fig. 5.10). Patients at low risk for postnatal uropathy are only followed with repeat ultrasound in 1–6 months. For higher-risk groups, recommendations are made for more frequent repeat ultrasound and, when appropriate, VCUG, diuretic renography, and prophylactic antibiotics. Boys with bilateral hydronephrosis and a distended bladder require early postnatal evaluation with a VCUG to rule out a posterior urethral valve. Unfortunately, there

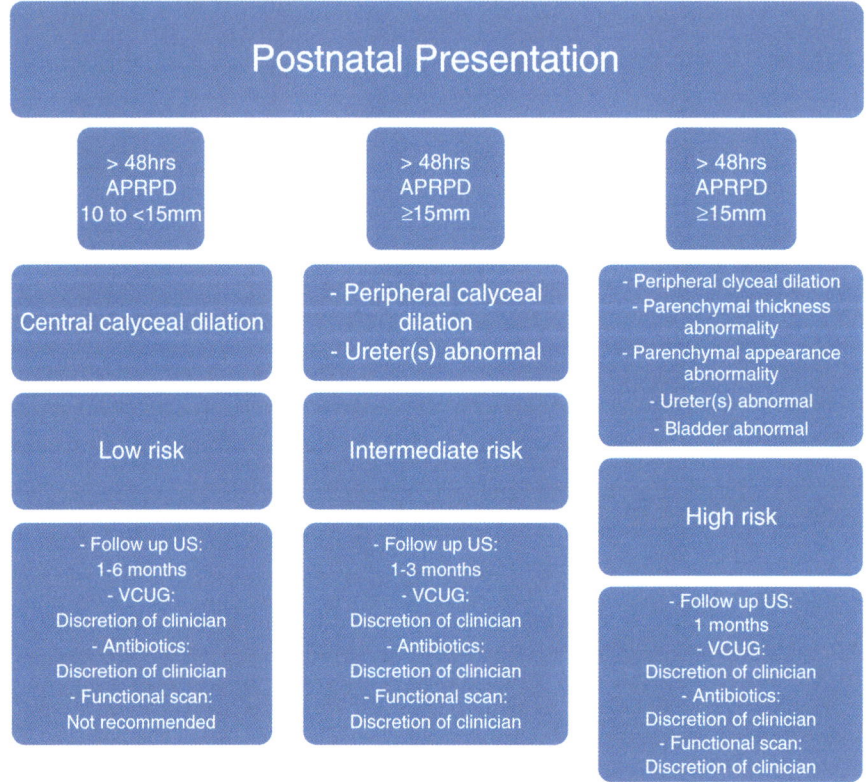

Fig. 5.10 SFU recommended risk stratification system and management schema for postnatal urinary tract dilation

are not enough data to support strong recommendations in many instances, and some decisions are left to the discretion of the specialist (Fig. 5.10) [6]. It is hoped that the new system will standardize data collection, provide risk assessment information to clinicians, and be a guide for future research. How well it will be universally adopted remains unclear.

Conclusion

Congenital hydronephrosis remains a clinical challenge with a wide gray zone. Identifying the select group of patients who will benefit from early intervention to prevent renal damage as a consequence of hydronephrosis requires careful follow-up and good clinical judgment. We recommend that the newly revised SFU classification and risk-based management proposal be used universally in the care of patients with congenital hydronephrosis. Future clinical care and research using the new SFU classification will help better understand the correlation between the SFU classification and outcomes.

References

1. Sadler T.W. Langman's medical embryology. 12th ed. Philadelphia: Lippincott Williams & Wilkins; 2012. Chapter 16, Urogenital system. p. 232–59.
2. Nguyen HT, Herndon CD, Cooper C, Gatti J, Kirsch A, Kokorowski P, et al. The Society for Fetal Urology consensus statement on the evaluation and management of antenatal hydronephrosis. J Pediatr Urol. 2010;6:212–31.
3. Liu DB, Armstrong 3rd WR, Maizels M. Hydronephrosis: prenatal and postnatal evaluation and management. Clin Perinatol. 2014;41:661–78.
4. Corteville JE, Gray DL, Crane JP. Congenital hydronephrosis: correlation of fetal ultrasonographic findings with infant outcome. Am J Obstet Gynecol. 1991;165:384–8.
5. Fernbach SK, Maizels M, Conway JJ. Ultrasound grading of hydronephrosis: introduction to the system used by the Society for Fetal Urology. Pediatr Radiol. 1993;23:478–80.
6. Nguyen HT, Benson CB, Bromley B, Campbell JB, Chow J, Coleman B, et al. Multidisciplinary consensus on the classification of prenatal and postnatal urinary tract dilation (UTD classification system). J Pediatr Urol. 2014;10:982–98.
7. Lee RS, Cendron M, Kinnamon DD, Nguyen HT. Antenatal hydronephrosis as a predictor of postnatal outcome: a meta-analysis. Pediatrics. 2006;118:586–93.
8. Koff SA, Campbell KD. The nonoperative management of unilateral neonatal hydronephrosis: natural history of poorly functioning kidneys. J Urol. 1994;152:593–5.
9. Ransley PG, Dhillon HK, Gordon I, Duffy PG, Dillon MJ, Barratt TM. The postnatal management of hydronephrosis diagnosed by prenatal ultrasound. J Urol. 1990;144:584–7. discussion 593–4.
10. Nguyen HT, Kogan BA. Upper urinary tract obstruction: experimental and clinical aspects. Br J Urol. 1998;81 Suppl 2:13–21.
11. Palmer LS, Maizels M, Cartwright PC, Fernbach SK, Conway JJ. Surgery versus observation for managing obstructive grade 3 to 4 unilateral hydronephrosis: a report from the Society for Fetal Urology. J Urol. 1998;159:222–8.
12. Dhillon HK. Prenatally diagnosed hydronephrosis: the Great Ormond Street experience. Br J Urol. 1998;81 Suppl 2:39–44.
13. Capello SA, Kogan BA, Giorgi Jr LJ, Kaufman Jr RP. Prenatal ultrasound has led to earlier detection and repair of ureteropelvic junction obstruction. J Urol. 2005;174:1425–8.
14. Carr M, Casale P. Campbell-Walsh urology. 10th ed. Philadelphia: Elsevier Saunders; 2011. Chapter 120, Anomalies and surgery of the ureter in children. p. 3212–35.
15. Thakre AA, Bailly Y, Sun LW, Van Meer F, Yeung CK. Is smaller workspace a limitation for robot performance in laparoscopy? J Urol. 2008;179:1138–42.
16. Tanagho EA, Pugh RC. The anatomy and function of the ureterovesical junction. Br J Urol. 1963;35:151–65.

Chapter 6
Vesicoureteral Reflux

Angela M. Arlen and Christopher S. Cooper

Abbreviations

AAP	American Academy of Pediatrics
BBD	Bladder-bowel dysfunction
DMSA	Dimercaptosuccinic acid
NICE	National Institute for Health and Clinical Excellence
RNC	Radionuclide cystography
US	Ultrasound
UTI	Urinary tract infection
UVJ	Ureterovesical junction
VCUG	Voiding cystourethrogram
VUR	Vesicoureteral reflux

Introduction

Vesicoureteral reflux (VUR) is one of the most common urologic diagnoses affecting children, with an estimated prevalence of 0.4–1.8 % in the general pediatric population [1] and 30 % in those with a history of febrile urinary tract infection [2]. Approximately 10–20 % of infants with antenatal hydronephrosis will be diagnosed with reflux [3].

Spontaneous resolution of primary reflux is common. Resolution is thought to result from remodeling of the ureterovesical junction (UVJ) involving an elongation of the ureter traversing the bladder wall with growth of the child. In addition, stabilization of bladder storage and voiding dynamics over the first several years of life may

A.M. Arlen, M.D. • C.S. Cooper, M.D., F.A.A.P., F.A.C.S. (✉)
Department of Urology, University of Iowa Hospitals and Clinics, University of Iowa Carver College of Medicine, 200 Hawkins Drive, 3RCP, Iowa City, IA 52242-1089, USA
e-mail: christopher-cooper@uiowa.edu

© Springer International Publishing Switzerland 2016
A.J. Barakat, H. Gil Rushton (eds.), *Congenital Anomalies of the Kidney and Urinary Tract*, DOI 10.1007/978-3-319-29219-9_6

result in lower intravesical pressures contributing to reflux resolution. Multiple factors impact the chance for spontaneous reflux resolution including the grade of reflux, gender, age, presence of voiding dysfunction, presence of renal parenchymal scarring, and bladder volume at the onset of VUR on voiding cystourethrogram (VCUG) [4, 5]. A risk-based approach considering multiple demographic, radiographic, and clinical factors should be employed to guide individualized patient management [6]. Surgical intervention may be necessary in children with persistent reflux, renal scarring, or recurrent febrile UTI.

Pathophysiology

VUR can be categorized as either primary or secondary. Primary VUR is frequently attributed to an abnormally short intravesical tunnel at the ureterovesical junction. Secondary VUR develops when abnormal lower urinary tract function and elevated intravesical pressures overcome an otherwise competent ureterovesical junction resulting in retrograde flow of urine.

Primary Vesicoureteral Reflux

Primary VUR is caused by failure of vesicoureteric junction to develop properly. Frequently, the ratio of the length of the ureter within the bladder wall to its diameter is reduced in refluxing ureters. This is thought to occur early during embryonic development of the ureter, at 6 weeks gestation [7].

Secondary Vesicoureteral Reflux (VUR)

Secondary VUR is found in disorders that result in abnormal urinary tract function and increased intravesical pressure such as neurogenic bladder or posterior urethral valves. The increased intravesical pressures in these conditions overcome what would otherwise be a competent ureterovesical junction (UVJ). The goals of management of pediatric neurogenic or otherwise severely compromised bladders include achieving low-pressure urinary storage and providing urinary continence while preserving upper tract function. In most cases reflux will resolve or improve by directly decreasing bladder pressure via anticholinergic therapy and/or intermittent catheterization. Children with secondary VUR require close monitoring with serial sonography as well as urodynamics. Congenital anomalies involving the UVJ such as periureteral bladder diverticula or complete ureteral duplication also predispose to reflux [8]. Secondary VUR may also be seen in children with no anatomic genitourinary or neurologic abnormality but suffer from bladder and bowel dysfunction [9]. The increased risk of urinary tract infections in these children is improved by identification and treatment of their bladder and bowel dysfunction. In addition, this treatment may result in resolution of the VUR.

Diagnosis

The diagnosis and subsequent management of VUR in young children have become increasingly controversial regarding which patients should be evaluated for reflux and when detected, which patients should be treated. While not all children are subject to the potentially harmful sequelae of reflux, in select patients, the prompt diagnosis and treatment of VUR may prevent recurrent pyelonephritis, renal scarring, and loss of function.

Initial Febrile Urinary Tract Infection

The diagnosis of VUR often follows the diagnosis of febrile UTI. Approximately 1/3 of children with febrile UTIs will have VUR demonstrated by VCUG. In a febrile child the diagnosis of a UTI requires a positive urine culture. The method of obtaining the urine specimen is critical for an accurate diagnosis of UTI. Urine specimens should be obtained through catheterization or suprapubic aspiration if a clean catch specimen is not feasible, as the diagnosis of UTI cannot be reliably established via urine culture collected in a bag [10]. To accurately establish the diagnosis of UTI, the AAP requires the presence of >50,000 colony-forming unites per mL of a uropathogen on catheterized specimen as well as pyuria and/or bacteriuria on urinalysis [10]. Approximately 15 % of children with UTI have renal scarring identified by DMSA scan, and this percentage increases as the number of UTIs increases [11]. Recurrent pyelonephritis is also associated with increased risk of subsequent hypertension and chronic kidney disease. The potential to minimize renal scaring and significant morbidity with prompt and appropriate antibiotic therapy emphasizes the need for early and accurate diagnosis of pediatric UTI [12].

Once the diagnosis of UTI is made, there is a lack of consensus regarding subsequent imaging. Recommendations for imaging after a UTI vary significantly between guideline committees [6, 10, 13, 14]. The NICE guidelines recommend routinely obtaining an ultrasound in children less than 6 months but limit sonography in those over 6 months of age to children with either a recurrent UTI or an atypical UTI as defined by being seriously ill, poor urine flow, abdominal or bladder mass, raised creatinine, septicemia, failure to respond to treatment within 48 h, or infection with a non-*E. coli* organism [14].

In 2011, the American Academy of Pediatrics (AAP) revised their practice guidelines regarding the diagnosis and management of initial febrile UTIs in infants and young children aged 2–24 months [10]. Unlike the NICE guidelines, the AAP recommends screening renal and bladder ultrasound for all of these children but no longer recommends routine VCUG after the initial febrile UTI in this age cohort. The recommendation to limit VCUG was based largely on a meta-analysis of several studies showing no benefit to antibiotic prophylaxis in children with VUR [15–18]. The validity of these studies, with the conclusion that it is not worth making the diagnosis of VUR, has been challenged by recent large, randomized controlled trials showing the benefit of prophylactic antibiotics in reducing recurrent febrile UTI in children with VUR [19, 20]. The Swedish Reflux Trial demonstrated that antibiotic prophylaxis significantly decreased the recurrent fUTI rates in girls with grade III or IV VUR. In addition, new renal damage in girls due to infection seen on DMSA renal scan was three times greater in the nontreatment group than the prophylaxis group [20, 21]. Likewise, the RIVUR trial also demonstrated a substantially reduced risk of recurrent UTI in children with VUR on antibiotic prophylaxis [19].

The AAP Section on Urology voiced strong disagreement with the omission of routine VCUG in the evaluation of young children following initial febrile UTI [22]. Rather, they recommended that VCUG remain as an accepted option at this time noting that some children with VUR benefit from early detection and treatment.

An alternative approach to the evaluation of children with febrile UTIs begins with a DMSA renal scan rather than a VCUG. The "top-down approach" in the management of febrile UTI attempts to identify which children may have clinically significant VUR by evaluating kidneys for pyelonephritis and/or scarring with DMSA scans. Prospective studies of children evaluated with DMSA scintigraphy at the time of their first febrile infection demonstrated that 60–80 % with febrile UTI have DMSA findings consistent with acute pyelonephritis. Acute DMSA abnormalities detected at acute febrile UTI persist in 36–56 % of affected kidneys with full recovery of renal function in the remainder [23, 24]. A positive DMSA scan performed within weeks of the onset of a febrile UTI used as an indication for VCUG may potentially reduce "unnecessary" VCUGs by 50 % compared to an approach obtaining VCUGs in all children with febrile UTI. The benefit of such an approach is not only a reduction in children undergoing VCUG but identification of reflux in a higher risk group with structural and/or functional renal abnormalities. It can therefore also avoid overtreatment of patients with clinically insignificant VUR.

Patient History/Physical Examination

Approximately 10–20 % of infants with a history of antenatal hydronephrosis will have VUR. Retroperitoneal ultrasound (US) should be obtained in all infants with prenatally detected hydronephrosis. The incidence of reflux appears to increase with the degree of sonographic dilation postnatally; however, the degree of dilation does not appear to correlate with the grade of VUR [3]. Ultrasound findings including hydroureter, duplication, and renal dysmorphia have been shown to correlate with diagnosis of VUR, allowing for more discrete use of VCUG in the antenatal period [8]. However, a large percentage of children with VUR, even high-grade reflux, will have a normal renal ultrasound.

The family history may identify a child at risk for VUR. A strong inheritance pattern exists with primary VUR, highlighting the importance of obtaining family history in children presenting with febrile UTI. It is most prevalent in Caucasians of Scandinavian descent and less common in those of African descent. The incidence of VUR in children of a parent that had VUR is about 50%, and the incidence in siblings is about 25%. Screening of siblings with reflux has demonstrated an increased prevalence of VUR on meta-analysis, with younger children more likely to be diagnosed [1]. Sibling screening remains controversial and is not uniformly performed; recommendations for screening are limited by the uncertainty of any potential benefit gained from identifying VUR in asymptomatic patients. A VCUG or radionuclide cystogram is recommended in siblings of children with VUR if they have evidence of renal cortical abnormalities or renal size asymmetry on ultrasound as well as if they have had a UTI [1].

While the majority of children with VUR will have an entirely normal physical examination, thorough examination of the back should be performed to exclude any sacral anomalies that may be indicative of occult spinal dysraphism (Fig. 6.1). Circumcision status of male patients should be determined as it impacts recurrent febrile UTI risk, particularly in boys under 12 months of age [25, 26]. Smith et al. demonstrated that circumcised males with high-grade VUR had fewer infections as well as a lower risk of new parenchymal scarring [27].

Imaging

As with any testing, the clinician should first ask if the results will alter the management of the child, and if the answer is "no," then the test should not be ordered. At present, it is reasonable to state that all imaging strategies fall short of the ultimate

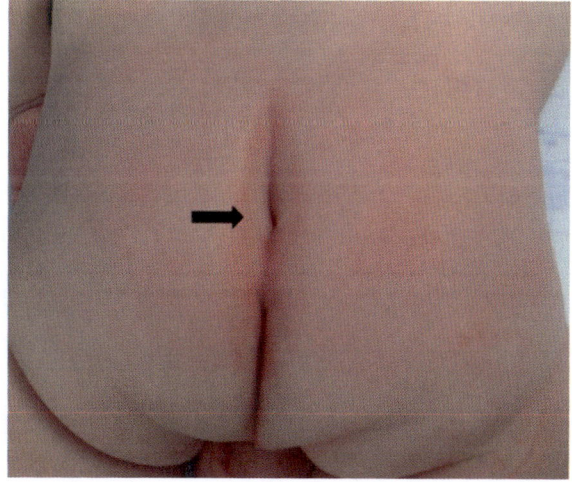

Fig. 6.1 Sacral dimple (*arrow*). When a sacral dimple is present, it requires further evaluation with spinal ultrasound and/ or plain films to exclude sacral anomalies

goal of being able to identify and test only those children who will benefit from VUR diagnosis and management.

Renal and Bladder Ultrasonography (US)

Parenchymal echogenicity or scarring, renal atrophy, alterations in corticomedullary differentiation, calyceal or ureteral dilation, and urothelial thickening have been associated with reflux [28–30]; however sonography is neither sensitive nor specific for VUR. Several recent publications focusing on the utility of retroperitoneal US as a diagnostic tool in children with febrile UTI have concluded that sonography is a poor screening test for pyelonephritis and VUR [31, 32].

Voiding Cystourethrogram (VCUG)

Contrast VCUG has long been a mainstay of VUR diagnosis. Advantages include the ability to grade the severity of reflux based on a standardized international scale, visualization of bladder anatomy, and assessment of the urethra during voiding [33]. VCUGs performed with a single cycle of filling and voiding show false-negatives up to 15–20 %; for improved sensitivity, cyclic VCUGs consisting of 2–3 voiding cycles are recommended [34, 35].

The International Reflux Study classified VUR along a 5-point scale defined by the degree of retrograde urine flow and accompanying distortion of the pyelocalyceal system (Figs. 6.2, 6.3, 6.4, 6.5, and 6.6) [33]. The VUR grading system conveys clinical significance regarding the chance for spontaneous resolution, the risk of breakthrough UTIs, and treatment outcomes. Higher-grade VUR is associated with decreased spontaneous resolution, higher rates of breakthrough UTIs, and renal scars [4, 20, 36–38]. A lower bladder volume at which reflux occurs during VCUG has been shown to be an independent risk factor that decreases the likelihood of spontaneous resolution and increases the risk of breakthrough febrile UTIs [4, 39].

Dimercaptosuccinic Acid (DMSA) Renal Scintigraphy

DMSA scintigraphy is considered the "gold standard" for documentation of acute inflammatory parenchymal changes associated with pyelonephritis and for documentation of the long-term sequelae of chronic irreversible renal scarring. Typical findings of acute pyelonephritis are photopenic defects associated with preservation of the normal renal contour. In contrast, irreversible renal scarring is represented by

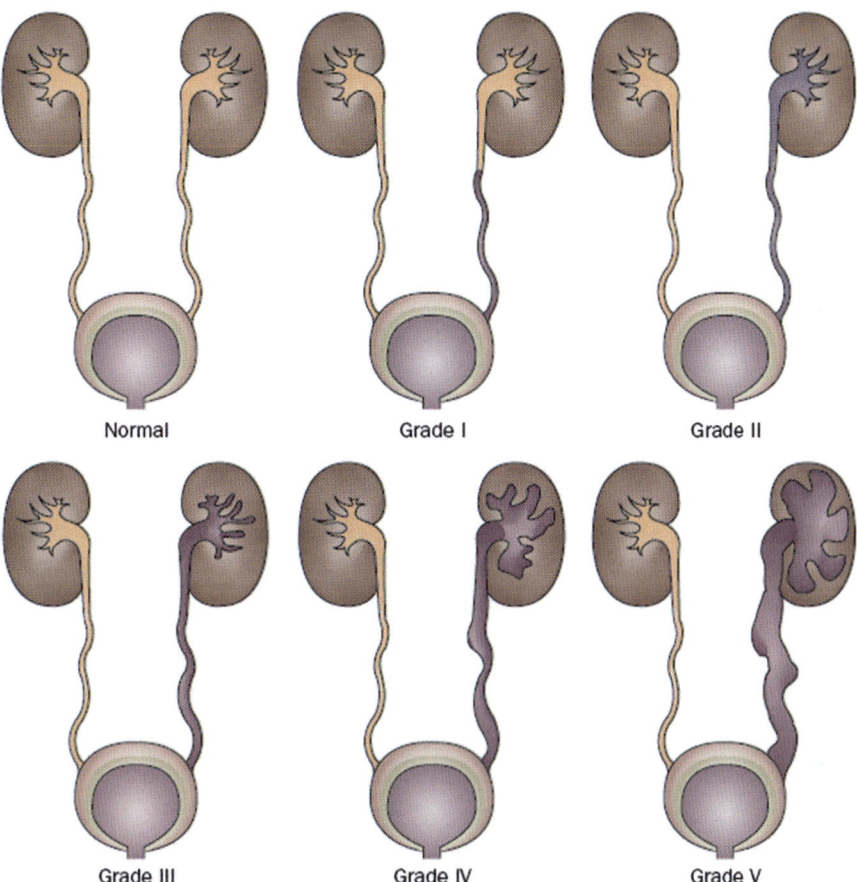

Fig. 6.2 Grade I VUR is reflux into the ureter only. Grade II involves reflux into a non-dilated pyelocalyceal system. Grade III is dilatation of the collecting system. Grade IV involves more extensive dilation with blunting of the calyces and tortuosity of the ureter, and grade V is massive dilation of the collecting system and severe tortuosity of the ureter. *With permission from Cooper CS. Diagnosis and management of vesicoureteral reflux in children. Nat Rev Urol doi:* 10.1038/ nrurol.2009.150. *Nature Publishing Group* [64]

focal defects associated with loss or contraction of the renal cortex. Unless one is using the "top-down approach" to determine which patients need further investigation with a VCUG, an early DMSA scan is not required in all patients suspected of having acute pyelonephritis. However, an acute DMSA scan can be useful in situations when the urine culture results or clinical presentation are equivocal. For example, patients with neuropathic bladders who perform intermittent catheterization are often chronically bacteriuric. Consequently, when they present with a fever and are found to have a positive urine culture, one cannot assume pyelonephritis is the cause of the fever. If the DMSA scan is negative, other sources of fever need to be evaluated. DMSA scintigraphy can also be used to evaluate for renal scarring in high-risk

Fig. 6.3 Left grade I
VUR, detected in a
7-year-old girl with
recurrent febrile urinary
tract infections and normal
renal-bladder ultrasound

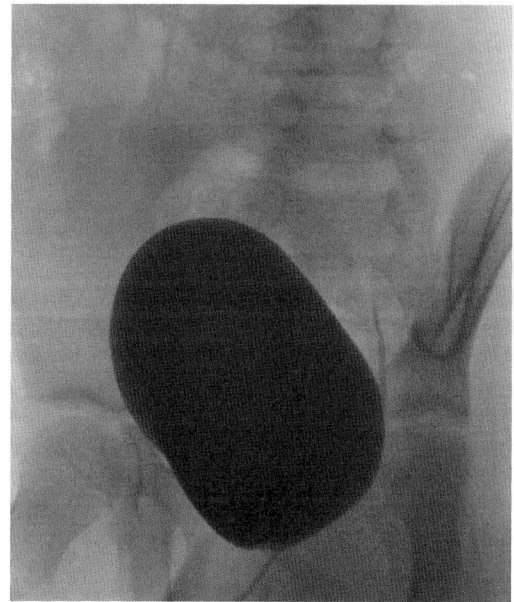

Fig. 6.4 Bilateral grade II
in a 14-month-old girl who
presented with urosepsis
necessitating
hospitalization. Note there
is no dilation of the
pyelocalyceal system on
either side

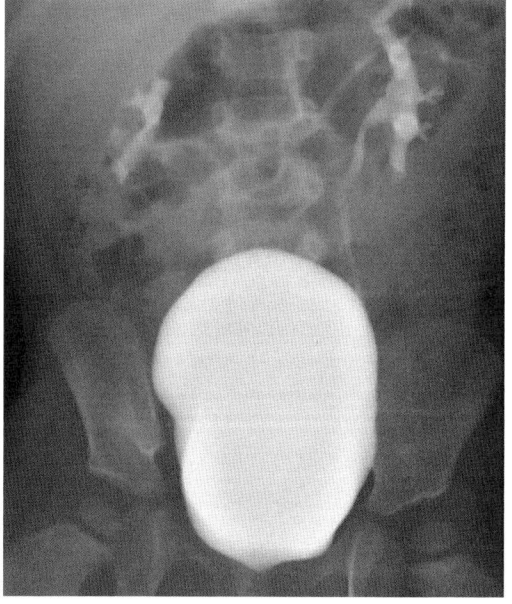

patients such as those with high-grade VUR or a history of recurrent episodes of
pyelonephritis. In those found to have renal scarring, it can provide differential renal
function which may influence management. While the presence of renal parenchymal scarring is known to affect VUR resolution rates, DMSA imaging may be

Fig. 6.5 Bilateral VUR (left grade III, right grade IV) detected in a 6-year-old child with recurrent febrile urinary tract infections. Note the mild dilation of the collecting system on the *left* and more pronounced dilation with blunting of the calyces on the *right*

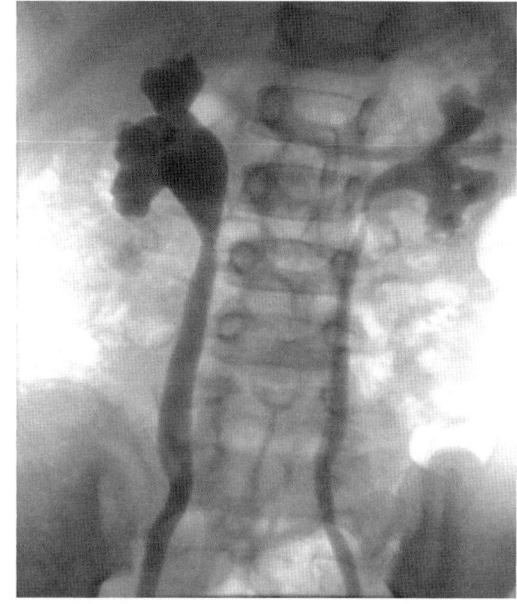

Fig. 6.6 Left grade V reflux diagnosed in a 2-day-old baby boy. In this case, left hydroureteronephrosis was detected prenatally and VCUG was obtained prior to discharge. Note the massive upper tract dilation and tortuosity of the ureter

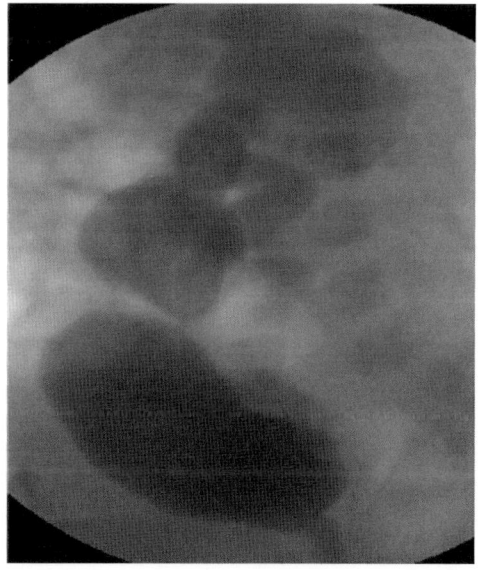

limited by expense, radiation exposure, possible need for sedation, and inconsistent availability. Although most children with febrile UTI do not undergo DMSA scans, the 2010 AUA Summary Guidelines do recommend DMSA imaging in children with primary VUR in whom ultrasound is abnormal, or there is greater concern for scarring due to breakthrough UTI, high-grade VUR, or elevated creatinine [6].

Additional Testing

Initial evaluation of the pediatric patient with VUR should include a careful general medical assessment including measurement of height, weight, and blood pressure, as well as serum creatinine if bilateral renal cortical abnormalities are found [6]. Urinalysis to detect proteinuria and bacteriuria is recommended. If there is concern for infection based on urinalysis, a catheterized urinalysis should be performed, and if positive a urine culture should be obtained.

Management

Despite being one of the most prevalent pediatric urologic diagnoses, optimal management of VUR remains controversial. Management goals include prevention of recurrent febrile UTI and renal injury while minimizing morbidity of treatment and follow-up. Options include observation with or without continuous antibiotic prophylaxis and surgical correction via endoscopic, open, or laparoscopic/robotic approaches (Fig. 6.7). Spontaneous resolution of VUR is dependent on initial grade of reflux, gender, age, voiding dysfunction, presence of renal scarring, and the bladder volume when VUR is first detected on VCUG. Various algorithms have been developed to predict spontaneous resolution based on a variety of factors [40–42].

Need for surgical correction is influenced by a child's risk for further infections, potential for renal scarring, and likelihood of spontaneous resolution, along with parental preferences. Ureteral reimplantation has high success rates, exceeding 95 %, and has been shown to reduce the occurrence of febrile UTI [5]. Endoscopic treatment of VUR is an outpatient procedure associated with decreased morbidity but lower long-term success rates closer to 70 % in some series [6].

Prophylactic Antibiotics

The use of prophylactic antibiotics may be considered a nonspecific approach to the prevention of recurrent UTIs (Table 6.1). Daily administration of low-dose (1/4–1/2 therapeutic dose) antibiotics in children with VUR is based on knowledge that spontaneous resolution rates for primary VUR are high, and sterile VUR is not thought to injure the kidneys. Maintenance of sterile urine until spontaneous reflux resolution avoids the morbidity of surgery and renal scarring.

Neither the revised AAP guidelines nor the NICE guidelines recommend routinely prescribing prophylactic antibiotics in infants and children following their first UTI [10, 14]. As might be expected, the benefit of prophylactic antibiotics is more easily demonstrated when used in specific populations known to be at high risk for recurrent UTI [20, 43]. The following factors are associated with a low risk of recurrent UTI and therefore make any benefit of prophylactic antibiotics more difficult to

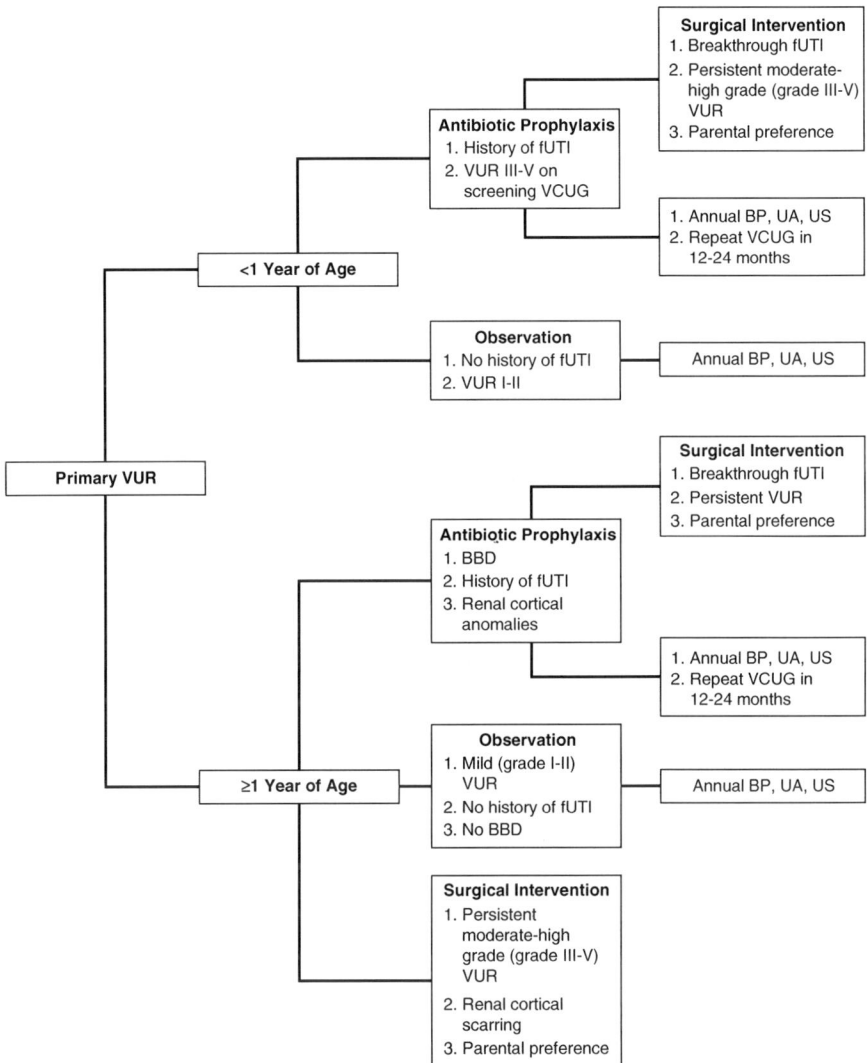

Fig. 6.7 Management algorithm for primary vesicoureteral reflux. It is important to note that circumcision should be offered to all male patients and that bladder-bowel dysfunction should be treated in all children, preferably prior to any surgical intervention. *BBD* bladder-bowel dysfunction, *BP* blood pressure, *fUTI* febrile urinary tract infection, *UA* urinalysis, *US* ultrasound, *VCUG* voiding cystourethrogram, *VUR* vesicoureteral reflux

demonstrate: circumcised boys, normal bladder and bowel function, no prior history of UTI, normal renal ultrasound or DMSA scan, a lack of anatomic abnormalities such as duplication or paraureteral diverticulum, and grade I or II VUR [6].

Continuous antibiotic prophylaxis appears to be generally safe and well tolerated but does incur cost and potential risks. Aside from a lack of efficacy, antibiotic

Table 6.1 Dosing of frequently prescribed prophylactic antibiotics

Antibiotic	Dose (mg/kg/day)	Contraindications
Sulfamethoxazole trimethoprim	2	<2 months of age
Nitrofurantoin	2	<2 months of age
Amoxicillin	5–20	
Cephalexin	5–10	

Note that infants under 2 months of age should be placed on daily amoxicillin or cephalexin

resistance is another concern regarding the use of prophylactic antibiotics. Multiple studies confirm that exposure to antibiotics increases the likelihood that any subsequent UTIs will be caused by bacteria resistant to the previously prescribed antibiotics [20, 43, 44].

The 2010 AUA Guidelines recommend prophylaxis in children <1 year of age with VUR and a history of fUTI based on greater morbidity of recurrent infection in this patient cohort [6]. In the absence of febrile UTI, antibiotic prophylaxis is recommended in children <1 year of age with VUR grades III–V who are identified through screening (hydronephrosis, sibling screening). Management of children >1 year of age should be based on the clinical context, including the presence of bladder-bowel dysfunction (BBD), patient age, VUR grade, presence of renal scarring, and parental preferences. Observation without antibiotic prophylaxis may be considered in children >1 year of age with VUR in the absence of BBD, recurrent febrile UTIs, and renal cortical abnormalities [6]. BBD is known to adversely affect UTI rate as well as spontaneous resolution in children with VUR, and treatment of BBD (timed voiding, management of constipation, and anticholinergics when indicated) should be implemented when this is identified, either by clinical history or urodynamic evaluation. Recommended follow-up in the AUA guidelines includes annual blood pressure and urinalysis assessment, retroperitoneal ultrasound every 12 months to monitor renal growth, and VCUG every 12–24 months to evaluate for improvement of resolution of VUR [6].

Operative Management

Families should be thoroughly counseled regarding various VUR management options and all children should undergo screening for and treatment of BBD since bladder and/or bowel dysfunction influences the risk of febrile UTI, spontaneous resolution, and operative success. Prevention of febrile UTI or pyelonephritis is one of the primary goals of surgical management. Surgical cure of VUR has been shown to reduce the occurrence of pyelonephritis although it has not been proven to significantly reduce renal injury [45]. Relative indications for surgical correction of VUR include persistent moderate- to high-grade reflux (grades III–V), low probability of spontaneous resolution, renal scarring, recurrent pyelonephritis, breakthrough febrile UTI while on continuous antibiotic prophylaxis, and parental preference [6, 45].

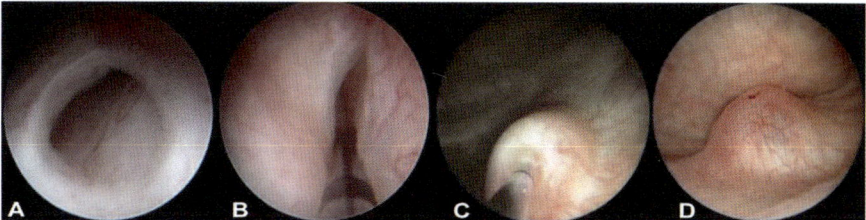

Fig. 6.8 Double HIT method. The bladder is emptied and ureteral orifice visualized, followed by hydrodistention (**a**). Proximal HIT is then performed with the needle inserted into the mid ureteral tunnel at the 6 O'clock position (**b**) and sufficient bulking agent is injected to produce a bulge which coapts the tunnel. Distal HIT (**c**) leads to coaptation of the ureteral orifice (**d**)

Endoscopic Injection Techniques

Initially described by Matouschek in 1981, endoscopic repairs correct reflux by injection of a bulking substance that allows elevation and coaptation of the ureteral orifice and detrusor tunnel [29]. O'Donnell and Puri further advanced the concept by performing subureteric injections using Teflon paste coining the term "STING" (subureteric teflon injection) [30]. Modifications to the initial injection method led to development of the double hydrodistention implantation technique (Double HIT), where total ureteral tunnel and orifice coaptation are achieved by two intramural injections [46–48] (Fig. 6.8).

Endoscopic injection is an outpatient procedure performed under general anesthesia with minimal postoperative pain and no need for urinary catheter drainage. Children should be kept on prophylactic antibiotics until appropriate postoperative studies are obtained. Renal-bladder ultrasound should be obtained 4–6 weeks postoperatively to assess for asymptomatic hydronephrosis secondary to obstruction. The AUA Reflux Guidelines recommend postoperative VCUG [6], but in practice there is wide variability in postoperative imaging dependent upon the individual patient and a given surgeon's clinical experience. The average resolution of VUR following a single endoscopic injection is 83 % based on aggregate data, though success rates have ranged from 70 to 95 % [6]. Considering the lower rate of success when compared to ureteral reimplantation, a follow-up VCUG to evaluate the success of the procedure seems prudent.

Ureteral Reimplantation

Various open ureteral reimplantation techniques have been described including both intravesical and extravesical approaches. More recently, robot-assisted laparoscopic ureteral reimplantation has been reported. The Cohen cross-trigonal reimplant is the most widely utilized intravesical ureteroneocystostomy technique and has reliable results and broad applicability (Fig. 6.9a). It maintains the same ureteral hiatus in the bladder wall. The ureter is advanced through a submucosal tunnel across the trigone toward the contralateral side; ureteral advancement across the back wall of the bladder rarely results in kinking or obstruction [45, 49, 50].

The technique utilized for extravesical ureteral reimplantation is the Lich-Gregoir or one of its modifications (Fig. 6.9b). In this procedure, the juxtavesical ureter is dissected, and a detrusor trough is created by incising the serosa and detrusor down to the mucosa. The bladder mucosa is not violated. The ureter is placed into the trough, and the detrusor is closed over the ureter, creating a flap valve mechanism similar to the cross-trigonal approach noted above; however, it is done without "opening" the bladder [51, 52].

Laparoscopic approaches to ureteral reimplantation were initially reported in the 1990s. More recently, robot-assisted laparoscopic approaches have been described, negating some of the longer operative times and technical difficulty associated with pure laparoscopy (Fig. 6.9c) [53]. Long-term studies are required to demonstrate cost and quality of life benefits of robotic surgery over standard open repairs.

Following ureteral reimplantation, children typically have an indwelling catheter overnight and are admitted for observation. Patients are discharged with narcotic pain medication (with or without anticholinergic) and are kept on prophylactic antibiotics until postoperative imaging is obtained. The estimated success rate of open ureteral reimplantation is 98 % for grades I–IV, with slightly higher success rates reported for the intra-versus extravesical approach. Ultrasound should be obtained 6–12 weeks postoperatively to assess for ureteric obstruction identified by hydroureteronephrosis greater than expected based on the previous degree of VUR. Due to high success rates of open repairs, postoperative VCUG can be limited to high-risk cases or those with postoperative pyelonephritis or new hydronephrosis [6].

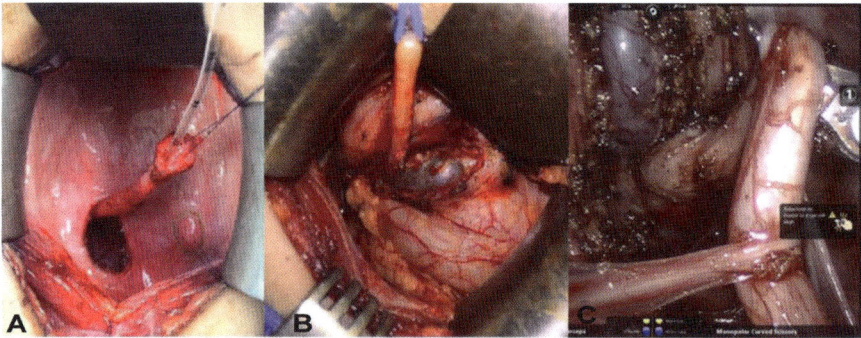

Fig. 6.9 Bilateral intravesical Cohen cross-trigonal reimplant; the ureters are mobilized to ensure the tunnel length is five times the ureteral diameter (**a**). Extravesical ureteral reimplant; the refluxing ureter is encircled with a vessel loop and a detrusor trough has been created by incising down to the mucosa (**b**). Robotic reimplantation is typically performed in an extravesical fashion; the camera port is placed in the umbilicus, and the procedure can be readily performed utilizing two 8 mm robotic ports without the use of an accessory port (**c**)

Referral to Specialist

While there is a natural tendency for reflux to improve or cease with time, there remains a subset of children with persistent VUR who are subject to the potentially harmful sequelae of reflux. Patients with an indication for surgical VUR correction including moderate- to high-grade reflux (grades III–V), low probability of spontaneous resolution, renal scarring, recurrent pyelonephritis, and/or breakthrough febrile UTI while on continuous antibiotic prophylaxis should be promptly referred to a pediatric urologist. Education and counseling play an important role in parental preferences of VUR management, with the pediatric urologist's opinion often cited as the chief determining factor [54]. Children with evidence of reflux nephropathy or elevated creatinine should be referred to both pediatric nephrology and urology.

Long-Term Sequelae and Follow-Up

VUR increases the risk of pyelonephritis, with higher febrile UTI rates in the affected population and increased risk of renal scarring and upper tract damage. Recurrent pyelonephritis is associated with renal scarring, hypertension, and chronic kidney disease. At least one-third of VUR patients have renal scars, and the presence of scarring implies parenchymal damage and increases the risk for long-term adverse sequelae [55]. The risk of renal scarring is significantly associated with a higher VUR grade [56]. Prenatally detected VUR is associated with diffuse rather than focal renal abnormalities, is characterized by renal dysplasia, and occurs more frequently in male [57, 58]. Postnatally acquired renal damage associated with VUR is the result of the acute inflammatory reaction from bacterial infection of the renal parenchyma and is more commonly found in girls [12, 59].

It remains unknown if poor renal outcome reflect intrinsic congenital dysplastic parenchymal abnormalities associated with but not caused by VUR or if delayed recognition of urinary tract infections and/or VUR played the primary role [12, 60]. The potential for significant morbidity has placed emphasis on early and accurate diagnosis of pediatric UTI as well as long term monitoring. It is anticipated that most children with normal renal function at the time of VUR diagnosis will do well in the long term; however for those with extensive kidney damage, especially when bilateral, monitoring should include blood pressure and excretory function assessment [61]. In one study with >10 years follow-up, children with unilateral renal scars had an 11 % chance of hypertension, and those with bilateral scarring had an incidence of 18.5 % [62]. While the incidence of significant comorbidities is often minimal at diagnosis, long-term follow-up with respect to disease-specific morbidity is necessary as decades may pass between the first episode of pyelonephritic damage and development of hypertension or end-stage renal disease [63].

Summary

VUR is the most common uropathy affecting children. Spontaneous resolution of primary reflux is common and is dependent upon initial grade of reflux, gender, age, voiding dysfunction, presence of renal scarring, and bladder volume at the onset of VUR. Management should be individualized and based on patient age, health, VUR grade, clinical course, renal scarring, and parental preference. While high grades of VUR are more likely to result in recurrent urinary tract infections and renal damage, low grade of reflux associated with recurrent febrile infections and/or other risk variables can also predispose to renal damage.

References

1. Skoog SJ, Peters CA, Arant Jr BS, Copp HL, Elder JS, Hudson RG, et al. Pediatric vesicoureteral reflux guideline panel summary report: clinical practice guidelines for screening siblings of children with vesicoureteral reflux and neonates/infants with prenatal hydronephrosis. J Urol. 2010;184:1145–51.
2. Sargent MA. What is the normal prevalence of vesicoureteral reflux? Pediatr Radiol. 2000;30:587–93.
3. Nguyen HT, Herndon CD, Cooper C, Gatti J, Kirsch A, Kokorowski P, et al. The Society for Fetal Urology consensus statement on the evaluation and management of antenatal hydronephrosis. J Pediatr Urol. 2010;6:212–31.
4. Knudson MJ, Austin JC, McMillan ZM, Hawtrey CE, Cooper CS. Predictive factors of early spontaneous resolution in children with primary vesicoureteral reflux. J Urol. 2007;178:1684–8.
5. Martin AD, Iqbal MW, Sprague BM, Diaz M, Rushton HG, Peters CA, et al. Most infants with dilating vesicoureteral reflux can be treated nonoperatively. J Urol. 2014;191:1620–6.
6. Peters CA, Skoog SJ, Arant Jr BS, Copp HL, Elder JS, Hudson RG, et al. Summary of the AUA guideline on management of primary vesicoureteral reflux in children. J Urol. 2010;184:1134–44.
7. Lopez PJ, Celis S, Reed F, Zubieta R. Vesicoureteral reflux: current management in children. Curr Urol Rep. 2014;15:447.
8. Lee NG, Rushton HG, Peters CA, Groves DS, Pohl HG. Evaluation of prenatal hydronephrosis: novel criteria for predicting vesicoureteral reflux on ultrasonography. J Urol. 2014;192:914–8.
9. Sillen U, Brandström P, Jodal U, Holmdahl G, Sandin A, Sjöberg I, et al. The Swedish reflux trial in children: V. Bladder dysfunction. J Urol. 2010;184:298–304.
10. Roberts KB. Urinary tract infection: clinical practice guideline for the diagnosis and management of the initial UTI in febrile infants and children 2 to 24 months. Pediatrics. 2011;128:595–610.
11. Shaikh N, Ewing AL, Bhatnagar S, Hoberman A. Risk of renal scarring in children with a first urinary tract infection: a systematic review. Pediatrics. 2010;126:1084–91.
12. Peters C, Rushton HG. Vesicoureteral reflux associated renal damage: congenital reflux nephropathy and acquired renal scarring. J Urol. 2010;184:265–73.
13. Stein R, Dogan HS, Hoebeke P, Kočvara R, Nijman RJ, Radmayr C, et al. Urinary tract infections in children: EAU/ESPU guidelines. Eur Urol. 2015;67:546–58.
14. National Collaborating Centre for Women's and Children's Health. National Institute for Health and Clinical Excellence (NICE) Guideline. Urinary tract infection in children: diagnosis, treatment

and long-term management. London: RCOG Press; 2007. http://www.nice.org.uk/nicemedia/pdf/CG54fullguideline.pdf.

15. Garin EH, Olavarria F, Garcia Nieto V, Valenciano B, Campos A, Young L. Clinical significance of primary vesicoureteral reflux and urinary antibiotic prophylaxis after acute pyelonephritis: a multicenter, randomized, controlled study. Pediatrics. 2006;117:626–32.

16. Montini G, Rigon L, Zucchetta O, Fregonese F, Toffolo A, Gobber D, et al. Prophylaxis after first febrile urinary tract infection in children? A multicenter, randomized, controlled, noninferiority trial. Pediatrics. 2008;122:1064–71.

17. Pennesi M, Traven L, Peratoner L, Bordugo A, Cattaneo A, Ronfani L, et al. Is antibiotic prophylaxis in children with vesicoureteral reflux effective in preventing renal scars? A randomized, controlled trial. Pediatrics. 2008;121:e1489–94.

18. Roussey-Kesler G, Gadjos V, Idres N, Horen B, Ichay L, Leclair MD, et al. Antibiotic prophylaxis for the prevention of recurrent urinary tract infection in children with low grade vesicoureteral reflux: results from a prospective randomized study. J Urol. 2008;179:674–9.

19. The RIVUR Trial Investigators, Hoberman A, Greenfield SP, Mattoo TK, Keren R, Mathews R, et al. Antimicrobial prophylaxis for children with vesicoureteral reflux. N Engl J Med. 2014;370:2367–76.

20. Brandstrom P, Esbjorner E, Herthelius M, Swerkersson S, Jodal U, Hansson S. The Swedish reflux trial in children: III. Urinary tract infection pattern. J Urol. 2010;184:286–91.

21. Brandström P, Nevéus T, Sixt R, Stokland E, Jodal U, Hansson S. The Swedish reflux trial in children: IV. Renal damage. J Urol. 2010;184:292–7.

22. Wan J, Skoog SJ, Hulbert WC, Casale AJ, Greenfield SP, Cheng EY, et al. Section on urology response to new guidelines for the diagnosis and management of UTI. Pediatrics. 2012;129:e1051–3.

23. Rushton HG. The evaluation of acute pyelonephritis and renal scarring with technetium 99m-dimercaptosuccinic acid renal scintigraphy: evolving concepts and future directions. Pediatr Nephrol. 1997;11:108–20.

24. Oh MM, Jin MH, Bae JH, Park HS, Lee JG, du Moon G. The role of vesicoureteral reflux in acute renal cortical scintigraphic lesion and ultimate scar formation. J Urol. 2008;180:2167–70.

25. Mingin GC, Hinds A, Nguyen HT, Baskin LS. Children with a febrile urinary tract infection and a negative radiologic workup: factors predictive of recurrence. Urology. 2004;63:562–5.

26. Shaikh N, Morone NE, Bost JE, Farrell MH. Prevalence of urinary tract infection in childhood: a meta-analysis. Pediatr Infect Dis. 2008;27:302–8.

27. Alsaywid BS, Saleh H, Deshpande A, Howman-Giles R, Smith GH. High grade primary vesicoureteral reflux in boys: long-term results of a prospective cohort study. J Urol. 2010;184:1598–603.

28. Hoberman A, Charron M, Hickey RW, Baskin M, Kearney DH, Wald ER. Imaging studies after a first febrile urinary tract infection in young children. N Engl J Med. 2003;348:195–202.

29. Carpenter MA, Hoberman A, Mattoo TK, Mathews R, Keren R, Chesney RW, et al. The RIVUR trial: profile and baseline clinical associations of children with vesicoureteral reflux. Pediatrics. 2013;32:e34–45.

30. Jahnukainen T, Honkinen O, Ruuskanen O, Mertsola J. Ultrasonography after the first febrile urinary tract infection in children. Eur J Pediatr. 2006;165:556–9.

31. Matouschek E. Die behandlung des vesikorenalen refluxes durch transurethrale einspritzung von Telfon paste. Urologe A. 1981;20:263–4.

32. O'Donnell B, Puri P. Treatment of vesicoureteral reflux by endoscopic injection of Teflon. Br Med J. 1984;289:7–9.

33. Lebowitz RL, Olbing H, Parkkulainen KV, Smellie JM, Tamminen-Möbius TE. International system of radiographic grading of vesicoureteric reflux. International Reflux Study in Children. Pediatr Radiol. 1985;15:105–9.

34. Gelfand MJ, Koch BL, Elgazzar AH, Gylys-Morin VM, Gartside PS, Torgerson CL. Cyclic cystography: diagnostic yield in selected pediatric populations. Radiology. 1999;21:118–20.

35. Papadopoulou F, Efremidis SC, Oiconomou A, Badouraki M, Panteleli M, Papachristou F, et al. Cyclic voiding cystourethrography: is vesicoureteral reflux missed with standard voiding cystourethrography? Eur Radiol. 2002;12:666–70.
36. Schwab CW, Wu H, Selman H, Smith GH, Snyder 3rd HM, Canning DA. Spontaneous resolution of vesicoureteral reflux: a 15-year perspective. J Urol. 2002;168:2594–9.
37. Sjostrom S, Sillen U, Bachelard M, Hansson S, Stokland E. Spontaneous resolution of high grade infantile vesicoureteral reflux. J Urol. 2004;172:694–8.
38. Lin KY, Chiu NT, Chen MJ, Lai CH, Huang JJ, Wang YT, et al. Acute pyelonephritis and sequelae of renal scar in pediatric first febrile urinary tract infection. Pediatr Nephrol. 2003;18:362–5.
39. Alexander SE, Arlen AM, Storm DW, Kieran K, Cooper CS. Bladder volume at onset of vesicoureteral reflux is an independent risk factor for breakthrough febrile urinary tract infection. J Urol. 2015;193:1342–6.
40. Estrada CR, Passerotti CC, Grahm DA, Peters CA, Bauer SB, Diamond DA, et al. Nomograms for predicting annual resolution rate of primary vesicoureteral reflux: results from 2,462 children. J Urol. 2009;182:1535–41.
41. Knudson MJ, Austin JC, Wald M, Makhlouf AA, Niederberger CS, Cooper CS. Computational model for predicting the chance of early resolution in children with vesicoureteral reflux. J Urol. 2007;178:1824–7.
42. Kirsch AJ, Arlen AM, Leong T, Merriman LS, Herrel LA, Scherz HC, et al. Vesicoureteral reflux index (VURx): a novel tool to predict primary reflux improvement and resolution in children less than 2 years of age. J Pediatr Urol. 2014;10:1249–54.
43. Craig JC, Simpson JM, Williams GJ, Lowe A, Reynolds GJ, McTaggart SJ. Antibiotic prophylaxis and recurrent urinary tract infection in children. N Engl Med. 2009;361:1748–59.
44. Conway PH, Cnaan A, Zaoutis T, Henry BV, Grundmeier RW, Keren R. Recurrent urinary tract infections in children: risk factors and association with prophylactic antimicrobials. JAMA. 2007;298:179–86.
45. Sung J, Skoog S. Surgical management of vesicoureteral reflux in children. Pediatr Nephrol. 2012;27:551–61.
46. Lackgren G, Kirsch AJ. Endoscopic treatment of vesicoureteral reflux. BJUI. 2010;105:1332–47.
47. Kirsch AJ, Perez-Brayfield M, Scherz HC. The modified STING procedure to correct vesicoureteral reflux: improved results with submucosal implantation within the intramural ureter. J Urol. 2004;171:2413–6.
48. Cerwinka W, Scherz HC, Kirsch AJ. Dynamic hydrodistention classification of the ureter and the double HIT method to correct vesicoureteral reflux. Arch Esp Urol. 2008;61:882–7.
49. Cohen SJ. Ureterozystoneostomie: eine neue antireflux Technik. Aktuelle Urol. 1975;6:1.
50. Retik AB, Colodny AH, Bauer SB. Pediatric urology. In: Paulson DF, editor. Genitourinary surgery, vol. 2. New York: Churchill Livingstone; 1984. p. 731–885.
51. Lich Jr R, Howerton LW, Davis LA. Recurrent urosepsis in children. J Urol. 1961;86:554–8.
52. Gregoir W, Van Regemorter G. Le reflux vesicoureteral congenital. Urol Int. 1964;18:122–36.
53. Casale P, Patel RP, Kolon TF. Nerve sparing robotic extravesical ureteral reimplantation. J Urol. 2008;179:1987–90.
54. Routh JC, Nelson CP, Graham DA, Lieu TA. Variation in surgical management of vesicoureteral reflux: influence of hospital and patient factors. Pediatrics. 2010;125:e446–51.
55. Mak RH, Kuo HJ. Pathogenesis of urinary tract infection: an update. Curr Opin Pediatr. 2006;18:148–52.
56. Stokland E, Hellström M, Jacobsson B, Jodal U, Sixt R. Renal damage one year after first urinary tract infection: role of dimercaptosuccinic acid scintigraphy. J Pediatr. 1996;129:815–20.
57. Sweeney B, Cascio S, Velayudham M, Puri P. Reflux nephropathy in infancy: a comparison of infants presenting with and without urinary tract infection. J Urol. 2001;166:648–50.
58. Silva JM, Diniz JS, Lima EM, Pinheiro SV, Marino VP, Cardoso LS, et al. Independent risk factors for renal damage in a series of primary vesicoureteral reflux: a multivariate analysis. Nephrology. 2009;14:198–204.

59. Swerkersson S, Jodal U, Sixt R, Stokland E, Hansson S. Relationship among vesicoureteral reflux, urinary tract infection and renal damage in children. J Urol. 2007;178:647–51.
60. Chesney RW, Carpenter MA, Moxey-Mims M, Nyberg L, Greenfield SP, Hoberman A, et al. Randomized Intervention for children with vesicoureteral reflux (RIVUR): background commentary of RIVUR investigators. Pediatrics. 2008;122:S233–9.
61. Jodal U, Smellie JM, Lax H, Hoyer PF. Ten-year results of randomized treatment of children with severe vesicoureteral reflux. Final report of the International Reflux Study in Children. Pediatr Nephrol. 2006;21:785–92.
62. Wallace DM, Rothwell D, Williams DI. The long-term follow-up of surgically treated vesicoureteric reflux. Br J Urol. 1978;50:479–84.
63. Cooper CS, Austin JC. Vesicoureteral reflux: who benefits from surgery? Urol Clin N Am. 2004;31:535–41.
64. Cooper CS. Diagnosis and management of vesicoureteral reflux in children. Nat Rev Urol. Doi: 10.1038/nrurol.2009.150.

Chapter 7
Congenital Anomalies of the Urethra

Kenneth I. Glassberg, Jason P. Van Batavia, Andrew J. Combs, and Rosalia Misseri

Abbreviations

BNI	Bladder neck incision
BNO	Bladder neck obstruction
CIC	Clean intermittent catheterization
CKD	Chronic kidney disease
EBC	Expected bladder capacity
ESRD	End-stage renal disease
HUN	Hydroureteronephrosis
LOC	Loss of compliance
LUT	Lower urinary tract
LUTO	Lower urinary tract obstruction
NBE	Nocturnal bladder emptying
PUV	Posterior urethral valve
PVR	Post-void residual

K.I. Glassberg, M.D. (✉)
Department of Urology, Columbia University Medical Center,
New York, NY, USA
e-mail: kglassberg@aol.com

J.P. Van Batavia, M.D.
Division of Urology, Children's Hospital of Philadelphia, Philadelphia, PA, USA

A.J. Combs, P.A-.C.
Division of Urology, Weill Cornell Medical College, New York, NY, USA

R. Misseri, M.D.
Department of Urology, Riley Hospital for Children, Indianapolis, IN, USA

Department of Urology, Indiana University School of Medicine, Indianapolis, IN, USA

© Springer International Publishing Switzerland 2016
A.J. Barakat, H. Gil Rushton (eds.), *Congenital Anomalies of the Kidney and Urinary Tract*, DOI 10.1007/978-3-319-29219-9_7

SNOB	Syndrome of nocturnal overdistention of the bladder
VA	Vesicoamniotic
VCUG	Voiding cystourethrogram
VUDS	Video urodynamic study
VUR	Vesicoureteral reflux
VURD	Vesicoureteral reflux dysplasia

Posterior Urethral Valve

Incidence

Posterior urethral valve represents the most common cause of congenital urethral obstruction and occurs in 1 in 5000–25,000 live male births [1–3]. Interestingly, the incidence of PUV appears to differ across different geographic locations and has been noted to be as high as 1 in 2375 newborn males in the country of Oman [4]. Reasons for global variation in live birth incidence rates include possible genetic and environmental factors, as well as differences in rates of prenatal diagnosis and elective termination which may decrease live birth rate without affecting the rate of in utero diagnosis. Despite the ability to diagnose PUV earlier and more accurately, one recent analysis of the Kids' Inpatient Database (KID) in the USA noted no significant change in the birth prevalence of PUV from 1997 to 2009 [5]. Reported rates of PUV diagnosis based on prenatal ultrasound screening are as high as 1 in 1250 suggesting that the true incidence may be higher than even the most generous estimates [6].

Classification [1]

According to the Young classification, there are three types of PUVs [7]. Type I is characterized by a bicuspid-type valve that usually originates from the distal lateral portion of the verumontanum at the floor of the urethra and extends anteriorly and distally to join in the midline. The vast majority of PUV (~95 %) seen clinically are type I. The valves here are obstructive to antegrade urine flow and balloon with urine-like sails during micturition. Type II valves are the rarest form of PUV arising from the verumontanum and coursing proximally along the posterior urethra toward the bladder neck. These valves are not obstructive and some authors recommend their removal from the nomenclature [8]. According to Young and coworkers [7], type III valves appear as a circumferential membrane distal to the verumontanum with a small central opening. They represent approximately 5 % of all PUVs and are thought to lie transversely across the urethra. Williams and Eckstein [9] suggested that these valves may represent a type of congenital urethral stricture.

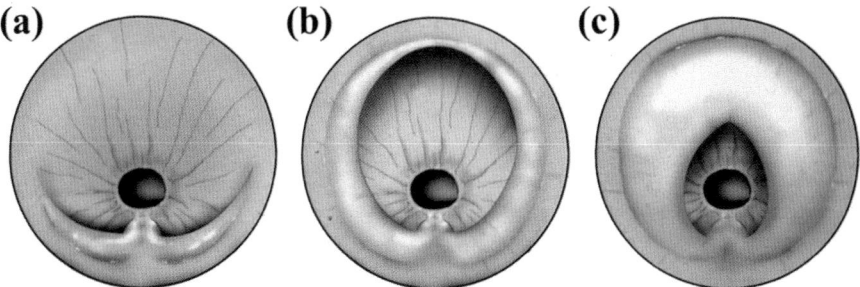

Fig. 7.1 Spectrum of normal plicae colliculi to full blown valve. (**a**) Normal urethra demonstrating prominent normal folds, i.e., plicae colliculi, arising from the verumontanum and inserting on the lateral wall. There is no evidence of anterior fusion. (**b**) "Minivalves": less obstructive valves, but pathologic since leaflets fuse anteriorly. (**c**) Obstructive posterior urethral valve arising from verumontanum fusing anteriorly and more distally. With permission from Glassberg KI, Horowitz M. Urethral valves and other anomalies of the male urethra, in Belman AB, King LR, Kramer SA {eds}: *Clinical Pediatric Urology*, ed 4. London, Martin Dunitz Ltd, 2002;pp:899; Chapt 28, Fig. 28.3. © Taylor and Francis [10]

Embryology/Anatomy

The normal male urethra contains a pair of lateral, small folds (plicae colliculi) that arise at the distal lateral edge of the verumontanum and continue distally onto the lateral walls of the urethra for a short distance (Fig. 7.1). Stephens [11] postulated that these folds represent the integration of the Wolffian duct into the cloaca. Stephens supported the belief that PUV results from the Wolffian duct integrating at a more anterior position resulting in a lack of posteromedial migration and formation of PUV as a consequence of the anterior fusion of these leaflets. Dewan and colleagues [12] believe that all PUVs are not in fact true valves but rather are a single obstructive membrane with a small posterior midline opening. Rather than referring to this condition as PUV, they proposed using the term "congenital obstructing posterior urethral membrane (COPUM)" for this entity [13].

The present authors agree with Dewan and colleagues that the term "posterior urethral valves" is misleading and that the condition is not two discrete valves but rather a singular obstructive membrane [14]. Therefore, the singular term "posterior urethral valve" is preferable to the plural "valves."

Genetic/Familial Posterior Urethral Valve

The genetic contribution to PUV is not well understood, and familial PUV is rare with few case reports in the literature. Findings from these case studies have been inconclusive with some suggesting an autosomal recessive inheritance and others supporting a more complex and less-defined mechanism of inheritance [15]. Regardless, no specific gene or genes implicated in PUV have been localized, and it is likely that PUVs represent a polygenetic condition [16].

Diagnosis

The diagnosis of PUV is usually made on the basis of findings on a voiding cysto-urethrogram (VCUG). The posterior urethra appears more dilated than the urethra distal to the valve. Often it will take on a shield-shaped appearance, lying between a well-defined muscular bladder neck and collapsed distal urethra. Almost always the distal roof of the posterior urethra will hang over the bulbar urethra distal to the valve due to the caudad bulging of the valve itself [9]. The hypertrophied bladder neck causes a prominent posterior lip, and sometimes an anterior lip as well, almost appearing as if the bladder neck is pinched (Fig. 7.2).

Prenatal Diagnosis

PUV should be suspected prenatally in all male fetuses with bilateral hydronephrosis and especially in those with a thick-walled bladder that is not seen to empty during ultrasound imaging. Additional in utero ultrasound findings that can be seen in fetuses

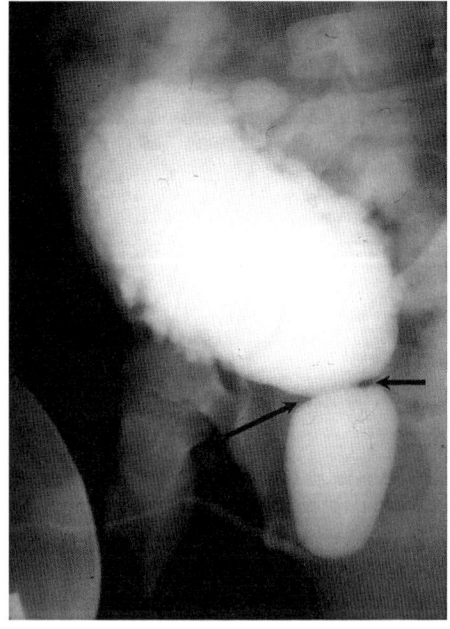

Fig. 7.2 Diagnosis of posterior urethral valves on voiding cystourethrogram. Note the shield-shaped posterior urethra that bulges over the bulbous urethra, the collapsed anterior urethra, and the prominent bladder neck outlines by posterior and anterior indentations (*arrows*). With permission from Glassberg KI, Horowitz M. Urethral valves and other anomalies of the male urethra, in Belman AB, King LR, Kramer SA {eds}: *Clinical Pediatric Urology*, ed 4. London, Martin Dunitz Ltd, 2002;pp:899; Chapt 28, Fig. 28.6. © Taylor and Francis [10]

Fig. 7.3 Antenatal
ultrasound demonstrating
the dilated bladder and
posterior urethra
mimicking a keyhole

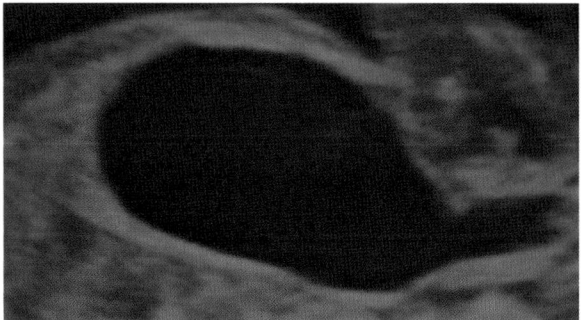

with PUV include dilated posterior urethra with bright echogenic lines representing the valve tissue as well as the "keyhole" sign—the dilated, thick-walled bladder appears to be the wider upper portion of the keyhole, and the dilated posterior urethra appears to be the lesser dilated lower portion (Fig. 7.3) [17]. The combination of renal hyperechogenicity, oligohydramnios, and bladder distension during prenatal ultrasound has also been shown to be a strong indicator of outlet obstruction [18].

Fetal urine makes up ~90 % of amniotic fluid, and thus obstruction secondary to PUV and/or dysplastic kidneys as a consequence of that obstruction can lead to decreased urine production/voiding and thus oligohydramnios. When severe, oligohydramnios can cause spontaneous abortion with the facial and limb features associated with Potter's syndrome, stillbirth, or respiratory distress at birth due to pulmonary hypoplasia.

Previously it appeared that those babies diagnosed in utero had a worse prognosis but that no longer holds true, as the majority of such neonates now are diagnosed in utero [19]. When the diagnosis is made before 20 weeks, it is often associated with massive hydronephrosis and poorly functioning kidneys with cysts and dysplasia, a scenario that is too late for vesicoamniotic (VA) shunting. Such fetuses will have severe pulmonary hypoplasia and if they survive the pregnancy often are stillborn or die soon after birth. While in utero bilateral hydronephrosis and bladder distention in a male should immediately make one consider PUV as a possible diagnosis, it actually will be the diagnosis in little more that 50 % of such cases [20]. However, if a keyhole sign were identified in association with bilateral hydronephrosis, then the diagnosis of PUV becomes very likely [17].

Prenatal Indicators for Intervention

The major causes of death in fetuses and neonates with PUV are complications from pulmonary hypoplasia and renal failure. Efforts and strategies to treat affected fetuses before these conditions cause catastrophic effects that have evolved over the past few decades. The rationale for fetal intervention is to prevent further renal damage from obstruction and to increase amniotic fluid to a level that allows proper lung development. Consideration must always be given to the fact that not all fetuses suspected of having PUV will actually have the condition. Additionally, any fetal intervention is also a procedure on the mother and can have deleterious effects on the fetus, mother, and/or pregnancy (i.e., induce premature labor).

As previously suggested, a major indication for fetal intervention is oligohydramnios, specifically evidence of decreasing amniotic fluid. An initial finding of oligohydramnios on first ultrasound makes prediction of intervention success difficult. However, decreasing amniotic fluid on successive ultrasounds with evidence of adequate renal function is often used as an indicator for intervention. In this situation, vesicoamniotic shunting likely decreases risk of pulmonary disease [21]. Optimal gestational timing for fetal intervention is between 20 weeks and 32 weeks, since severe oligohydramnios prior to 20 weeks is likely incompatible with life and after 32 weeks, early delivery is preferable to intervention.

In addition to the development of oligohydramnios, fetal urine parameters may also play a role in determining outcomes and likelihood of in utero renal damage. Glick and associates [22] found that aspirated fetal bladder urine with high sodium concentration and high osmolarity compared to serum values had worse renal function. Additionally they found that low amniotic fluid status and low hourly urine output were also predictors of poor renal function. The following amniotic fluid values have been shown to be associated with poor renal function [22–24]:

Total protein	>20 mg/dL
B$_2$-microglobulin	>4.0 mg/dL
Sodium	>100 mg/dL
Chloride	>90 mg/dL
Calcium	>8 mg/dL
Osmolarity	>200 mOsm

No study has determined how many of these urine values are necessary to eliminate intervention as a viable option although it seems reasonable to infer that the more elevated values present, the less likely that intervention will be effective.

Prenatal Interventions

Options for fetal intervention include percutaneous or endoscopic placement of a vesicoamniotic (VA) shunt, open fetal cystostomy, and fetal urethroscopy with valve laser ablation [25, 26]. Early studies on fetal interventions showed high fetal mortality rates. The results of the randomized, prospective PLUTO trial, in addition to prior published retrospective reviews and case series, have been discouraging, and as a result fetal VA shunting has not gained general acceptance [27]. While there is the suggestion that survival may be slightly improved with VA shunting, the short- and long-term outcomes in terms of renal function appear poor. In fact, the major criticism of fetal intervention to date has been the lack of evidence for improvement of renal function compared to controls. To this end, one recent study suggests that there may be a future role for fetal cystoscopy with valve laser ablation in preference to shunting [26]. When comparing fetal cystoscopy with laser ablation, VA shunting and no intervention, both intervention arms had higher overall survival at 6 months compared with the no-intervention arm. Fetal cystoscopy was effective at improving both survival and renal function at 6 months when compared to controls, while VA shunting was only associated with an improvement in survival at 6 months when compared to controls [26]. Complications from fetal cystoscopy included urological fistulas (8.8 %) and need for second intervention for recurrent lower urinary tract obstruction (LUTO) (6 %). Future randomized trials must confirm these results before definitive recommendations can be made. In addition, these interventions are quite risky and should be performed in centers with experienced fetal surgeons after multidisciplinary consultation with the parents of the affected fetus.

Presentation

The use of prenatal ultrasound has increased the frequency of diagnosis of PUV in utero. Earlier studies have documented a high neonatal mortality of approximately 50 % with deaths usually resulting from respiratory failure, acidosis, renal failure, or sepsis. The outlook for children with PUV has dramatically improved as a result of the in utero diagnosis. While some of the decrease in mortality has been related to elective termination of the more severely affected fetuses, the major factor has been the early intervention and proactive management that early detection allows for. Improvement in the management of pulmonary hypoplasia has also decreased mortality in these children.

Affected children with renal failure may appear lethargic, present with intrauterine growth failure, and feed poorly. The bladder might be distended and palpable, the kidneys hydronephrotic and palpable, and the urine stream might appear weak or dribbling. Urinary ascites can be a cause of abdominal distension or even elevation of the diaphragm causing respiratory distress (Fig. 7.4). Obstructed urine can leak from the renal fornices, accumulate perirenally and retroperitoneally, and because of transudation lead to the urinary ascites (Fig. 7.5). The clinical course and outlook for these neonates will be discussed in the section on "Pop-off Phenomena."

Initial Management

Since most infants with PUV are identified prenatally, a pediatric urologist should be consulted antenatally and notified when the delivery will occur. Once the diagnosis of PUV becomes a valid possibility, the baby should have a urethral catheter placed in the bladder. Not infrequently the urethra will be difficult to catheterize, particularly at the bladder neck where the catheter needs to negotiate its high-riding posterior lip. It is helpful to use either a soft coude-tip catheter or a straight catheter manually bent at the tip in the fashion of a coude prior to insertion. If there is still difficulty passing the catheter, it is worthwhile to try to deflect the catheter anteriorly with a small finger in the rectum. Feeding tubes seem to pass more easily than do Foley catheters. We usually try to pass an 8 Fr first as it is stiffer than the 5 Fr,

Fig. 7.4 Flat plate of the distended abdomen of a newborn with a posterior urethral valve and urinary ascites. Note the "ground-glass" appearance of the abdomen and the centrally located bowel gas. With permission from Glassberg KI, Horowitz M. Urethral valves and other anomalies of the male urethra, in Belman AB, King LR, Kramer SA {eds}: *Clinical Pediatric Urology*, ed 4. London, Martin Dunitz Ltd, 2002;pp:899; Chapt 28, Fig. 28.23. © Taylor and Francis [10]

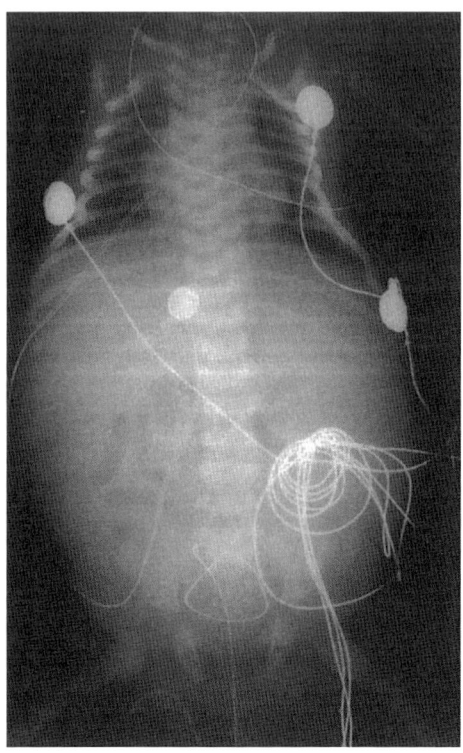

Fig. 7.5 Another image from the same MRI study, showing compression of the left renal parenchyma from the urinoma

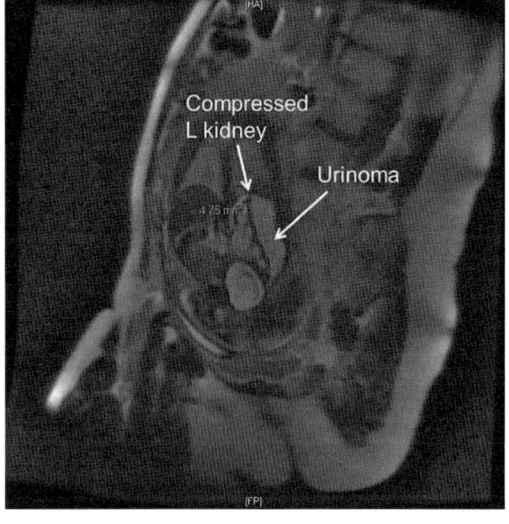

but if that does not work, it is then worthwhile to try the 5 Fr. A bladder ultrasound or KUB may be useful to confirm positioning.

Once the catheter is in place and the neonate is stable, he can be sent to the radiology department for a VCUG. While no studies exist as to what duration of catheterization lends a significantly increased risk of later urethral stricture, it is generally believed that the sooner cystoscopy is performed and the valves ablated the better.

With improvements in instrumentation and improved optics, most patients are currently treated with transurethral ablation. For boys with severe hydronephrosis, some have reported better long-term outcomes when these infants are temporarily diverted; however, most feel that primary valve ablation is the treatment of choice [27, 28]. For those who believe temporary diversion is best or when the child is too small to allow for transurethral resection, vesical and supravesical diversion of the obstructed bladder may be considered.

Transurethral Valve Ablation

In the twenty-first century, valve ablation is most commonly accomplished transurethrally. Typically, a 7.5 Fr or 8.5 Fr scope is used in infants. The distal urethra may require gentle dilation to allow for passage of the scope. The valve leaflets are more easily seen emanating from the verumontanum and extending distally to fuse anteriorly when the bladder is full and when gentle suprapubic pressure is applied. The goal of valve ablation is the disruption of the leaflets therefore eliminating the obstruction (Fig. 7.6).

When using a small pediatric resectoscope to incise valves, a right-angle hook, narrow loop electrode, or hook-shaped cold knife should be used. While many prefer incising at the 4–5 o'clock and 7–8 o'clock positions using a hook-shaped cold

Fig. 7.6 Endoscopic view of posterior urethral valves. Note the small catheter perforating the valve leaflet on the left

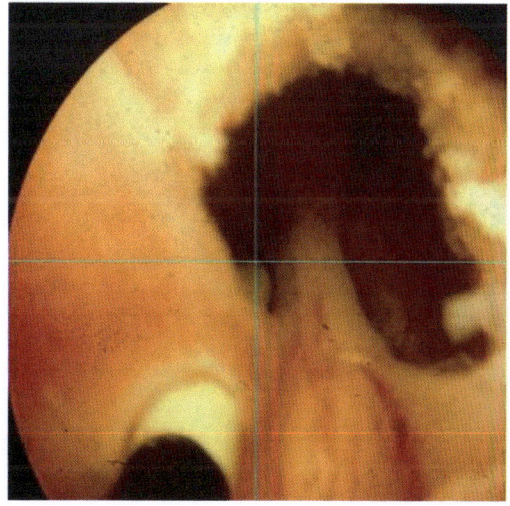

knife or with the cutting current set at 20–25 W pure cut, others have advocated incising at the 12 o'clock position, while others advocated cutting at the 4, 8, and 12 o'clock positions. With a full bladder, gentle pressure to the suprapubic area should yield full stream at the end of the procedure. A small urethral catheter is left in place for 1–2 days following the procedure or until an elevated nadir creatinine.

Postoperatively, serum electrolytes and creatinine should be obtained 24 h after catheter removal and certainly prior to discharge. A renal ultrasound is useful in the postoperative period to look for improvement in hydronephrosis.

Post-ablation VCUG

A postoperative imaging study, usually a VCUG, is typically performed 6–8 weeks following the valve ablation to determine its success. Follow-up renal ultrasound and serum creatinine and electrolytes should be performed at the same time of the imaging study or sooner, based on the child's renal function and clinical presentation.

On VCUG the posterior urethra might still appear dilated although usually not to the degree seen on pre-ablation images. One anticipates better filling of the distal urethra compared to the preoperative VCUG. Residual dilation usually results from the previously overstretched posterior urethra. A persistent dilation may represent residual obstructive valve tissue or development of an iatrogenic stricture (Fig. 7.7).

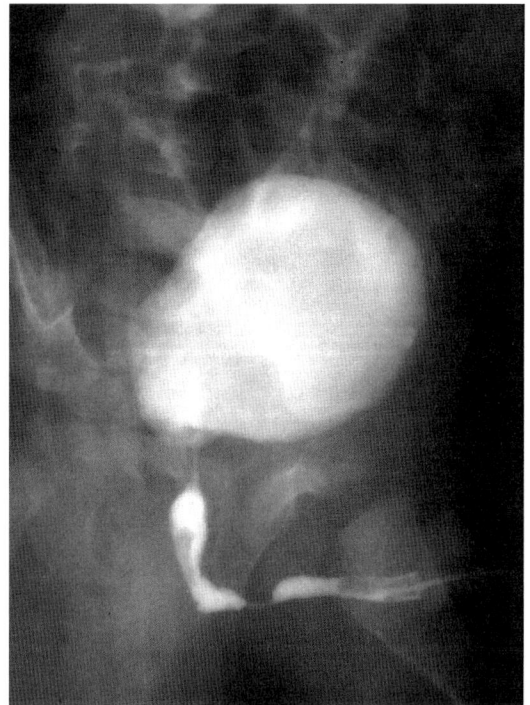

Fig. 7.7 Six months after valve ablation, anterior urethra stricture is seen, although none was seen on initial post-valve ablation VCUG. Optical urethrotomy was unsuccessful and formal urethroplasty was eventually required to correct the obstruction

When residual dilation is present, the urologist has the option of repeating cystoscopy to make sure there is no residual valve tissue or to perform urodynamic studies to assess for elevated voiding detrusor pressures. If a video urodynamic study (VUDS) reveals elevated detrusor pressures during voiding that are not related to increased external urethral sphincter activity, it can help further identify if there is residual valve tissue, secondary bladder neck obstruction, or a urethral stricture. Videourodynamics also gives insight into bladder compliance and stability making it superior to VCUG.

Vesicostomy

A vesicostomy may be useful in neonates whose urethra cannot accommodate a cystoscope or in those whose serum creatinine rises despite adequate valve resection. This allows for continuous bladder emptying into a diaper. When performing a vesicostomy, the bladder is incised near the dome and a stoma is created approximating the bladder to the skin. The vesicostomy should be approximately 24 Fr or large enough to allow passage of the surgeon's fifth digit to insure drainage and prevent stenosis and prolapse.

Ultimately, the timing of closure is dictated by the surgeon's philosophy, but usually it is done just prior to the expected time of potty training. As indicated by the findings on the pre-closure VUDS, we initiate oxybutynin therapy with or without alpha-blockers a few weeks prior to vesicostomy closure and tend to continue the medication as we follow the child post-closure urodynamically. Careful follow-up with renal ultrasounds, serum electrolytes, and creatinine is essential as some children may have poor bladder dynamics after closure of the vesicostomy. Urodynamic reevaluations should be performed after the bladder has healed.

Supravesical Diversions (Fig. 7.8)

The use of supravesical diversion remains controversial and is rarely used. Some urologists feel that the failure of the creatinine to improve after bladder drainage or valve ablation is related to a secondary ureterovesical obstruction and advocate supravesical diversion [29]. With the advent of smaller drainage tubes and the availability of skilled interventional radiologists, percutaneous tube placement may be considered prior to performing a diversion. A *cutaneous pyelostomy* allows for urine to drain directly from the renal pelvis onto the patient's flank. This procedure is usually reserved for patients with a dilated renal pelvis.

High cutaneous loop ureterostomy is used when the renal pelvis is not large enough for a cutaneous pyelostomy to be performed. Through a flank incision, the ureter is brought to skin level and a vertical ureterotomy is made. As loop

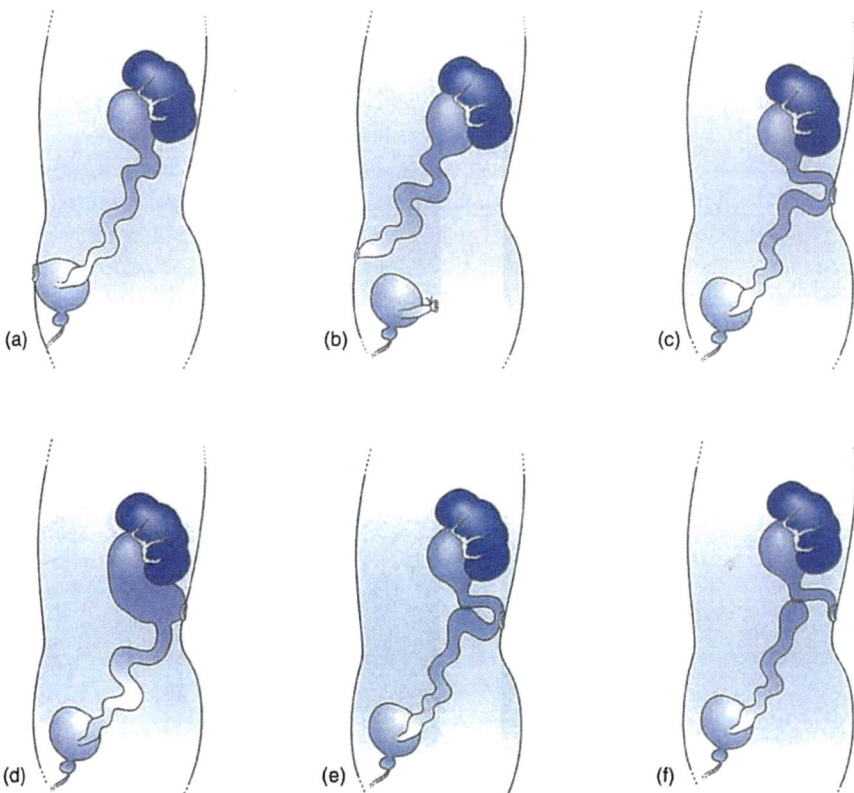

Fig. 7.8 Various temporary diversions for posterior urethral valves with some of historical note: (**a**) cutaneous vesicostomy, (**b**) cutaneous ureterostomy, (**c**) cutaneous loop ureterostomy, (**d**) cutaneous pyelostomy, (**e**) ring ureterostomy, (**f**) Sober-Y-ureterostomy. With permission from Glassberg KI, Horowitz M. Urethral valves and other anomalies of the male urethra, in Belman AB, King LR, Kramer SA {eds}: *Clinical Pediatric Urology*, ed 4. London, Martin Dunitz Ltd, 2002;pp:899; Chapt 28, Fig. 28.11. © Taylor and Francis [10]

ureterostomies maintain continuity of part of the ureter, there is a decreased likelihood of disruption of ureteral blood supply, decreasing the risk of stenosis and possibly making closure of the ureterostomy simpler.

Pelvioureterostomy-en-Y (*Sober loop ureterostomy*) allows some urine to drain into the bladder while some drains onto the flank. This avoids completely defunctionalization of the bladder [30]. The procedure is more time consuming than other forms of diversion and should not be the procedure of choice in critically ill patients. It is best used in patients with redundant tortuous ureters.

End cutaneous ureterostomy is best performed on a ureter that is sufficiently thick walled and dilated. A lower abdominal incision is made and an extraperitoneal dissection is performed.

The distal ureter is transected and brought to the anterior abdominal wall at the right or left lower quadrant. The ureter is spatulated and then sewn to a V-shaped skin incision to decrease the risk of stomal stenosis. Bilateral end ureterostomies may be brought to the midline or either lower quadrant.

Percutaneous nephrostomy tube is typically performed with ultrasound guidance by interventional radiologists. Ghali and colleagues [31] propose placement of a percutaneous nephrostomy tube prior to formal supravesical diversion. In addition, tube placement allows for antegrade nephrostogram and pressure flow studies to confirm ureterovesical junction obstruction. This minimally invasive technique is also particularly useful in septic or otherwise critically ill children. Despite the ease of the procedure, tubes may become dislodged and formal diversion may be more difficult secondary to inflammatory reaction to the tube placement.

Surgical Complications

Transurethral resection of posterior urethral valves may result in urethral stricture or sphincteric incontinence. The reported incidence of stricture varies from 2 to 50 %, with some authors finding an increased incidence with the use of cautery [32–34]. The use of appropriately sized resectoscopes, limited cautery, and good visualization with care to identify the external sphincter during resection are essential to avoid these complications. As with any urologic procedure, there is also a risk of urinary tract infection. A preoperative urine culture should be obtained and treated appropriately prior to any intervention.

Early or late prolapse of the dome or posterior bladder wall may occur in up to 17 % of patients of cutaneous vesicostomies [35]. To prevent prolapse, the most cephalad portion of the bladder or the urachus should be used as the site for the vesicostomy. The stomal opening itself should be no larger than 2 cm and should calibrate to 24 Fr. Excessive mucosal eversion may be mistaken for prolapse and despite its appearance, no intervention is necessary for excessive eversion.

Stomal stenosis rates are reported in 3–12 % [35] and should be suspected if the vesicostomy does not appear to be draining well and there is evidence of large amounts of residual bladder urine or when large amounts of urine are voided by urethra. Prolonged, severe dermatitis may contribute to stomal stenosis and may be prevented by air-drying the skin or applying topical ointments used for diaper rash. Fungal superinfections may occur and are treated with antifungal creams and powders.

As in cutaneous vesicostomy, chronic skin irritation and dermatitis are also a common complication of pyelostomy and ureterostomy. Less common complications include stomal stenosis and prolapse of the renal pelvis. Chronic bacteriuria is the most common complication in this group, occurring in approximately two-thirds of patients. Stomal stenosis occurs in 11–70 % of patients undergoing end cutaneous ureterostomies [36].

Persistent Hydroureteronephrosis (HUN) and Valve Bladder Syndrome

Whether initial treatment includes primary valve ablation alone, temporary diversion, or total ureteral reconstruction with reimplantation at the time of valve ablation, some will achieve significantly reduced hydronephrosis while others will have persistent dilatation [37, 38]. Intuitively it seems that there must be some relationship between the bladder and the upper tracts that does not lead to uniform improvement once the obstruction is gone. We evaluated 13 renal units with persistent HUN following valve ablation and classified each unit into one of the following three types: [37]

Type 1: *Unobstructed* with the bladder empty and during bladder filling
Type 2: *Unobstructed* with the bladder empty, but *obstructed* during bladder filling
Type 3: *Obstructed* with the bladder empty and during bladder filling

Only one of the first 13 units classified fell into the type 3 category and reimplantation corrected the HUN (Table 7.1) [37]. Similar reports have also shown the low occurrence of type 3 [39, 40]. The majority however fell into the type 2 variety leading to the conclusion that elevated pressure in the bladder or thickening of the detrusor was the etiology of the obstruction. This was later confirmed with urodynamic investigation and, once available, videourodynamics [37].

Early on we noted high urinary output in these patients and a urine specific gravity of less than 1.010 and serum osmolality of less than 300 mOsm even after a 14-h fast [41]. By 1979, it became evident that the major cause of persistent HUN in valve boys was the thick-walled, high-pressure, noncompliant bladder that was made worse by the large urine output these ureters and bladders had to contend with [41]. In that same year, Bauer and associates [42] published urodynamic findings in 8 of 62 boys with a history of PUV in whom lower urinary tract symptoms persisted. Of the eight, one had high voiding pressure, two had uninhibited contractions, one had a small capacity bladder, and three could not generate a sustained voluntary voiding contraction, representing a condition now referred to as "myogenic failure." The following year, Mitchell [43] also reported the same findings associated with persistent HUN following valve ablation, i.e., nephrogenic diabetes insipidus and noncompliant bladders. He coined the term "valve bladder syndrome" and that term has stuck.

At this point we started to investigate our patients with DTPA scans and made a number of observations. First of all if the child was not asked to void at the beginning of the study, isotope-filled urine in the upper tracts could not reach the bladder

Table 7.1 Whitaker pressure findings in 12 dilated renal units

Type 1 ↓BE↓BF	Type II ↓BE↑BF	Type III ↑BE↑BF
4	7	1

↓ = decreased, ↑ = increased, BE = bladder empty, BF = bladder filling

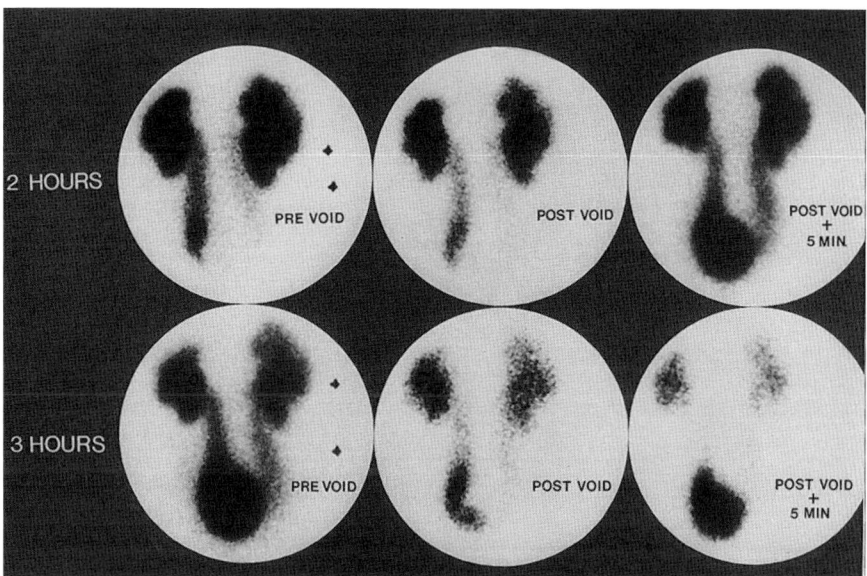

Fig. 7.9 DTPA renal scan in a 12-year-old boy, 11 years after valve ablation and in the pre-furosemide washout scan era. At 2 h, the isotope is not seen in area of bladder because the full bladder has obstructed drainage from the upper tracts. Immediately after voiding and complete emptying, the bladder refills and reobstructs the upper tracts. The same phenomenon is seen at 3 h when voiding is repeated. With permission from Glassberg KI, Schneider M, Haller JO, Moel D, Waterhouse K. Observations on persistently dilated ureter after posterior urethral valve ablation. Urology 1982; 20: 20-8. © Elsevier [37]

and was held up in the kidney (Fig. 7.9). Once the child voided, the isotope-filled urine refilled the bladder within seconds. With a second urination, most often 5 min after the first, the child could easily void an additional large amount of urine and dramatic lessening of HUN becomes apparent. Each time the bladder is refilled, it again obstructed the upper tracts. These children were carrying a large urine volume in their upper tracts secondary to the obstruction, which was related to a poorly compliant bladder associated with large urine output. Obviously they would do better by emptying frequently but more important was the necessity to double and triple void [37].

Rapid upper tract dumping of urine into the bladder after voiding makes any determination of an elevated post-void residual (PVR) obtained by catheterization or delayed ultrasound questionable. In these patients real-time bladder ultrasound obtained immediately after voiding or direct visualization by fluoroscopy serves as the best tool for assessing the true PVR.

Eleven years after the 1979 report by Bauer and colleagues on abnormal urodynamic parameters in PUV boys particularly in those with lower urinary tract (LUT) symptoms, the same group urodynamically evaluated another 41 valve boys [42, 44]. They found 2 with high-pressure voiding; 10 with hyperreflexia; 11 had a small, poorly compliant bladder; and myogenic failure was identified in another 14.

In a subsequent study, we evaluated 20 patients with VUDS at a mean of 31 months following valve ablation who had persistent HUN in 32 renal units [45]. All 20 had varying degrees of bladder malfunction and all required anticholinergics. Another 7 had secondary bladder neck obstruction and will be discussed in the next section. Three boys with 5 dilated units were not compliant in taking their medication and the hydronephrosis did not improve. Correcting abnormal parameters lessened the degree of hydronephrosis in 26 of the 32 units; it resolved completely in 14 units and decreased significantly in another 12.

Urodynamics in the Valve Patient: General Considerations

Early valve identification and ablation is just the first step in the management of boys with congenital urethral obstruction. A significant number (nearly 40 % in our experience) will have secondary bladder neck obstruction either as an immediate consequence of the initial obstruction or develop it over time as the result of residual bladder/voiding dysfunction. Upward of 80 % of all valve patients are likely to have some degree of residual bladder dysfunction as a consequence of the earlier obstruction. This can include detrusor overactivity; external sphincter hyperactivity, usually in response to detrusor overactivity; impaired detrusor compliance; impaired contractility; impaired proprioception; inadequate emptying; myogenic failure; VUR; UTI; and progressive upper tract deterioration leading to renal failure. UDS plays a crucial role in the identification of these issues, helps in formulating a road map for their care, and assesses progress on what will be a long journey for many of these boys.

VUDS are not only the initial study of choice after valve ablation, but they should be considered for use whenever fluoroscopic imaging is being contemplated. The primary indications for obtaining VUDS after the initial assessment are follow-up in patients with significant reflux, worsening or new onset hydronephrosis, and prior to any planned surgical intervention (augmentation, reflux correction, bladder outlet enhancement). It should also be considered for those without a history of reflux who develop a febrile UTI. In those situations where fluoroscopy is not available or desirable, real-time ultrasound monitoring of the kidneys during UDS, done before bladder filling, at capacity and again post-void, can yield valuable information on the effect bladder dynamics and treatment is having on the upper tracts.

As the child matures, uroflowmetry with simultaneous patch pelvic floor electromyography or uroflow/EMG is the noninvasive study of choice in patients. The uroflow component reveals pattern of flow, volume voided, and both peak and average flow rates and can suggest, though not prove, the presence of obstruction. Real-time bladder ultrasound is invaluable in making sure the patient is adequately filled prior to voiding and for measuring post-void residual, which should be done immediately after voiding. The pelvic floor EMG assesses increased muscle recruitment in response to urgency/bladder overactivity and for pelvic floor muscle activity during voiding to screen for synergistic versus discoordinate voiding. More recently, this has been shown help tease out whether detrusor overactivity is present based a short

EMG lag time, where basically flow, in the presence of urgency, begins instanta-
neously with pelvic floor relaxation [46]. Uroflow/EMG is also a useful tool in monitoring objectively response to therapy, particularly those on medication for detrusor
overactivity and secondary bladder neck obstruction. The reader will find a good
review on urodynamic practices by Schafer et al. [47] and another on urodynamic
testing in children by Drzewiecki et al. [48].

Urodynamics in the Valve Patient: Specific Considerations

Detrusor Compliance and Overactivity

Detrusor compliance is the mathematical expression (Δvolume/ΔPdet expressed as
mL/cm H_2O) of the bladder's ability to accommodate increasing volumes of stored
urine. We grade compliance as normal if ≥ 30 mL/cm H_2O, mild loss of compliance
(LOC) 20–29 cm/H_2O, moderate LOC 10–19 cm H_2O, and severe LOC ≤ 9 cm H_2O
[49]. It is generally accepted that there is a minimum threshold of a change of at least
10 cm/H_2O before compliance is felt to be compromised. But like most things in
urodynamics, there is a lot of subjectivity to the analysis. For example, although a
LOC that starts at 400 mL and progresses to a change of 40 cm H_2O at 600 mL during
urodynamics may seem ominous, it is of little concern if the child is on clean intermittent catheterization (CIC) and documented catheterization volumes rarely if ever
exceed 350 mL, while a progressive change of 9–10 cm H_2O in an infant's 40-mL
capacity bladder, though barely meeting the threshold required, is worrisome.

The presence of VUR or a bladder diverticulum may be suspected when during
the course of filling there is loss of compliance that suddenly levels off, despite
continuation of filling, suggesting the gain of compliance through one of these
pop-off mechanisms.

It is important to be aware of factors that can falsely influence compliance measurements. Too rapid a fill rate can falsely suggest impaired compliance or detrusor overactivity that may not be present when the child fills more naturally. Filling should follow
the guidelines detailed in the previous section and stopped periodically to see if the rise
in pressure falls back to baseline or remains steady indicating true LOC. Pressures that
rise rapidly and are unrelated to filling are indicative of an active detrusor contraction.
However they do need to meet a minimum threshold change of at least 10–15 cm H_2O
to be considered detrusor overactivity. We also consider a contraction of essentially any
magnitude significant, if it causes urgency or leakage of urine.

While the compliance value at capacity is what generally is reported, it is
also important to note when loss of compliance began, e.g., early, mid fill, terminal, or after expected bladder capacity is exceeded, as the earlier loss of compliance is noted, the more likely it is that significant changes in the detrusor
matrix have occurred.

Even though detrusor storage pressures greater than 40 cm H_2O are known to have
a greater association with upper tract deterioration, it is a misconception to think that

all storage pressures below that level are safe. The goal of therapy in those with impaired compliance is to lower storage pressures as close to normal as possible.

Secondary Bladder Neck Obstruction (2°BNO)

Consideration of 2°BNO in boys with a history of PUV as a real phenomenon has slowly grown over the past 50 years. In 1975, McGuire and Weiss reported on two children who could not void following undiversion of temporary loop ureterostomies [50]. When treated with phenoxybenzamine, a long-acting alpha-blocker, at 5 mg QD, both boys voided subsequently and the hydroureteronephrosis improved. Weiss felt that the beneficial effect on the hydronephrosis resulted from the alpha-blocker preventing an abnormal detrusor pressure rise during bladder filling and/or lower outlet resistance during voiding [51]. On the basis of what we now know, it is likely that the lowering of outlet resistance at the bladder neck with alpha blockers is what led to the lowering of the abnormally elevated detrusor pressures during bladder filling.

2°BNO is characterized by elevated voiding pressures and diminished urine flow parameters and often associated with incomplete emptying. However, it is important to recognize that uroflow parameters alone can be deceiving as there are some boys who generate very high voiding pressures that can overcome the obstruction to yield relatively normal uroflow parameters, while a depressed flow might also be the result of impaired contractility. To accurately make the diagnosis of 2°BNO, one must analyze both detrusor voiding pressures and uroflow parameters and rule out the existence of urethral stricture or residual valve tissue. This is typically done by VUDS, as neither imaging studies nor endoscopy are highly reliable in identifying 2°BNO on the basis of appearance alone.

We diagnose the presence of unequivocal 2°BNO based on meeting one of the following three criteria (when voiding with a relaxed EMG and without radiographic evidence of residual valve or stricture): (1) Pdet > 100 cm H_2O regardless of flow, (2) Pdet > 80 cm H_2O and Qave < 10 cc/s, and (3) Pdet > 60 cm H_2O and Qave < 5 cc/s. We also treat those boys whose pressure flow findings are equivocal if there is associated upper tract dilation that is not resolving and/or impaired emptying.

In 2009 we reviewed our experience with alpha-blocker therapy in 28 valve boys with suspected 2°BNO, 14 of whom met the unequivocal criteria and 14 in whom the diagnosis was equivocal [52]. All had either resolution or improvement over time in reflux or hydronephrosis if either was previously present.

Androulakakis et al. [53] proposed that myogenic failure was secondary to BNO and recommended treatment with either alpha-blockers or bladder neck incision (BNI). Abraham et al. [54] believed that 2°BNO could be diagnosed on the basis of elevated post-void residuals that were greater than 10% of the expected bladder capacity (EBC) for age. After treatment with terazosin, another alpha-blocker, mean PVR fell from 15.7% of capacity (i.e., 34% EBC) to 2.4 cc as determined by ultrasound. Previously, Kajbafzadeh et al. [55] treated 24 boys diagnosed with PUV at a mean age of 1.8 years with primary valve ablation and another 22 at a mean age of

1.8 years, both with valve ablation and BNI. Of the 24 with valve ablation alone on a follow-up 4.5-year post-ablation, 38 % had hypercontractility, 25 % detrusor overactivity, and 21 % developed myogenic failure. Noteworthy, of the valve ablation/BNI group, none had any of these complications. Ten valve patients who have undergone the combined surgery and who are now over 21 years of age were recently reevaluated, and none have incontinence and all have normal ejaculation (personnel communication, Kajbafzadeh 2015). Similar findings were reported by Taskinen et al. in 2012 in Finish men who had BNI prior to 1970 [56]. These findings suggest that the chance of developing a dry ejaculate following BNI is no different than if BNI had not been done.

The majority of patients with 2°BNO respond well to alpha-blocker therapy of which there are several to choose from. Presently we prefer tamsulosin for its selectivity and low side effect profile. However, this use of alpha-blockers is currently off label and parents need to be so informed. We do monitor blood pressure in our older patients, both pre- and on therapy and have not experienced any associated hypotension in the well child (Fig. 7.10a, b).

The general starting dosing scheme we follow is age 3–12 months 0.05 mg (0.5 mL), 12–24 months 0.075 mg (0.75 mL), 2–5 years 0.1 mg (1 mL or 1/4 cap), 5–12 years 0.2 mg (1/2 cap), and 12–16 years 0.2 mg to start and then after 2–3 weeks if well tolerated increase to a full cap (0.4 mg), 16 years and older 0.4 mg. Further adjustments in dosing are made after 3–6 months based on clinical needs and urodynamic improvements as measured either on UDS or uroflow/PVR. The average effective dose in our children 7 years and older is 0.4 mg.

Myogenic Failure

Myogenic failure, sometimes referred to as a hypocontractile, acontractile, or underactive bladder, is a term used most specifically for the bladder that cannot sustain an effective voluntary detrusor contraction to fully empty the bladder that sometimes develops in older boys with a history of PUV. The diagnosis is made urodynamically. Failure to empty is not in and of itself proof of myogenic failure. A sustained detrusor contraction of normal magnitude may result in retention if there is an obstructive process that remains unaddressed. Upper tract dumping with rapid bladder refill can be read as failure to empty depending on method used to measure PVR. Likewise, flow patterns, specifically intermittent flow, while suggestive of, are not proof of it.

Holmdahl et al. reported in 1995 and 1996 that with increasing age, the instability often disappeared and hypocompliant bladders became hypercompliant [57, 58]. The authors believed that growth of the prostate and nephrogenic diabetes insipidus also contributed to large bladder size. De Gennaro et al. [59] also hypothesized that the myogenic failure that developed in older valve patients represented decompensation of the bladder after years of increased detrusor pressure, decreased compliance, and pronounced instability. Bladder neck obstruction may also be an additional cause of myogenic failure [53, 60].

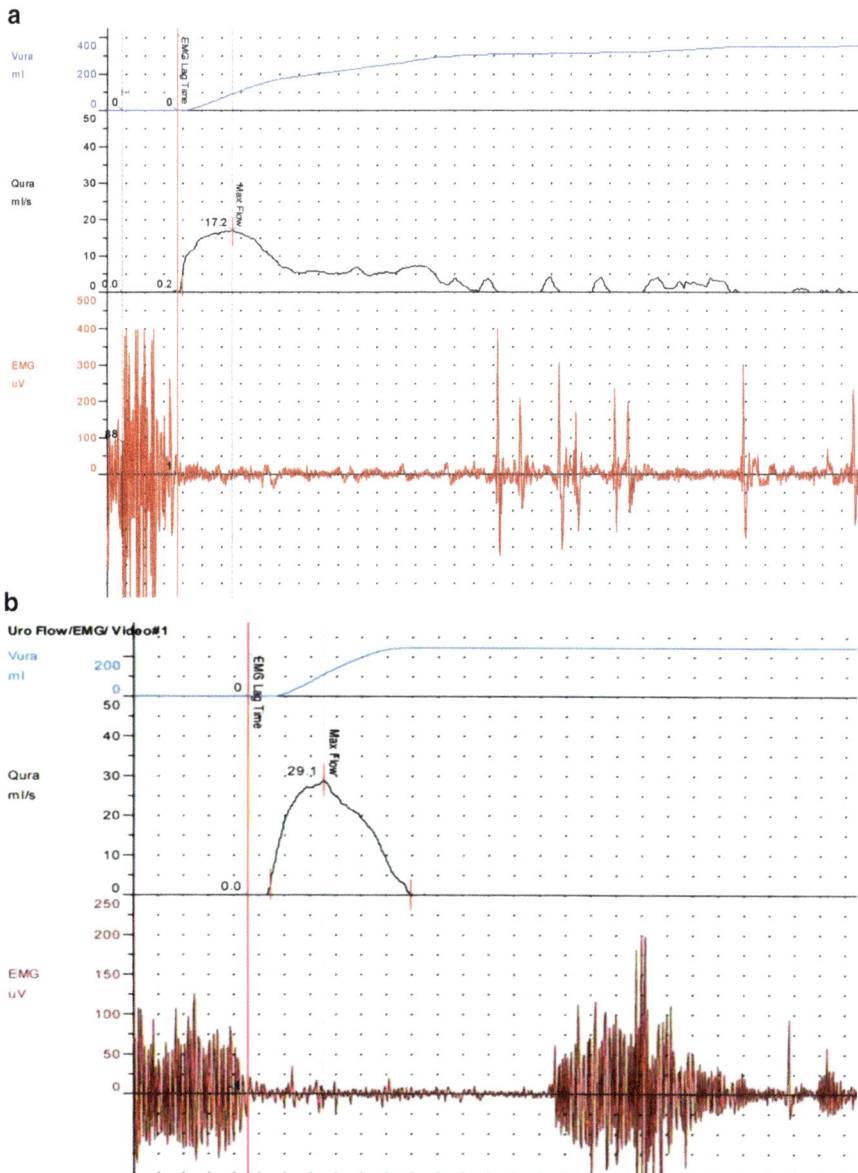

Fig. 7.10 An 11-year-old boy with persistent urgency and occasional wetting despite long-term oxybutynin therapy. (**a**) Screening uroflow/EMG on oxybutynin therapy, note short EMG lag time indicative of overactivity, a deceptively normal Qmax of 17.2 mL/s, but a grossly abnormal Qave of 5.6 mL/s and straining at the end to empty. Because upper tracts were normal, it was decided to treat suspected 2°BNO empirically instead of repeating VUDS that were negative for urethral obstruction when last done several years prior. (**b**) Uroflow/EMG repeated 3 months later after adding tamsulosin to his oxybutynin therapy. Note normalization of EMG lag time and flow pattern, Qmax now 25.7 mL/s and Qave 17.9 mL/s; urgency and wetting completely resolved thus supporting diagnosis of 2°BNO

Table 7.2 Incidence of myogenic failure being diagnosed on UDS obtained years following valve ablation

Series	No. of patients	No. myogenic failure (%)
Peters et al. [44]	41	14 (34)
Parkhouse and Woodhouse [32]	42	4 (9.5)
Jaureguizar et al. [61]	21	0 (0)
Kim et al. [49]	31	0 (0)
De Gennaro et al. [59]	65	17 (26)
Jaureguizar et al. [62]	59	3 (5)
Misseri et al. [60]	51	0 (0)

Misseri et al. [60] reviewed our data of posterior urethral valve boys evaluated urodynamically and in whom abnormal findings were appropriately and aggressively treated with follow-up continued into the teenage years [60]. None developed true myogenic failure although a few had anticholinergic therapy-induced myogenic failure that resolved following discontinuation of medication. In other studies, however, the incidence of myogenic failure was as high as 34 % [44, 60]. It is not clear from these studies just how aggressive treatment had been and whether or not patients were on anticholinergic therapy at the time myogenic failure was diagnosed. Over 2 decades we have been prescribing anticholinergic therapy for newborn valves, particularly the more severely affected ones, prior to neonatal discharge. One cautionary note to be aware of is that an anticholinergic-induced form of myogenic failure can occasionally occur but usually disappears with cessation of the medication [28]. If lowering the dose does not solve the problem or bladder hyperactivity requires the use of medication, CIC might be the better option as opposed to stopping therapy. The disparity in incidences of myogenic failure lends oneself to consider whether it is truly the natural progression of the valve condition as some suggest or is it a consequence of treatment failure (Table 7.2).

Temporary Diversion and the Defunctionalized Bladder

Veenema reported that the diverted bladder became smaller and hypertonic with time [63, 64]. Schmaelzle et al. [65] also demonstrated that in dogs following diversion, bladder capacity decreased to 12.5 % of prediversion volumes. However, once undiverted, bladder capacity returned to 88 % of prediversion volumes. In addition, compliance, response to muscarinics, and muscarinic receptor density normalized as well.

Tanagho recommended caution when advising supravesical diversion, and if diversion had to be done, to reverse it as soon as possible [66]. Others found that these bladders did well following undiversion [66–68]. Jayanthi et al. [69] studied 30 valve patients who had temporary diversion, 10 with cutaneous pyelostomy, and 20 with vesicostomy. Only one of the 20 with a vesicostomy later required an augmentation, while 7 of the 10 treated with cutaneous pyelostomy required augmentation [69]. Duckett [70] suggested that the

Table 7.3 Bladder compliance[a] and percentage of expected bladder capacity for age[b] following three forms of initial therapy

Initial management	Moderately impaired	Severely impaired	Percent with impairment (%)	Expected bladder capacity for age following therapy (%)
Valve ablation (n = 20)	8	4	60	90
Pyelostomy (n = 4)	0	1	25	123
Vesicostomy (n = 5)	1	0	20	196

[a]Compliance = $\Delta V/\Delta P$; severely impaired < 10 mL/cm; moderately impaired 10–20 mL/cm; mildly impaired 21–30 mL/cm (none had mildly impaired compliance)
[b]Based on Koff's formula [expected volume for age (in ounces) = age + 2 (in ounces)]. Based on data in Kim et al. [49]

vesicostomy patients did better because some urine always stays behind in the bladder after vesicostomy even though the bladder itself drains to the skin. However, it is possible that those with the worst bladders to begin with underwent supravesical diversion.

Subsequently Kim et al. [49] reported that our patients who underwent either vesicostomy or pyelostomy ended up with larger bladders and with better compliance and less overactivity (Table 7.3). On the other hand, Podesta et al. [71, 72] in two similar studies demonstrated worse bladders in those who underwent vesicostomy or supravesical diversion as compared to primary ablation.

The balance of the evidence in the literature suggests that temporary proximal diversion does not harm the bladder. The problem with most studies that compare outcomes of valve patients treated with primary ablation, temporary vesicostomy, and temporary supravesical diversion is that those temporarily diverted tend to be those initially with the worst serum creatinines, the worst bladders, and the most hydroureteronephrosis. Perhaps the most notable study on this subject was the one done by Jaureguizar et al. [62] in which they compared outcomes of patients treated with temporary cutaneous pyelostomy with a group treated by primary valve ablation alone. Surprisingly, those who were diverted ended up with better bladder compliance and grew taller.

In the end, proximal diversion is now seldom performed in our practices as similar results can be obtained from aggressive pharmacologic therapy agents. Most evidence suggests that temporary diversion causes little harm to the bladder and, if diverted patients are treated aggressively with anticholinergics both before and after undiversion, and the outlook for these bladders will be better.

Bladder Histology

The majority of studies on histologic changes to the bladder as a consequence of in utero outlet obstruction are from animal models. Historically, it was thought that partial bladder obstruction induced detrusor muscle hypertrophy with replacement of smooth muscle tissue with fibrotic connective tissue [73]. Numerous studies over the past few decades have shown that other factors also play a role in bladder changes from obstruction including diminished blood flow to the developing bladder, diminished mitochondrial enzyme activity, reduced nerve density with decreased autonomic detrusor innervation, changes in collage-type ratios, and downregulation of bladder angiotensin-II receptors [74–78].

Studies show that obstructed fetal bladders are associated with marked increase in bladder wall thickness as compared to normal fetal controls [79, 80].

Pop-Off Mechanisms

Early studies on the presence of urinary extravasation (i.e., perirenal urinomas, urinary ascites, or bladder perforation) and unilateral VUR with renal dysplasia (the VURD syndrome) suggested a protective role for renal function in patients with these conditions at diagnosis [81–84]. Despite the low numbers and short follow-up, these early reports supported the concept of the "pop-off" mechanism for conserving renal function. By affording a pressure sink, these pop-off mechanisms allow either relief of pressure damage to the kidneys or one kidney to take the full damage of that pressure and allow protection of the contralateral kidney. In 1988, Rittenberg and colleagues [85] formerly proposed three anatomical associations (i.e., pressure "pop-off" mechanisms) found to be protective in PUV: (1) unilateral VUR and renal dysplasia syndrome (VURD), (2) large congenital bladder diverticula, and (3) urinary extravasation with or without ascites. The authors noted that among 71 boys with PUV, those with a "pop-off" mechanism were more likely to have a lower serum nadir creatinine than patients with no "pop-off" mechanism. A patent urachus likely represents another "pop-off" mechanism although there are few reports in the literature [18, 86]. In addition to preservation of renal function, presence of a "pop-off" mechanism has been shown to be significantly associated with favorable bladder outcome on urodynamic studies [18].

Urinomas

The incidence of urinary extravasation at presentation in boys with PUV ranges from 3 to 17 % [87–89]. Urinary extravasation occurs most commonly in the kidney and is thought to occur from urine being forced across a renal fornix due to high intraluminal pressure or forniceal rupture. Kay and associates [81] were among the first to suggest a protective role of urinary ascites in the neonate with obstructive uropathy. Heikkila and associates [88] were the first to retrospectively compare outcomes of PUV patients with urinomas to those without urinomas. The authors concluded that kidney function is similar in PUV patients regardless of urinoma status (whether manifested as perirenal urinoma or urinary ascites). Wells and coworkers [89] on the other hand found that boys with urinomas at presentation had significantly lower serum creatinine at >5 years of follow-up compared to boys without urinomas. Interestingly, none of the boys with urinomas in their study progressed to ESRD or required transplant compared to 9 % of the boys without urinomas. Given the widely differing results and conclusions of these two recent studies—the largest and only comparative studies to date on the topic—it is difficult to draw a definitive conclusion on the protective role of urinomas in boys with PUV. Therefore, the role urinary extravasation plays as a "pop-off" mechanism requires further study and longer follow-up.

Vesicoureteral Reflux and the VURD Syndrome

At least half to 72 % of PUV patients have VUR at presentation [39, 90]. Interestingly, unilateral VUR is more common on the left (75–80 %) and approximately 1/3 of boys will have bilateral VUR [82, 84, 90, 91]. Early studies showed a high rate of mortality and CKD in boys with bilateral VUR [92, 93]. With treatment of the PUV, up to 39 % of boys with grade 3 or higher VUR will show spontaneous resolution of VUR [39, 90]. Thus the VUR is thought to be secondary to the outlet obstruction in most of these boys.

The concept of VUR leading to a unilateral dysplastic kidney while at the same time protecting or sparing the nonrefluxing kidney was first proposed by Hoover and Duckett in 1982 [82]. A year later, Greenfield and colleagues [84] confirmed good contralateral renal function and "excellent" long-term prognosis in patients with the VURD. In 1988, Rittenberg and associates described the VURD syndrome in nine patients and included it as one of three renal protective factors in boys with PUV [85]. Since these publications, the VURD syndrome has been shown to be present in as many as 20–26 % of all boys presenting with PUV (Fig. 7.11a–c) [91, 94].

The protective nature of the VURD syndrome suggested by these earlier reports with limited follow-up were called into question by Cuckow and coworkers [91] and Narasimhan and colleagues [95] who reported that the VURD syndrome does not offer a protective effect on renal function in the long term. Hoag and coworkers also found similar rates of renal impairment after 57–77 months of follow-up between the two groups [94].

While early reports supported the benefits of the "pop-off" mechanism, recent studies call these conclusions into question, and the VURD syndrome is less likely to be indicative of positive clinical outcome than originally believed. In fact, the protective effect of these "pop-off" mechanisms is extremely variable and likely dependent on other factors on an individual basis. Whether or not there is a benefit in terms of bladder function as suggested by Kaefer and colleagues needs to be confirmed by more robust future studies [18].

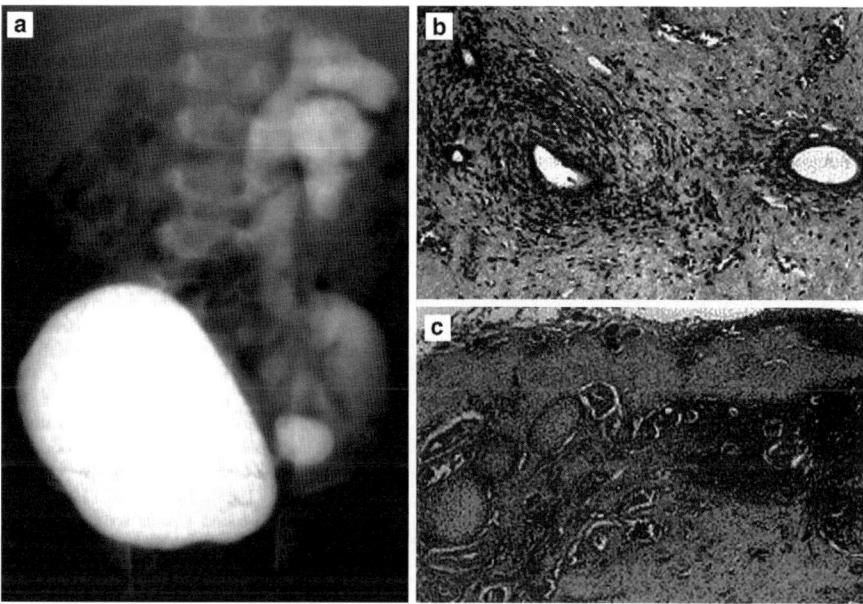

Fig. 7.11 (**a**) Cystogram of a child with a posterior urethral valve and grade V left reflux, a large paraureteric diverticulum, and a nonfunctioning left kidney. (**b**) Primitive ducts, the sine qua non of dysplasia, and loose parenchymal tissue are seen in one area (×100). (**c**) Cartilage is identified in another area (×40). With permission from Glassberg KI, Horowitz M. Urethral valves and other anomalies of the male urethra, in Belman AB, King LR, Kramer SA {eds}: *Clinical Pediatric Urology*, ed 4. London, Martin Dunitz Ltd, 2002;pp:899; Chapt 28, Fig. 28.3. © Taylor and Francis [10]

Prognostic Indicators

Aside from pop-off phenomenon, other findings have been investigated for prognostic value. Hubert et al. found a higher incidence of CKD in patients without identifiable pyramids on ultrasound at the time of diagnosis [95, 96]. Also, a nadir creatinine in the first year of life <0.8 mg% seems to be an excellent prognostic sign that CKD will not develop in the future [97–99].

Dineen et al. [100] studied concentrating ability and found 59 % of boys with a history of PUV to have a mild concentrating defect (unable to concentrate >800 mOsm/kg) and 16 % had a severe defect (unable to concentrate >300 mOsm/kg) [100]. If urinary osmolality was >800 mOsm/kg, the GFR was likely to be >80 mL/min per 1.73 m², and if <400 mOsm/kg, the creatinine clearance was more likely to be <60 mL/min per 1.73 m². Incontinence itself has been identified as a prognostic indicator as well. Incontinence at 5 years of age was found to be associated with a 46 % incidence of renal failure, while continence by 5 years was associated with only a 5 % incidence of renal failure [93].

In conclusion one can say that there is a list of prognostic indicators. Favorable prognostic signs include in utero presentation after 24 weeks in those with a normal ultrasound before 24 weeks, ultrasound appearance of at least one pyramid in the kidney, nadir serum creatinine <0.8 mg% before age 1 year, absence of VUR, and continence at age 5 years.

Incontinence

Incontinence has been reported in 19–81 % of 5-year-old boys with a history of PUV [42, 93, 101–103]. It invariably disappears, possibly due to the growth of the prostate, disappearance of detrusor overactivity, and increase in bladder capacity [58, 104, 105]. One additional cause of incontinence is loss of normal sensation in the chronically overdistended bladder [106]. Smith et al. [103] found decreasing incontinence with age (81 % of 5-year-olds, 46 % of 10-year-olds, and 1 % of 20-year-olds). Obviously it is not the incontinence that is bad for the kidneys; it is that incontinence is a reflection of poor bladder function and secondary nephrogenic diabetes insipidus, findings that often are accompanied by persistent HUN. Correcting the cause of incontinence likely does play a role in preventing the later development of myogenic bladder.

Overnight Bladder Drainage

Koff et al., in 2002, first reported on the utility of using overnight bladder emptying by indwelling catheter, overnight intermittent catheterization, or frequent overnight voiding/double voiding for the valve patient with persistent HUN [107]. They found significant improvement or resolution of the hydronephrosis equivalent to that achieved with augmentation. He also found that some bladders had improved function, compliance, and capacity. He postulated that the problem was a consequence of bladders with impaired compliance/high-pressure storage of urine particularly in the circumstance of high renal output overnight or what he later termed SNOB (syndrome of nocturnal overdistention of the bladder). Our experience with nocturnal bladder emptying has been similar to Koff's. Nocturnal bladder emptying (NBE) is likely needed only until the abnormal bladder dynamics are corrected and the urine output is normalized (usually after renal transplant).

Augmentation Cystoplasty

The incidence of augmentation among valve patients varies tremendously between centers. Holmdahl [105] suggests holding off on augmentation since compliance may increase with time and the need for augmentation may disappear. Overnight catheterization has also been shown to be effective in normalizing detrusor pressures in the small, poorly compliant bladder. To put augmentation in perspective in valve boys, one of the present authors (KIG) has managed more than 200 boys with a history of PUV and has only had to resort to bladder augmentation in three patients. We strongly believe that in every boy considered for augmentation secondary BNO be ruled out and that a period of overnight bladder drainage be tried first. Lastly, before removing a dilated ureter at the time of a nephrectomy, one should keep in mind that that ureter might serve a future useful purpose should either an augmentation or catheterizable channel become necessary.

Long-Term Outcomes and Transitional Care

The follow-up of the valve patient into childhood is quite variable. In utero diagnosis likely will result in reduced or delayed development of end-stage renal disease (ESRD) because the most severely affected fetuses often are aborted and treatment in the others is instituted earlier. Ability to father a child is difficult to interpret on the basis of current literature and the paucity of long-term studies. Because the incidence of LUT symptoms in adults varies so greatly in the literature between institutions, conclusions regarding long-term bladder function are hard to make.

Renal Function and ESRD

While the ultimate goal in treating boys with PUV is preservation of renal function, many neonates and infants already show signs of deterioration of renal function prior to intervention. Hennus et al. reported mean rates of CKD and ESRD after neonatal intervention of 5–32 % and 0–20 %, respectively, after follow-up times ranging from 1 to 12 years [108]. Other studies have reported a 20–50 % rate of ESRD by 18 years of age in PUV patients [19, 93, 103]. In fact, the incidences of both CKD and development of ESRD is likely to continue to rise throughout early to mid-adulthood.

Holmdahl and Sillen [109] noted that the incidence of ESRD and renal insufficiency in PUV patients at age 5–11 years was 8 % and 21 %, respectively, while at age 31–44 years, they were 21 % and 17 %, respectively. Interestingly, 50 % of the adult men with ESRD had a GFR of 40–50 mL/min (stage 3 CKD) at the time of discharge after initial valve ablation during infancy. These men later progressed to ESRD in adulthood at a median age of 30, although no patient over the age of 37 in the study developed ESRD. Heikkila and colleagues reported a lifetime risk of ESRD of 28.5 %, and interestingly, one-third of cases were diagnosed after 17 years of age [110]. Approximately one-third to one-half of all ESRD in PUV patients occur in early adulthood, and the incidence of ESRD presenting after the middle to end of the fourth decade of life is rare [109, 110].

Given that the risks of CKD and even ESRD do not appear to go away and may first be detected when these boys reach early adulthood or even later, long-term monitoring during childhood and adolescence for signs of renal deterioration with blood pressure measurements, serum creatinine, and urinalysis (particularly proteinuria) should be performed by pediatric urologists in conjunction with pediatricians and pediatric nephrologists. Nadir serum creatinine, especially in the first year of life, and presence of bladder dysfunction are two important predictors of renal outcomes in boys as they transition through childhood and adolescence [97, 102, 111]. In adult men with a history of PUV, one important predictor of CKD/ESRD is the onset and magnitude of proteinuria [112]. No patient in this series with proteinuria of <50 mg/mmol creatinine progressed to ESRD after a minimal follow-up of 5 years.

Renal Transplantation in PUV Patients

ESRD in both children and adults can be treated with dialysis and/or renal transplantation. PUV patients present a challenge for transplantation compared to patients with ESRD from medical diseases secondary to the possibility of bladder damage and/or dysfunction. Historical series noted worse outcomes and higher graft failure following renal transplant in children with PUV [113–115]. Reinberg and associates [114] noted only 50 % graft survival at 5 years in boys with PUV compared to 73 % for children who underwent transplantation secondary to VUR and 75 % for a control group of children with ESRD from non-urologic etiologies. Similar reports were presented by Groenewegen and colleagues [115]. Despite these earlier findings, more recent studies have shown better graft survival and renal function [116–119]. In 1997, Salomon and colleagues [117] reported equivalent graft survival between 66 children with PUV and 116 controls (54 % vs. 50 % at 10 years, respectively). Interestingly, they noted that children with PUV had a significantly higher serum creatinine than controls at 10 years after transplantation.

Several authors have attempted to define the role, if any, of the bladder dysfunction in future graft failure. Salomon and colleagues [120] noted significantly worse renal function in PUV boys with bladder dysfunction compared to those without bladder dysfunction. Of note, bladder dysfunction was loosely defined in their study, and the majority of children did not undergo urodynamic studies. In contrast to this study, other authors found no negative effect of the bladder on graft function and overall graft survival [116, 121]. Despite these findings, we agree with those authors who support the complete evaluation of bladder function especially with urodynamic studies in any PUV patient with voiding symptoms prior to renal transplantation.

Despite these similar success rates, several studies have shown that the risk of posttransplantation complications is higher in PUV boys compared with controls [122, 123]. In 1996, higher risk of UTI after transplantation in PUV boys than controls was reported [122]. Mendizabal and associates [123] reported that boys with

PUV had a greater risk of posttransplantation urologic complications including urethral and/or ureterovesical strictures, stone formation, hematuria, bladder outlet obstruction, and UTI compared with non-PUV children.

VUR After Transplantation

VUR in transplanted kidneys is directly related to surgical technique for ureteroneocystostomy which in turn is dependent on surgeon preference and institution protocol. Interestingly, a recent study by Routh and associates [124] suggests that VUR is more common in transplanted kidneys in PUV boys even when performing a nonrefluxing anastomosis compared with non-PUV children (52% vs. 14%, respectively, $p < 0.0001$). The authors noted; however, that the long-term outcomes in terms of graft survival and function did not differ between PUV and non-PUV children [124].

LUT Symptoms

Three long-term large studies based on questionnaires demonstrate why it is so hard to make any conclusions. Two of the three studies showed that Lower urinary tract (LUT) symptoms were an infrequent finding in adults with history of PUV (12 and 13%), while the third showed that they were present in greater than 50% of men [109]. Even more confusing was that in the respective control groups without a history of PUV, the incidence of LUT symptoms was equivalent to, or even higher than, the incidence of LUT symptoms in the adults with a history of PUV.

Schober et al. [125] used VCUG and ultrasound rather than questionnaires to evaluate valve men at age 17–51. Sixty-nine percent were found to have incomplete emptying, 41% a thickened bladder wall, and 21% voided small volumes. None of the patients were reported to have a large capacity bladder. In conclusion, whether or not LUT symptoms are prevalent in the adult valve population, most of the symptoms are mild and it is those who have incontinence that are most likely to complain.

Fertility

Semen analysis findings in adults with a history of PUV have varied from normal to abnormal among a number of recent studies. Prolonged liquefaction time, high percent of abnormal forms, and preponderance of pyospermia, bacterial growth, and decreased motility among young men with PUV and LUT symptomatology have been described [125–127]. Contributing to increased infertility could be the increased incidence of cryptorchidism in association with PUV (16%), reflux of urine into the ejaculatory ducts, and an increased incidence of epididymo-orchitis. Paternity, however, has been reported to be high in numerous studies even among those who have undergone renal transplantation. Taskinen et al. [128] found a 49% incidence of paternity among Finnish men with a history of PUV with a mean age of 38 years, a percentage similar to the same age range for men without a history of PUV.

Erectile Dysfunction

Even though there is decreased libido and episodes of sexual activity in men with renal failure, both normalize with transplantation [129], Taskinen et al. [128] found no difference in erectile function when men with a history of PUV were compared to controls, although there was a significantly higher incidence of complaints about achievement of orgasm during sexual activity.

Quality of Life

The only LUT symptom that Taskinen et al. found to decrease quality of life was incontinence, but fortunately that was an infrequent finding [56, 128]. Bladder augmentation and its high association with the need for CIC very much bothered these men, similar to men on CIC without augmentation. CKD and its associated symptoms also can lower quality of life.

Other Urethral Anomalies

Anterior Urethral Valves

Anterior urethral valves occur very infrequently and may be located anywhere along the anterior urethra. Children with anterior urethral valves present with symptoms similar to those of boys with PUV. Boys may present with antenatal hydronephrosis, penile ballooning, or in older boys, voiding dysfunction. As with PUV, the diagnosis is also made on VCUG. A renal ultrasound should be performed to complete the evaluation. In most cases, an anterior urethral valve is actually a congenital urethral diverticulum with the lip of the diverticulum preventing antegrade flow of urine. The bulging diverticulum may further obstruct the urethra by compressing the lumen. Cystourethroscopy may miss the valve due to the retrograde flow of fluid during the procedure.

The obstruction is most commonly relieved endoscopically. The distal lip is incised using a hook or right-angle wire electrode (Fig. 7.12). Rushton et al. found vesicostomy to be a good temporizing procedure if the child is too small or too ill [130]. If

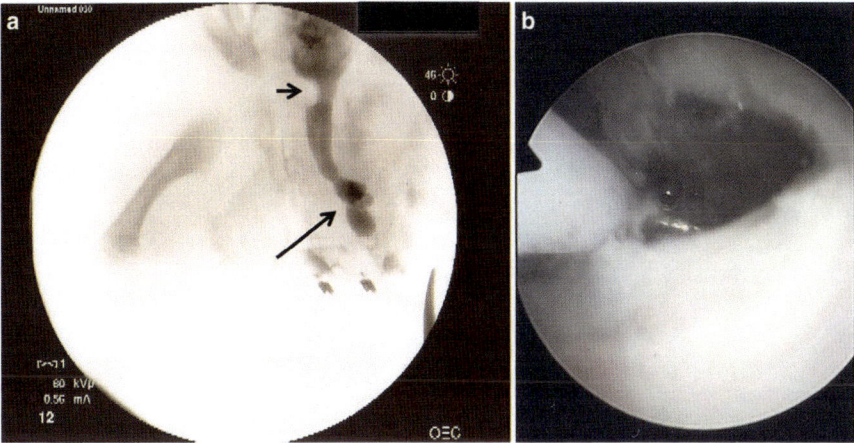

Fig. 7.12 Anterior urethral valves. (**a**) Expression cystourethrogram under anesthesia in a 15-day-old boy. Urine fills the urethra up until the site of the distal obstructing lip (*long arrow*). Note the bladder neck collar as seen frequently in patients with PUV (*short arrow*). Hemostatic is at the tip of the penis. (**b**) Right-angle wire electrode has engaged the distal lip. (**c**) The incision has been made with a cutting current and obstruction relieved

endoscopic management is unsuccessful, the redundant tissue of the diverticulum may be excised and the urethra reconfigured in two layers over an 8 or 10 Fr catheter.

Congenital Urethral Strictures

Another rare congenital urethral anomaly is congenital urethral stricture. Similar to boys with PUV, these patients may be identified antenatally with hydroureteronephrosis, a distended bladder, and/or oligohydramnios. The stricture may be too long or tight to treat endoscopically and a vesicostomy is often necessary soon after birth [131]. Sequential urethral dilation has been described with some success [132].

Urethral Duplication

Though rare, the duplicated urethra is typically in the sagittal plane with an orthotopic appearing meatus and a second meatus ventral or dorsal to it. The more ventrally located urethra is usually the more dominant one. In addition to the duplicated urethra being hypospadiac or epispadiac, the duplication may be to the right or left of the orthotopic appearing meatus or the duplication can be complete or incomplete. Patients can present with two streams, usually one more dominant than the other, incontinence depending upon where the secondary urethra connects to the urinary tract. A VCUG is helpful in determining the extent and anatomy of the duplicated urethras [133]. A retrograde urethrogram may be necessary to further delineate the abnormality. The accessory urethra may be blind ending, it may join the orthotopic urethra along its course, or it may be in continuity with the bladder. The complete form of duplication includes both urethras arising independently from the bladder with the normal caliber ventral channel exiting at the orthotopic site on the glans and the accessory channel opening in an epispadiac position.

Congenital Anterior Urethral Diverticula

Congenital diverticula of the anterior urethra are rare and usually diagnosed on a VCUG or cystoscopy obtained because of dysuria or post-void bleeding or post-void dribbling of blood or urine. They include syringocele and lacuna magna.

Syringoceles

Maizel et al. [134] named cystic dilatations of the main duct of Cowper's bulbar urethral glands as Cowper's syringoceles and based on radiographic appearance divided them into four types: (1) simple syringocele with minimal duct dilatation, (2) perforate syringocele represented by a bulbous duct with a patulous ostium, (3) imperforate syringocele appearing as a radiolucent bulge in the urethra on VCUG that can also be associated with a mass in the perineum or hydronephrosis, and (4) ruptured syringocele with only a membrane remaining. Both the perforate and ruptured syringoceles appear as a diverticulum when identified endoscopically. Bulging symptomatic cysts can be managed endoscopically with an incision.

Lacuna Magna

This entity was first described as a small diverticulum in the glanular urethra by Mogagni in 1719 [135]. In 1950, Guerin described a flap of tissue overlying a lacuna in the glans of urethra that became known as the valve of Guerin and described as almost a septum between the canalized ingrowth of ectodermal tissue and the advancing anterior urethra [136]. Sommer and Stephens referred to this finding as a lacuna magna and that it could be associated with dysuria and post-void dribbling of blood [137]. This diverticulum may be present in 30% of normal boys and is usually asymptomatic [138]. It can be seen filled with contrast on a VCUG, sometimes appearing as a teardrop or a blind-ending small canal in the roof of the distal urethra and must be differentiated from a drop of contrast-filled urine near the tip of the penis [139].

Congenital Urethral Polyps

Benign, congenital urethral polyps arise from the roof of the verumontanum and can be associated with a stalk, which allows it to flip back into the bladder or fall forward into the membranous urethra. Histologically they are composed of fibrous and muscular tissue that is covered with transitional epithelium. Congenital polyps of the anterior urethra are extremely rare. They usually present in young boys who already are out of diapers and who suddenly develop obstructive symptoms including hesitancy and retention. In a series reported by Gleason and Kramerthe, mean age at diagnosis was 8.9 years with 50 % presenting with voiding complaints and none with hydronephrosis [140]. The diagnosis usually can be made on VCUG with a radiolucent filling defect located in the posterior urethra and sometimes seen flipped proximally through the bladder neck into the bladder. Treatment is accomplished with a resectoscope and loop.

Congenital Megalourethra

Congenital megalourethra is divided into two types: scaphoid and fusiform, the former associated most commonly with prune belly syndrome (Fig. 7.13). A megalourethra is a diffuse dilation of the anterior urethra that results in a very large and abnormally formed phallus. Unlike an anterior urethral valve or stricture, there is no narrowing distally. In the fusiform variety, the corpora spongiosum and cavernosum are poorly formed. This form is more severe and may be associated with urinary tract anomalies leading to oligohydramnios and poor lung function [141]. The penile deformity is often associated with voiding dysfunction and later erectile dysfunction.

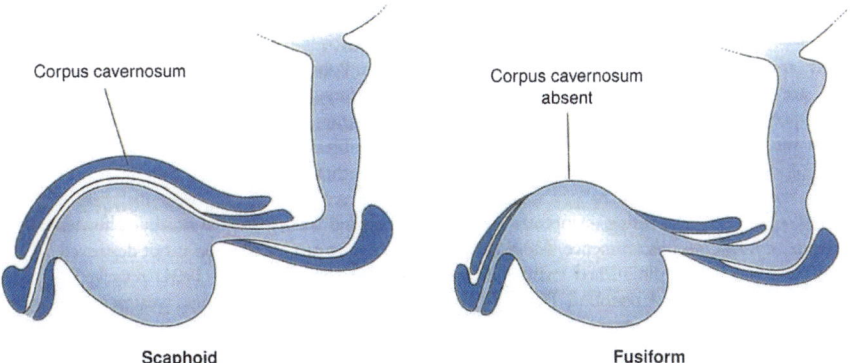

Corpus cavernosum

Corpus cavernosum absent

Scaphoid   Fusiform

Fig. 7.13 Types of megalourethra (*left*) scaphoid; (*right*) fusiform. With permission from Glassberg KI, Horowitz M. Urethral valves and other anomalies of the male urethra, in Belman AB, King LR, Kramer SA {eds}: *Clinical Pediatric Urology*, ed 4. London, Martin Dunitz Ltd, 2002;pp:899; Chapt 28, Fig. 28.28. © Taylor and Francis [10]

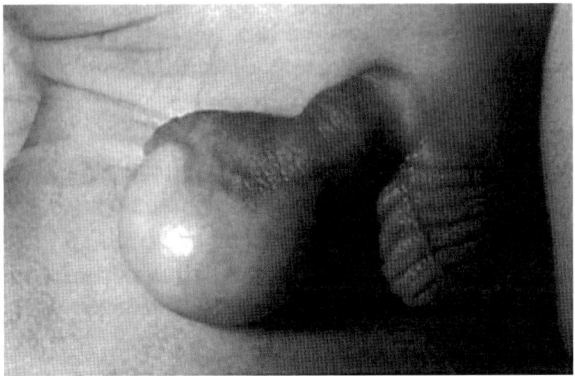

Fig. 7.14 Scaphoid megalourethra. Note how the penis bulges and elongates in this segment lacking corpus spongiosum. With permission from Glassberg KI, Horowitz M. Urethral valves and other anomalies of the male urethra, in Belman AB, King LR, Kramer SA {eds}: *Clinical Pediatric Urology*, ed 4. London, Martin Dunitz Ltd, 2002;pp:899; Chapt 28, Fig. 28.29. © Taylor and Francis [10]

The deformity is typically corrected by excising the redundant urethra and reconstructing it over an appropriately sized catheter. Excessive skin is also excised. The scaphoid megalourethra involves a defect of the corpus spongiosum along the ventral surface of the pendulous urethra. The corporal bodies are not affected. The penis may appear floppy and elongated when not voiding (Fig. 7.14). With voiding, the urethra bulges ventrally and becomes tense. It is not associated with hydronephrosis nor is a contributing cause to the large bladder or dilated upper tract in prune belly syndrome. Surgery involves degloving the penis to expose the baggy urethra. The excess width is excised and the urethra is subsequently closed. Excess penile skin is excised as well.

Urethral Atresia

Urethral atresia is a rare diagnosis and is fatal in the vast majority of cases. It is a congenital defect characterized by complete obstruction of the urethra. In the largest published series of six cases, Gonzalez and associates describe urethral atresia as caused by a membrane at the distal end of the prostatic urethra that leads to a hypoplastic distal urethra [142]. Long-term survival past the antenatal period is dependent on (1) a patent urachus or vesicocutaneous fistula which allows drainage of the bladder and protection of the kidneys, (2) in utero bladder perforation which leads to drainage of the bladder and fetal ascites, or (3) early diagnosis (i.e., imaging findings from fetal ultrasound or MRI) and prenatal intervention with vesicoamniotic shunt. Without one of these three conditions, urethral atresia is incompatible with life.

References

1. Atwell JD. Posterior urethral valves in the British Isles: a multicenter BAPS review. J Pediatr Surg. 1983;18:20–4.
2. King LR. Posterior urethra. In: Kelalis PP, King LR, Belman AB, editors. Urology. 2nd ed. Philadelphia, PA: WB Saunders; 1985. p. 527–58.
3. Casale A. Posterior urethral valves and other obstructions of the urethra. In: Gonzales ET, Bauer SB, editors. *Pediatric urology practice*. Philadelphia, PA: Lippincott, Williams, and Wilkins; 1999. p. 223–44.
4. Rajab A, Freeman NV, Patton M. The frequency of posterior urethral valves in Oman. Br J Urol. 1996;77:900–4.
5. Lloyd JC, Wiener JS, Gargollo PC, Inman BA, Ross SS, Routh JC. Contemporary epidemiological trends in complex congenital genitourinary anomalies. J Urol. 2013;190(4 suppl):1590–5.
6. Gunn TR, Mora JD, Pease P. Antenatal diagnosis of urinary tract abnormalities by ultrasonography after 28 weeks gestation: incidence and outcome. J Obstet Gynecol. 1995;172:479–86.
7. Young HH, Frontz WA, Baldwin JC. Congenital obstruction of the posterior urethra. J Urol. 1919;3:289–354.
8. Krishnan A, DeSouza A, Konijeti R, Baskin LS. The anatomy and embryology of posterior urethral valves. J Urol. 2006;175:1214–20.
9. Williams DI, Eckstein HB. Obstructive valves in the posterior urethra. J Urol. 1965;93:236–46.
10. Glassberg KI, Horowitz M. Urethral valves and other anomalies of the male urethra. In: Belman AB, King LR, Kramer SA, editors. Clinical pediatric urology. 4th ed. London: Martin Dunitz Ltd; 2002. p. 899.
11. Stephens FD. Congenital intrinsic lesions of the posterior urethra. In: Stephens FD, editor. Congenital malformations of the urinary tract. New York: Praeger; 1983. p. 95–125.
12. Dewan PA, Zappala PG, Ransley PG, Duffy PG. Endoscopic reappraisal of the morphology of congenital obstruction of the prostatic urethra. Br J Urol. 1992;70:439–44.
13. Dewan PA. Congential obstructing posterior urethral membrane (COPUM): further evidence for a common morphological diagnosis. Pediatr Surg Int. 1993;8:45–50.
14. Dewan PA, Keenan RJ, Morris LL, Le Quesne GW. Congenital urethral obstruction: Cobb's collar or prolapsed congenital obstruction posterior urethral membrane (COPUM). Br J Urol. 1994;73:91–5.
15. Weber S, Mir S, Schlingmann KP. Gene locus ambiguity in posterior urethral valves/prune-belly syndrome. Pediatr Nephrol. 2005;20:1036–42.
16. Livne PM, Delaune J, Gonzales ET. Genetic etiology of posterior urethral valves. J Urol. 1983;130:781–4.
17. Mahoney BS. Ultrasound evaluation of the fetal genitourinary system. In: Callen PW, editor. Ultrasonography in obstetrics and gynecology. 3rd ed. Philadelphia PA: WB Saunders; 1994. p. 400–10.
18. Kaefer M, Keating MA, Adams MC, Rink RC. Posterior urethra valves, pressure pop-offs and bladder function. J Urol. 1995;154:708–11.
19. Reinberg Y, de Castano I, Gonzales R. Influence of initial therapy on progression of renal failure and body growth in children with posterior urethral valves. J Urol. 1992;148:532–3.
20. El-Ghoniemi A, Desgrippes A, Lutton D. Outcome of posterior urethral valves: to what extent is it improved by prenatal diagnosis? J Urol. 1999;162:846–8.
21. Lome LG, Howat JM, Williams DI. The temporarily defunctionalized bladder in children. J Urol. 1972;107:46.
22. Glick PL, Harrison MR, Globus MS, Adzick NS, Filly RA, Callen PW, et al. Management of the fetus with hydronephrosis. II: prognostic criteria and selection for treatment. J Pediatr Surg. 1985;20:376–87.
23. Harrison MR. Fetal surgery. In fetal medicine (special issue). West J Med. 1993;159:341–9.

24. Harrison MR. Fetal surgical therapy. Lancet. 1994;343:897–902.
25. Estes JM, MacGilliuray TE, Hedrick MH, Adzick NS, Harrison MR. Fetoscopic surgery for the treatment of congenital anomalies. J Pediatr Surg. 1992;27:950–4.
26. Ruano R, Sananes N, Sangi-Haghpeykar H, Hernandez-Ruano S, Moog R, Becmeur F, et al. Fetal intervention for severe lower urinary tract obstruction: a multicenter case-control study comparing fetal cystoscopy with vesicoamniotic shunting. Ultrasound Obstet Gynecol. 2015;45:452–8.
27. Morris RK, Malin GL, Quinlan-Jones E, Hernandez-Ruano S, Moog R, Becmeur F, et al. Percutaneous vesicoamniotic shunting versus conservative management for fetal lower urinary tract obstruction (PLUTO): a randomized trial. Lancet. 2013;382:1496–506.
28. Glassberg KI. The valve bladder syndrome: 20 years later. J Urol. 2001;166:1406–14.
29. Casale A. Chapter 126: posterior urethral valves. In: Wein AJ, Kavoussi LR, Novick AC, et al., editors. Campbell-Walsh urology. 10th ed. Philadelphia, PA: Elsevier Saunders; 2012.
30. Sober I. Pelviouretorostomy-en-Y. J Urol. 1972;107:473–5.
31. Ghali AM, El Malki T, Sheir KZ, Ashmallah A, Mohsen T. Posterior urethral valves with persistent high serum creatinine: the value of percutaneous nephrostomy. J Urol. 2000;164:1340–4.
32. Parkhouse HF, Woodhouse CR. Long-term status of patients with posterior urethral valves. Urol Clin North Am. 1990;17:373–8.
33. Saran O, El-Ghoneimi A, Hafez A, et al. Surgical complications of posterior urethral valve ablation: 20 years experience. J Pediatr Surg. 2010;45:2222–6.
34. Babu R, Kumar R. Early outcome following diathermy versus cold knife ablation of posterior urethral valves. J Pediatr Urol. 2013;9:7–10.
35. Skoog SJ. Pediatric vesical diversion. In: Graham SD, Glenn JF, editors. Glenn's urologic surgery. 5th ed. Philadelphia, PA: Lippincott Williams & Wilkins; 1998. p. 871–8.
36. Burstein JD, Firlit CF. Complications of cutaneous ureterostomy and other cutaneous diversion. Urol Clin North Am. 1983;10:433–43.
37. Glassberg KI, Scheider M, Haller JO, Moel D, Waterhouse K. Observations on persistently dilated ureter after posterior urethral valve ablation. Urology. 1982;20:20–8.
38. Hendren WH. A new approach to infants with severe obstructive uropathy: early complete reconstruction. J Pediatr Surg. 1970;5:184–99.
39. Lal R, Bhatnagar V, Mitra DK. Upper-tract changes insipidus associated with posterior urethral valves. Pediatr Surg Int. 1998;13:396–9.
40. Tietjen DN, Gloor JM, Hussman DA. Proximal urinary diversion in the management of posterior urethral valves: is it necessary? J Urol. 1997;158:1008–10.
41. Glassberg KI, Schneider M, Waterhouse RK. Observations of the dilated ureter following posterior urethral valve ablation. Read at annual meeting of the American Urological Association, New York, 13 May 1979
42. Bauer SB, Dieppa RA, Libib KK, Retik AB. The bladder in boys with posterior urethral valves: a urodynamic assessment. J Urol. 1979;121:769–73.
43. Mitchell ME: Valve bladder syndrome. Read at the annual meeting of the north central section, American Urological Association, Hamilton, Bermuda, 1980
44. Peters CA, Bolkier M, Bauer SB, et al. The urodynamic consequences of posterior urethral valves. J Urol. 1990;144:122–6.
45. Donohoe JM, Weinstein RF, Combs AJ, Misseri R, Horowitz M, Schulsinger D, et al. When can persistent hydronephrosis in posterior urethral valve disease be considered residual stretching? J Urol. 2004;172:706–11.
46. Combs AJ, Van Batavia JP, Horowitz M, Glassberg KI. Short pelvic floor EMG lag time I: novel non-invasive approach to documenting the presence of detrusor over activity in children with LUTS. J Urol. 2013;189:2282–6.
47. Schaeffer W, Abrams P, Liao L, Mattiasson A, Pesce F, Spangberg A, et al. Good urodynamic practices: uroflowmetry, filling cystometry and pressure-flow studies. Neurourol Urodyn. 2002;21:261–74.
48. Drzewiecki BE, Bauer S. Urodynamic testing in children: indications, technique, interpretation and significance. J Urol. 2011;186:1190–7.

49. Kim YH, Horowitz M, Combs AJ, Nitti VW, Libretti D, Glassberg KI. Comparative urodynamic findings after valve ablation, vesicostomy or proximal diversion. J Urol. 1996;156:673–6.
50. McGuire EJ, Weiss RM. Secondary bladder neck obstruction in patients with urethral valves: treatment with phenoxybenzamine. Urology. 1975;5:756–8.
51. Weiss RM. Comments. In: Glassberg KI (ed) Persistent ureteral dilatation following posterior urethral valve ablation. Dialogues in Pediatric Urology. 1982;5:6
52. Combs AJ, Horowitz M, Glassberg KI. Secondary bladder neck obstruction in boys with a history of posterior urethral valves. Presented at annual meeting of American Urological Association, Chicago, 2009
53. Androulakakis P, Karramanolakis DK, Tssahouridis G, Stefanidis AA. Palaeodimos: myogenic decompensation in boys with a history of posterior urethral valves is caused by secondary bladder neck dysfunction. BJU Int. 2005;96:140–3.
54. Abraham MK, Rasheed A, Sudutsanan B, Puzhankara R, Kedari PM, Unnithan GR, et al. Role of alpha adrenergic blocker in the management of posterior urethral valves. Pediatr Surg Int. 2009;25:1113–5.
55. Kajbafzadeh AM, Payabvash S, Karimian G. The Effects of bladder neck incision on urodynamic abnormalities of children with posterior urethral valves. J Urol. 2007;178:21442–9.
56. Taskinen S, Heikkila J, Rintala R. Effects of posterior urethral valves on long term bladder and sexual function. Nat Rev Urol. 2012;9:699–706.
57. Holmdahl G, Sillen U, Bachelara M, et al. The changing urodynamic pattern in valve bladders during infancy. J Urol. 1995;153:463–7.
58. Holmdahl G, Sillen U, Hanson E, Hermansson G, Hjälmås K. Bladder dysfunction in boys with posterior urethral valves before and after puberty. J Urol. 1996;155:694–8.
59. De Gennaro M, Mosiello G, Capitunucci ML, Silveri M, Capozza N, Caione P. Early detection of bladder dysfunction following posterior urethral valves. Eur J Pediatr Surg. 1996;6:163–5.
60. Misseri R, Combs AJ, Horowitz M, Donohoe JM, Glassberg KI. Myogenic failure in posterior urethral valve disease: real or imagined. J Urol. 2002;168:1844–8.
61. Jaureguizar E, López Pereira P, Martínez Urrutia MJ, Bueno J, Espinosa L, Navarro M. The prognosis of patients with posterior urethral valves according to the initial treatment and their urodynamic behavior. Cir Pediatr. 1994;7(3):128–31.
62. Jaureguizar E, Lopez Pereira P, Martinez Urrutia M, Meseguer C, Navarro M. Does neonatal pyeloureterostomy worsen bladder function in children with posterior urethral valves? J Urol. 2000;164:1031–3.
63. Veenema RJ, Carpenter FG, Root WS. Residual urine, an important factor in the interpretation of cystometrogram, an experimental study. J Urol. 1952;68:237–43.
64. Nesbit RM. Transurethral resection. In: Campbell MF, Harrison JH, editors. Urology. 2nd ed. Philadelphia, PA: W. B. Saunders Co; 1963. p. 2612.
65. Schmaelzle JF, Cass AS, Hinman Jr F. Effect of disuse and restoration of function and vesical capacity. J Urol. 1969;101:700–5.
66. Tanagho EA. Congenitally obstructed bladders: fate after prolonged defunctionalization. J Urol. 1974;111:102–9.
67. Egami K, Smith ED. A study of the sequelae of posterior urethral valves. J Urol. 1982;127:84–7.
68. Khoury AE, Houle AM, Mclorie GA, Churchill RM. Cutaneous vesicostomy effect on bladder's eventual function. In: Hussman D, McConnel J, editors. Subject of controversy: bladder dysfunction. Dialogues in Pediatric Urology. 1990;13:4
69. Jayanthi VR, McLorie GA, Khoury AE, Churchill BM. The effect of temporary cutaneous diversion on ultimate bladder function. J Urol. 1995;154:889–92.
70. Duckett Jr JW. Are valve bladders congenital or iatrogenic? J Urol. 1997;79:271–5.
71. Podesta ML, Ruarte A, Gargiulo C, Medel R, Castera R. Urodynamic findings in boys with posterior urethral valves after treatment with primary valve ablation or vesicostomy and delayed ablation. J Urol. 2000;164:139–44.
72. Podesta M, Ruarte C, Gargiuli C, Castera R, Herrera M. Bladder function associated with posterior urethral valves after primary valve ablation or proximal urinary diversion in children and adolescents. J Urol. 2002;168:1830–5.

73. Keating MA. The noncompliant bladder: principles in pathogenesis and pathophysiology. Prog Urol. 1994;8:348–60.
74. Gosling JA, Gilpin SA, Dixon JS, Gilpin CJ. Decrease in autonomic innervations of human detrusor muscle in outflow obstruction. J Urol. 1986;136:501–4.
75. Speakman MJ, Brading AF, Gilpin CJ, Dixon JS, Gilpin SA, Gosling JA. Bladder outflow obstruction: a cause of denervation supersensitivity. J Urol. 1987;138:1461–6.
76. Hsu TH, Levin RM, Wein AJ, Haugaard N. Alterations of mitochondrial oxidative metabolism in rabbit urinary bladder after partial outlet obstruction. Mol Cell Biochem. 1994;141:21–6.
77. Wu C, Thiruchelvam N, Sui G, Woolf AS, Cuckow P, Fry CH. Ca2+ regulation in detrusor smooth muscle from ovine fetal bladder after in utero bladder outflow obstruction. J Urol. 2007;177:776–80.
78. Yamada S, Takeuchi C, Oyunzul L, Ito Y. Bladder angiotensin-II receptors: characterization and alteration in bladder outlet obstruction. Eur Urol. 2009;55:482–90.
79. Kim KM, Kogan BA, Massad CA, Huang YC. Collagen and elastin in the obstructed fetal bladder. J Urol. 1991;146:528–31.
80. Freedman AL, Qureshi F, Shapiro E. Smooth muscle development in the obstructed fetal bladder. Urology. 1997;49:104–7.
81. Kay R, Brereton RJ, Johnson JH. Urinary ascites in the newborn. Br J Urol. 1980;52:451–4.
82. Hoover DL, Duckett Jr JW. Posterior urethral valves, unilateral reflux and renal dysplasia: a syndrome. J Urol. 1982;128:994–7.
83. Greenfield SP, Hensle TW, Berdon WE, Geringer AM. Urinary extravasation in the newborn male with posterior urethral valves. J Pediatr Surg. 1982;17:751–6.
84. Greenfield SP, Hensle TW, Berdon WE, Wigger HJ. Unilateral vesicoureteral reflux and unilateral nonfunctioning kidney associated with posterior urethral valves—a syndrome? J Urol. 1983;130:733–8.
85. Rittenberg MH, Hulbert WC, Snyder 3rd HM, Duckett JW. Protective factors in posterior urethral valves. J Urol. 1988;140:993–6.
86. Bureau M, Bolduc S. Allantoic cysts and posterior urethral valves: a case report. Ultrasound Obstet Gynecol. 2011;38:116–8.
87. Patil KK, Wilcox DT, Samuel M, Duffy PG, Ransley PG. Management of urinary extravasation in 18 boys with posterior urethral valves. J Urol. 2003;169:1508–11.
88. Heikkila J, Taskinen S, Rintala R. Urinomas associated with posterior urethral valves. J Urol. 2008;180:1476–8.
89. Wells JM, Mukerji S, Chandran H, Parashar K, McCarthy L. Urinomas protect renal function in posterior urethral valves—a population based study. J Pediatr Surg. 2010;45:407–10.
90. Scott JES. Management of congenital posterior urethral valves. Br J Urol. 1985;57:71–7.
91. Cuckow PM, Dinneen MD, Risdon RA, Ransley PG, Duffy PG. Long-term renal function in the posterior urethral valves, unilateral reflux and renal dysplasia syndrome. J Urol. 1997;158:1004–7.
92. Johnston JH. Vesicoureteral reflux with urethral valves. Br J Urol. 1979;51:100–4.
93. Parkhouse HF, Barratt TM, Dillon MG, Duffy PG, Fay J, Ransley PG. Long-term outcomes of boys with posterior urethral valves. Br J Urol. 1988;62:59–62.
94. Hoag NA, MacNeily AE, Abdi H, Figueroa V, Afshar K. VURD syndrome—does it really preserve long-term renal function? J Urol. 2014;191:1523–6.
95. Narasimhan KL, Mahajan JK, Kaur B, Mittal BR, Bhattacharya A. The vesicoureteral reflux dysplasia syndrome in patients with posterior urethral valves. J Urol. 2005;174:1433–5.
96. Hubert WC, Rosenberg HK, Cartwright PC, Duckett JW, Snyder HM. The predictive value of ultrasonography in evaluation of infants with posterior urethral valves. J Urol. 1992;148:122–4.
97. Warshaw BI, Hymes LC, Trulock RS, Woodard JR. Prognostic features in infants with obstructive uropathy due to posterior urethral valves. J Urol. 1985;133:240–3.
98. Lyon RP, Marshall S, Baskin LS. Normal growth with renal insufficiency owing to posterior urethral valve of long-term diversion, a twenty year follow-up. Urol Int. 1992;48:125–9.

99. Denes ED, Barthold JS, Gonzales R. Early prognostic values of serum creatinine levels in children with posterior urethral valves. J Urol. 1996;157:1441–3.
100. Dineen M, Dhillon HK, Ward HC, Duffy PG, Ransley PG. Antenatal diagnosis of posterior urethral valves. Br J Urol. 1995;72:364–9.
101. Churchill BM, Krueger RP, Fleischer MH, Hardy BE. Complications of urethral valve surgery and their prevention. Urol Clin North Am. 1983;10:519–30.
102. Connor JP, Burbige KA. Long-term urinary continence and renal function in neonates with posterior urethral valves. J Urol. 1990;144:1209–11.
103. Smith GHH, Canning DA, Schulmam S, Snyder HM, Duckett JW. The long term outcome of posterior urethral valves treated with primary valve ablation and observation. J Urol. 1996;155:1730–4.
104. Johnston JH, Kulatilake AE. Posterior urethral valves: results and sequelae. In: Johnston JH, Sholtmeijer RJ, editors. Problems in pediatric urology. Amsterdam, The Netherlands: Excerpta Medica; 1972. p. 161–9.
105. Holmdahl G. Bladder dysfunction in boys with posterior urethral valves. Scand J Urol Nephrol. 1997;188:1–36.
106. Williams DI. Congenital valves of the posterior urethra. Br J Urol. 1954;26:623–7.
107. Koff SA, Mutabagani KH, Jayanthi VR. The valve bladder syndrome: pathophysiology and treatment with nocturnal bladder emptying. J Urol. 2002;167:291–7.
108. Hennus PM, van der Heijden GJ, Bosch JL, de Jong TP, de Kort LM. A systemic review on renal and bladder dysfunction after endoscopic treatment of infravesical obstruction in boys. Plos One. 2012;7(9):e44663.
109. Holmdahl G, Sillen U. Boys with posterior urethral valves: outcome concerning renal function, bladder function and paternity at ages 31 to 44 years. J Urol. 2005;174:1031–4.
110. Heikkila J, Holmberg C, Kyllonen L, Rintala R, Taskinen S. Long-term risk of end stage renal disease in patients with posterior urethral valves. J Urol. 2011;186:2392–6.
111. Ansari MS, Gulia A, Srivastava A, Kapoor R. Risk factors for progression to end-stage renal disease in children with posterior urethral valves. J Pediatr Urol. 2010;6:261–4.
112. Neild GH, Thomson G, Nitsch D, Woolfson RG, Connolly JO, Woodhouse CR. Renal outcome in adults with renal insufficiency and irregular asymmetric kidneys. BMC Nephrol. 2004;5:12.
113. Churchill BM, Sheldon CA, McLorie GA, Arbus GS. Factors influencing patient and graft survival in 300 cadaveric pediatric renal transplants. J Urol. 1988;140:1129–33.
114. Reinberg Y, Gonzalez R, Fryd D, Mauer SM. The outcome of renal transplantation in children with posterior urethral valves. J Urol. 1988;140:1491–3.
115. Groenewegen AA, Sukhai RN, Nauta J, Sholtmeyer RJ, Nijman RJM. Results of renal transplantation in boys treated for posterior urethral valves. J Urol. 1993;149:1517–20.
116. Rajagopalan PR, Hanevold CD, Orak JD, Cofer JB, Bromber JS, Baliga P, et al. Valve bladder does not affect the outcome of renal transplants in children with renal failure due to posterior urethral valves. Transplant Proc. 1994;26:115–6.
117. Salomon L, Fontaine E, Gagnadoux MF, Broyer M, Beurton D. Posterior urethral valves: long-term renal function consequences after transplantation. J Urol. 1997;157:992–5.
118. Indudara R, Joseph DB, Perez LM, Diethelm AG. Renal transplantation in children with posterior urethral valves revisited: a 10 year followup. J Urol. 1998;160:1201–3.
119. Kamal MM, El-Hefnawy AS, Soliman S, Shokeir AA, Ghoneim MA. Impact of posterior urethral valves on pediatric renal transplantation: a single-center comparative study of 297 cases. Pediatr Transplant. 2011;15:482–7.
120. Salomon L, Fontaine E, Guest G, Gagnadoux MF, Broyer M, Beurton D. Role of the bladder in delayed failure of kidney transplants in boys with posterior urethral valves. J Urol. 2000;163:1282–5.
121. Ross J, Kay R, Novick AC, Hayes JM. Long-term results of renal transplantation into the valve bladder. J Urol. 1994;151:1500–4.
122. Mochon M, Kaiser BA, Dunn S, Palmer J, Polinsky MS, Schulman SL, et al. Urinary tract infections in children with posterior urethral valves after kidney transplantation. J Urol. 1992;14:1874–6.

123. Mendizabal S, Zamora I, Serrano A, Sanahuja MJ, Roman E, Dominguez C, et al. Renal transplantation in children with posterior urethral valves. Pediatr Nephrol. 2006;21:566–71.
124. Routh JC, Yu RN, Kozinn SI, Nguyen HT, Borer JG. Urological complications and vesicoureteral reflux following pediatric kidney transplantation. J Urol. 2013;189:1071–6.
125. Schober JM, Dulabon LM, Gor RA, Woodhouse CR. Pyospermia in an adult cohort with persistent lower urinary tract symptoms and a history of ablated posterior urethral valve. J Pediatr Urol. 2010;6:614–8.
126. Puri A, Gaul KK, Kumar A, Bhatnagar V. Semen analysis in post-pubertal patients with posterior urethral valves: a pilot study. Pediatr Surg Int. 2002;18:140–1.
127. Lopez Pereira P, Miguel M, Martinez Urrutia MJ, Moreno JA, Marcus M, Lobata R, et al. Long-term bladder function, fertility and sexual function in patients with posterior urethral valves treated in infancy. J Pediatr Urol. 2013;9:38–41.
128. Taskinen S, Heikkila J, Santila P, Rintala R. Posterior urethral valves and adult sexual function. BJU Int. 2012;110:E392–6.
129. Palmer BF. Sexual dysfunction in uremia. J Am Soc Nephrol. 1999;10:1381–8.
130. Rushton HG, Parrott TS, Woodard JR, Walther M. The role of vesicostomy in the management of anterior urethral valves in neonates and infants. J Urol. 1987;138:107–9.
131. Currarino G, Stephens FD. An uncommon type of bulbar urethral stricture, sometimes familial, of unknown cause: congenital versus acquired. J Urol. 1981;126:658–62.
132. Passerini-Glazel G, Araguna F, Chiozza L, Artibani W, Rabinowitz R, Firlit CF. The P.A.D.U.A. (Progressive Augmentation by Dilating the Urethra Anterior) procedure for the treatment of severe urethral hypoplasia. J Urol. 1988;140:1247–9.
133. Effmann EL, Lebowitz RL, Colodny AH. Duplication of the urethra. Radiology. 1976;119:179–85.
134. Maizels M, Stephens ED, King LR, Firlit CF. Cowper's syringocele: a classification of dilatations of Cowper's gland duct-based upon clinical characteristics of 8 boys. J Urol. 1983;129:111–4.
135. Morgagni GB. Adversaria anatomica omnia. Padua: J Comipus; 1719. part I, article 10, p. 51.
136. Guerin A. In: Chameror C (ed). ElementsdeChurgurieoperatoire, Paris, 60: 749
137. Sommer JT, Stephens FD. Dorsal urethral diverticulum of the fossa navicularis: symptoms, diagnosis, and treatment. J Urol. 1980;124:94–7.
138. Bellinger MF, Purchi GS, Duckett JW, Cromie WJ. Lacuna magna: a hidden case of dysuria and bloody spotting in boys. J Pediatr Surg. 1983;18:163–6.
139. Seskin FE, Glassberg KI. Lacuna magnum in 6 boys with post-void bleeding and dysuria: alternative approach to treatment. J Urol. 1994;152:980–2.
140. Gleason PE, Kramer SA. Genitourinary polypsin children. Urology. 1994;144:106–9.
141. Kester RR, Mooppan UM, Ohm HK, Kim H. Congenital megalourethra. J Urol. 1990;143:1213–5.
142. Gonzalez R, DeFilippo R, Jednak R, Barthold JS. Urethral atresia: long-term outcome in 6 children who survived the neonatal period. J Urol. 2001;165:2241–4.

Chapter 8
Duplication Anomalies of the Kidney and Ureters

Orchid Djahangirian and Antoine Khoury

Abbreviations

IVP	Intravenous pyelogram
UP	Ureteropyelostomy
UTI	Urinary tract infection
UU	Ureteroureterostomy
VCUG	Voiding cystourethrogram
VUR	Vesicoureteral reflux

Embryology

An overview of the embryologic origins will aid in the understanding of the events leading to the formation of duplication anomalies. Both, the ureter and kidney begin their formation at around 4 weeks of gestation. The kidney originates from the intermediate mesoderm, which evolves through a few steps (pronephros, mesonephros) to finally involute and become the metanephros. The ureter, on the other hand, originates from the Wolffian duct. It branches off the latter as a ureteric bud, which contacts the condensating metanephric mesenchymal blastema (metanephros) at 5 weeks of gestation. This

O. Djahangirian, M.D.
Department of Urology, University of California, Irvine, CA, USA

Department of Urology, Children's Hospital of Orange County,
505 S Main St #100, Orange, CA 92868, USA

A. Khoury, M.D., F.R.C.S.C., F.A.A.P. (✉)
Department of Urology, University of California, Irvine, CA, USA

Children's Hospital of Orange County, Orange, CA, USA
e-mail: aekhoury@uci.edu

© Springer International Publishing Switzerland 2016
A.J. Barakat, H. Gil Rushton (eds.), *Congenital Anomalies of the Kidney and Urinary Tract*, DOI 10.1007/978-3-319-29219-9_8

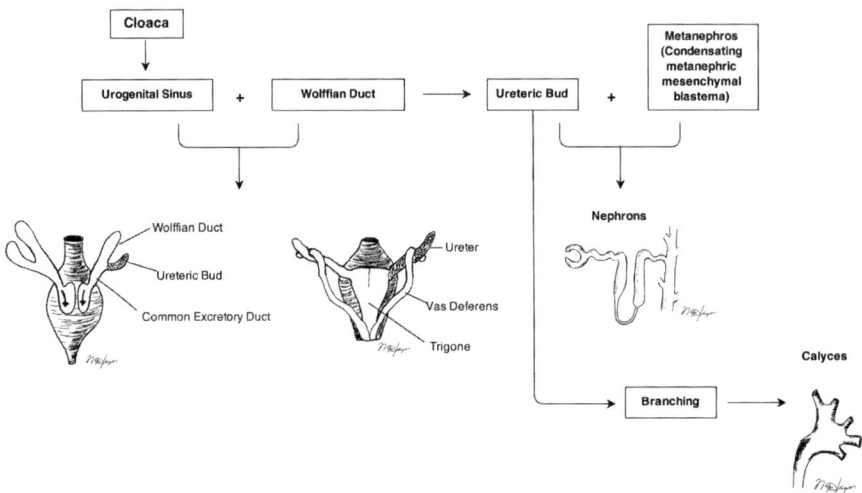

Fig. 8.1 Genitourinary embryology flowchart. © Nikta Khajeh with permission

mesenchymal–epithelial interaction is necessary for the creation of nephrons [1, 2], and the branching of the ureteric bud creates the renal pelvis, calyces and collecting ducts. Renal ascent and medial rotation is complete by week 8 of gestation.

Simultaneously, the primitive cloaca (endoderm) divides into the anorectal canal and the urogenital sinus. The two common excretory ducts, the Wolffian ducts caudal to the takeoff of the ureteric buds, fuse in the midline and join the urogenital sinus to form the primitive trigone. As the ureteric buds fuse with the primitive bladder, they migrate laterally and cephalad to become the future ureteral orifices, whereas the Wolffian duct orifices migrate caudally in the medial position to end at the utricle (as the future ejaculatory ducts). Figure 8.1 summarizes these events.

Pathogenesis

Ureteral anomalies arise from abnormal timing or location of the takeoff of the ureteric bud from the Wolffian duct. If the ureteric bud takes off from a more caudal position, or an earlier time, it will fuse with the primitive bladder earlier, and thus have more time to migrate to a more cranial and lateral position than normal. These ureteral orifices are often refluxing as the length of the submucosal trajectory of the ureter is shortened [3]. Alternatively, when the ureteric bud takes off at a more cranial position, or in a delayed fashion, it has less time to migrate once fused with the urogenital sinus, placing the ureteral orifice at a more caudal and medial position. These ureteral orifices are often obstructive or associated with ureteroceles or present as ectopia causing urinary incontinence.

If the collecting system is a complete duplicated system, two ureteric buds will have formed and branched off the Wolffian duct at two distinct sites. Following the Weigert–Meyer rule [1, 4], the caudal ureteric bud will drain the lower moiety of the kidney and

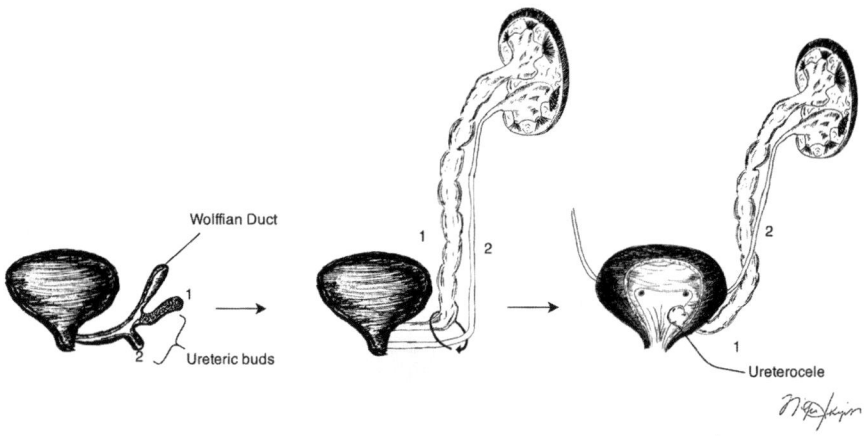

Fig. 8.2   Weigert–Meyer rule. © Nikta Khajeh with permission

fuse in the bladder as the most lateral and cephalad ureteral orifice (Fig. 8.2). On the other hand, the cranial ureteric bud connecting to the upper moiety of the kidney will end up as the most caudal ureteral orifice. The ectopic medial site of this ureteral orifice follows the path of Wolffian duct structures in males and remnants in females. Urinary incontinence does not ensue in males because the ureter inserts into structures proximal to the external urinary sphincter, such as the bladder neck or posterior urethra, the seminal vesicle, the utricle, the ejaculatory duct or the vas. However, in females, insertion can occur in the urethra, vestibule, vagina, cervix, uterus, or Gartner's duct (a Wolffian duct remnant), bypassing the external sphincter mechanism, thus leading to incontinence [3]. The difference between complete duplication (explained above) and incomplete duplication arises when a single ureteric bud branches early on or late, creating a bifidity, as depicted in Fig. 8.3.

A ureterocele is defined as a cystic dilatation of the distal ureter, as shown in Fig. 8.4. A few theories for the origins of ureteroceles exist. One of the more accepted theories states that they result from the persistence or incomplete dissolution of Chwalla's membrane, which transiently obstructs the ureteral orifice at its insertion in the urogenital sinus at 37 weeks of gestation [4]. Another theory explains the ballooning of the distal ureter by a deficiency or absence of muscle layers, shown in 90 % of the specimens in one study [5]. Renal dysplasia is hypothesized to occur in cases where the ureteric bud interacts with the metanephric blastema at more polar locations, as Mackie and Stephens demonstrated, whereas the middle of the blastema is most conductive to normal nephron formation [6].

Classification

Ureterocele nomenclature can be confusing. Many different classifications exist, without any consensus. It should be noted whether it is associated with a duplex or simple system. Stephens' nomenclature anatomically describes the anomaly (Table 8.1) [7]. The two types of ureteroceles are depicted in Figs. 8.5 and 8.6.

Fig. 8.3 Incomplete
ureteral duplication. ©
Nikta Khajeh with
permission

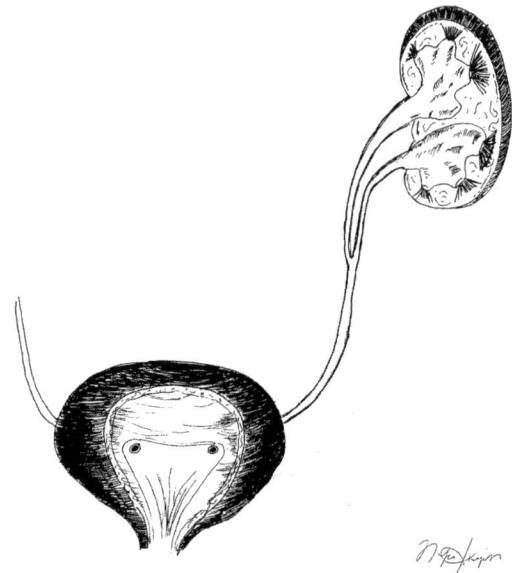

Table 8.1 Classification of ureteroceles in duplex systems

Ureterocele	Description
Intravesical stenotic	Inherently small obstructive ureteral orifice
Non-obstructed	Large, spherical ureteral orifice without obstruction
Extravesical sphincteric	Large or normal outside the bladder, proximal to external sphincter, with ureterocele extension into bladder neck and urethra. Sphincter and bladder neck's compression of the distal ureter results in obstruction
Sphincterostenotic	Comparable to sphincteric, with a stenotic ureteral orifice
Cecoureterocele	Large orifice in bladder with blind cecum extending into urethral submucosa. Urethral obstruction occurs when cecum fills with urine

A classification created by Churchill et al. for ectopic ureteroceles provides a functional grading system that aids in management decisions [8]. All patients presenting with this entity are divided into three functional grades:

Grade I: only one renal moiety is in jeopardy.
Grade II: the two ipsilateral renal moieties of a duplicated system are in jeopardy.
Grade III: all ipsilateral and contralateral renal moieties are in jeopardy.

In this classification, a renal unit is defined as being in jeopardy by the presence of moderate to severe hydronephrosis, grade 3 vesicoureteral reflux or higher, or the absence of visualization of the renal moiety on nuclear scintigraphy.

Fig. 8.4 Ureterocele.
© Nikta Khajeh with
permission

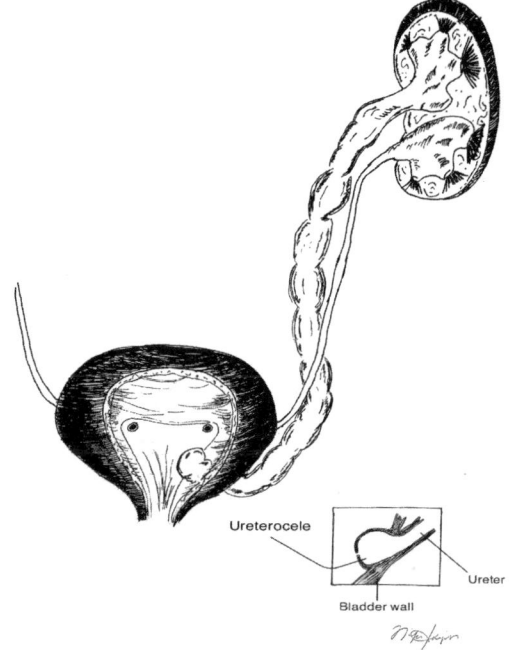

Fig. 8.5 Intravesical
ureterocele. © Nikta
Khajeh with permission

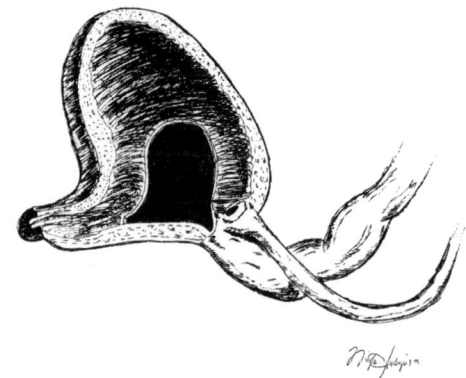

Epidemiology

Ureteral duplications are present in 0.75 % of the general population. Most commonly, they are not associated with an ectopic ureter or ureterocele, implying their benign nature [9, 10]. Approximately 1 % of them present with hydronephrosis and/or renal scarring [11]. Females are affected 2–4 times more commonly, but laterality is equal in frequency. Only 17–33 % of the cases are bilateral [12]. The anomaly is thought to be genetically transmitted with variable penetrance [13]. There is a 12 % incidence in the progeny of a person with this anomaly [14]. Incomplete duplication

Fig. 8.6 Extravesical
ureterocele. © Nikta
Khajeh with permission

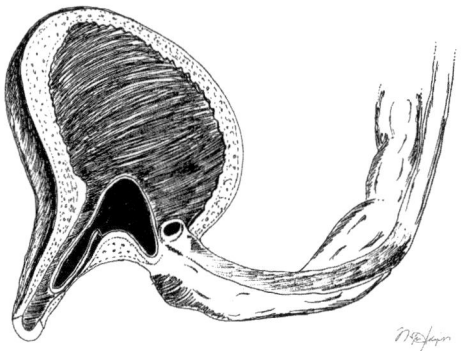

is reported to be three times more common than complete duplications [15, 16]. Ectopic ureters occur in the setting of complete duplication 70–80% of the time. Twenty percent of patients with ectopic ureters have bilateral involvement [17].

Ureteroceles occur four times more frequently in females than in males [18, 19]. Eighty percent of ureteroceles are associated with the upper moiety of a duplex system. The remainder is single system ureteroceles. Fifteen percent of cases are bilateral [20].

Clinical Presentation

Most patients with a duplication anomaly are now diagnosed prenatally with the wide use of antenatal ultrasonography, detecting those who would have remained asymptomatic. The minority associated with an ectopic ureter or ureterocele will be diagnosed with the presence of hydronephrosis or vesicoureteral reflux (VUR), and/ or urinary incontinence.

Four common complications of complete ureteral duplication occur: VUR, ectopic ureterocele, ectopic ureteral insertion, and ureteropelvic junction obstruction of the lower moiety [21, 22]. The most common problem with duplication anomalies is VUR in the lower moiety [23]. Afshar et al. demonstrated a significant difference between VUR in duplicated systems as compared to single systems. In that study spontaneous resolution of grade 3 and higher VUR was rare in patients with a duplicated system, with 69% undergoing surgical correction [24]. In newborn girls, an extravesical ureterocele may present with bladder outlet obstruction [15]. A completely prolapsed ureterocele can present as an introital mass. A more common presentation associated with duplicated system anomalies is the occurrence of urinary tract infection (UTI). Forty-five percent of patients were diagnosed in this manner before the age of 3 years [25]. In older children, undetected anomalies can present with abdominal pain or renal colic [26].

Ureteroceles and ectopic ureters in boys can present with irritative or obstructive voiding symptoms [15]. Ectopic ureter should be suspected in a boy presenting with bacterial epididymo-orchitis. In girls, one should suspect the existence of an ectopic ureter when presenting with the complaint of primary constant daytime and night-time enuresis. These girls will classically have a normal voluntary voiding pattern, accompanied by continuous urinary leakage with no dry interval [27–30]. Rarely, asymptomatic cases in childhood can go unnoticed until adulthood and the onset of sexual activity [15].

Evaluation

Ultrasonography

This modality diagnoses many anomalies in utero and should be repeated after birth to better define the anatomy, ideally past the first 48–72 h of life where dehydration can underestimate the degree of hydronephrosis [31]. Duplex kidneys and hydroureterone-phrosis are well imaged by this modality. Figure 8.7 shows an example of an ectopic dilated upper moiety ureter at the level of the bladder (Fig. 8.7a) and at the level of the kidney (Fig. 8.7b). The hydronephrosis can be caused by obstruction or VUR. The state of the parenchyma must also be assessed with hyperechoic changes signifying dyspla-sia. Imaging of the bladder should be included in this survey, as a ureterocele might be evident, as seen in Fig. 8.8, depending on the volume of the bladder at that time.

According to the American Academy of Pediatrics (AAP) and the Canadian Urological Association (CUA) guidelines, all children with the antenatal diagnosis of hydronephrosis should undergo a postnatal ultrasound. This should be carried out before discharge from the hospital, along with a serum creatinine level, if the hydro-nephrosis is bilateral or in a solitary kidney [32]. It is reasonable to keep neonates on prophylactic antibiotics until further evaluation, due to the risk of infection in a hydronephrotic system [33].

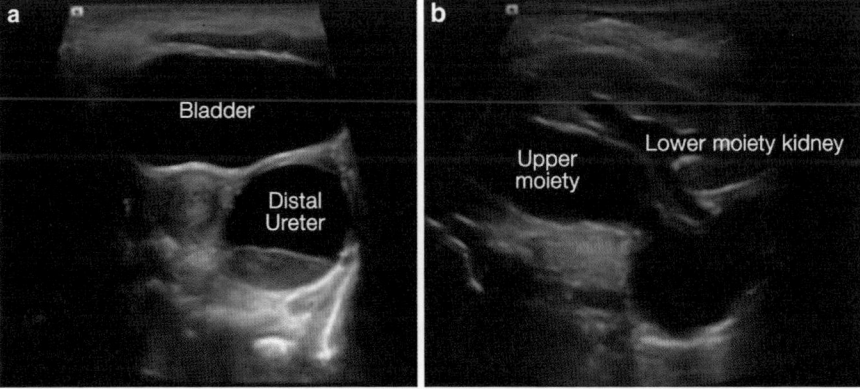

Fig. 8.7 Ectopic ureteral insertion of upper moiety. (**a**) Dilated ureter at bladder; (**b**) dilated ureter at kidney

Fig. 8.8 Intravesical ureterocele by ultrasonography

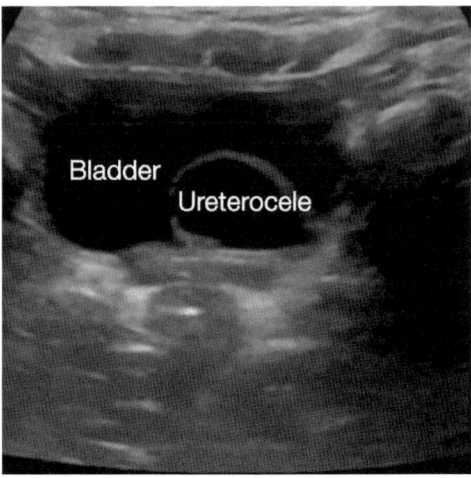

Table 8.2 Indications for VCUG

Hydroureter
Duplex kidney
Abnormal parenchymal echogenicity
Abnormal bladder
Bilateral hydronephrosis

Voiding Cystourethrogram (VCUG)

Indications to perform a voiding cystourethrogram (VCUG) within 1 month of life are listed by the AAP and CUA guidelines in Table 8.2. The presence of bilateral hydronephrosis and suspicion of bladder outlet obstruction warrant urgent evaluation before discharge from the hospital [32]. The CUA guidelines also recommend a VCUG in infants with persistent high-grade hydronephrosis. If this is negative, nuclear scintigraphy would be the next step. For low-grade hydronephrosis, VCUG is not necessary but should be performed if the child develops a UTI [32].

VCUG allows visualization of a ureterocele as a filling defect near the trigone (Fig. 8.9). To improve the yield of the study, early images during the filling phase should be taken and a feeding tube used to avoid distortion from the Foley catheter balloon. VUR can be present in the ipsilateral lower moiety as a result of the lateral displacement of the ureteral orifice and can be detected by performing a VCUG. If a large enough ureterocele is able to distort the trigone, contralateral VUR or obstruction can ensue [34]. The "drooping lily sign" is defined by the inferior and lateral displacement of the refluxing lower moiety by the upper moiety [6]. Figure 8.10 portrays this radiological appearance on a retrograde pyelogram.

Fig. 8.9 VCUG
demonstrating an
intravesical ureterocele
(filling defect at the base of
the bladder)

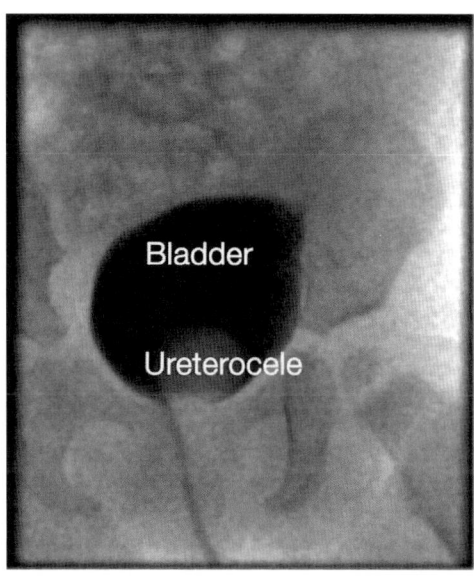

Fig. 8.10 "Drooping lily"
configuration of lower
moiety seen on retrograde
pyelogram

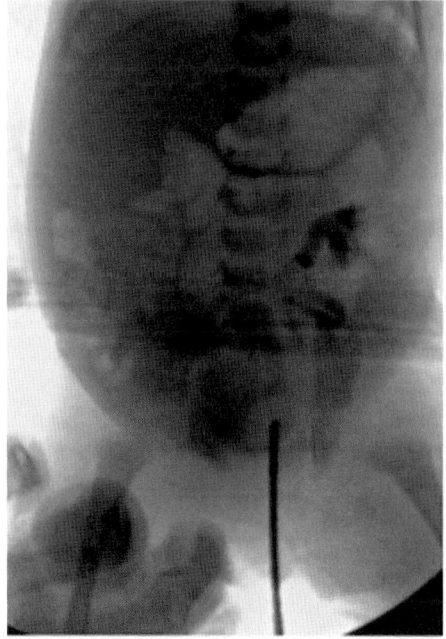

Intravenous Pyelogram (IVP)

Intravenous pyelogram (IVP), although rarely used in recent years, can aid in the diagnosis of ectopic ureters when all other tests have failed to define the anatomy. A functioning upper moiety leading to a ureterocele creates a contrast-filled "cobra head" at the ureterovesical junction [15].

Renal Scintigraphy

Renal scans play an important role in determining function in a renal parenchymal segment and assessing the presence of obstruction. Technetium 99 m (99mTc) labeled dimercaptosuccinic acid (DMSA) acts as a cortical tracer. It can help detect poorly functioning parenchyma in occult duplication anomalies, as well as cortical defects due to scarring [35–37]. 99mTc mercaptoacetyltriglycine (MAG3) and diethylene triamine pentoacetic acid (DTPA) efficaciously assess the presence of obstruction. However, they also provide a good evaluation of split renal function, such that a DMSA scan is not necessary if a MAG3 scan has already been performed to assess drainage [38, 39]. These tests should be delayed to 4–6 weeks of life, as the immature kidney renders the results uninterpretable. Other confounding factors include dehydration, infravesical obstruction, VUR [40], largely dilated renal pelvis and renal insufficiency.

Other Radiological Modalities

CT scanning can help define more complex anatomies. Magnetic resonance (MR) urography has become useful in cases where dysplastic renal moieties or ectopic ureters were unsuccessfully imaged by other means [41, 42]. Magnetic resonance urography has been shown to be comparable to MAG3 scans to depict obstruction and assess split renal function [43].

Cystoscopy

Cystocopy is therapeutic when puncture of a ureterocele is performed, However, it rarely changes the management when looking for ectopic ureteral orifices.. In more than half the cases, the orifice cannot be found. Intravenous indigo carmine, as it is excreted, can aid in localizing the ectopic ureter. If found, the orifice can be cannulated and a retrograde pyelogram performed [9]. Dye tests can also be used as less invasive tests in older girls whose source of continuous urinary incontinence is thought to be due to an ectopic ureter. The bladder is instilled with indigo carmine and a pad is examined to assess wetness and its color. Clear leakage indicates ectopia. Alternatively, a cotton swab or tampon can be inserted in the vagina after indigo carmine is administered intravenously or pyridium by mouth. Coloring of the swab indicates ectopic ureter insertion in the vagina [15].

Management

General Guidelines

While there are no black and white guidelines for management of infants and children with duplication anomalies that can be applicable to every patient, there are certain principles that are critical when deciding on the best course of management for any particular patient. The main goals of the treatment path chosen are the following:

1. Diminish the risk of urinary tract infections.
2. Preserve renal function when applicable and feasible without harm.
3. Correct obstructive or refluxing defects.
4. Promote urinary continence and bladder emptying.
5. Protect normal ipsilateral and contralateral renal units.

The following criteria are important to define before deciding on the type and timing of management:

1. Risk for urinary tract infections.
2. Patient age.
3. Degree of ureteral dilation and potential for urinary stasis.
4. Obstructed or refluxing system, or both.
5. Impact of a large ureterocele on ipsilateral or contralateral ureter or bladder outlet.
6. Renal parenchymal status and overall renal function.

We will address some of the common scenarios that the clinician encounters when managing patients with duplication anomalies.

Ectopic Ureter in Duplex System: Nonfunctioning Moiety

If the affected moiety is nonfunctioning and the associated ureter is massively dilated, partial nephrectomy is recommended, as urinary stasis or VUR may predispose the child to recurrent UTIs. This should be accomplished with a subtotal ureterectomy, by taking down the ureter as far distally as possible, usually to the pelvic brim where the ureters intertwine. The distal ureteral stump should be tied off in a refluxing system, and decompressed and left open in an obstructive system [11]. This is usually curative with only 10 % of patients requiring a second operation to complete a distal ureterectomy [44]. In those instances, to avoid ischemia to the normal ureter caused by separation of the common ureteral wall, the diseased ureter can be split open along its axis and its edges trimmed, leaving the blood supply intact. With ectopic ureters inserting near the sphincteric mechanism, care should be exercised and the dissection limited to avoid the risk of causing urinary incontinence.

Ectopic Ureter in Duplex System: Functioning Moiety

If the affected moiety is functioning, its ureter can be drained in the normal ipsilateral ureter or renal pelvis in an end-to-side fashion by a distal ureteroureterostomy (UU) or a proximal ureteropyelostomy (UP). The so-called "yo-yo effect," where urine cycles between the two ureters rather than drain in the bladder, has been shown to be clinically insignificant except when the obstructed ureter is massively dilated [45–48]. In general, we prefer not to perform a UU or UP in children who present following multiple UTIs as the obstructed system is frequently colonized and may result in further infections after surgery, requiring partial nephrectomy as a secondary procedure.

In cases where one or both ureters are refluxing, common sheath reimplantation may be the preferred option as long as the size disparity between the ureters is not significant [49]. This often requires tapering of the ureter for adequate submucosal tunnel creation. Ellsworth et al. demonstrated a 98 % success rate for common sheath reimplantation [12]. If the obstructed upper moiety ureter is massively dilated, a UU can be performed at the level of the pelvic brim, with reimplantation of the normal caliber lower moiety ureter and excision of the distal upper moiety ureter. Distal UU, with reimplantation of the recipient ureter only in the presence of VUR, was performed with a 94 % success rate [48].

Partial upper pole nephrectomy always remains an option, as the contribution of that moiety typically maximizes at 10–15 % of the total renal function and 43 % of renal moieties removed in this setting have abnormal histology [50, 51]. Figure 8.11 shows an algorithm for the management of the ectopic ureter.

Ureterocele in a Duplex System: Nonfunctioning Moiety

In cases where the affected moiety is nonfunctioning, a partial nephrectomy and subtotal ureterectomy is indicated. This alone will decompress the ureterocele and restore normal trigonal anatomy. However, persistent or new ipsilateral or contralateral reflux is possible. Studies have demonstrated reflux rates of 20 % after

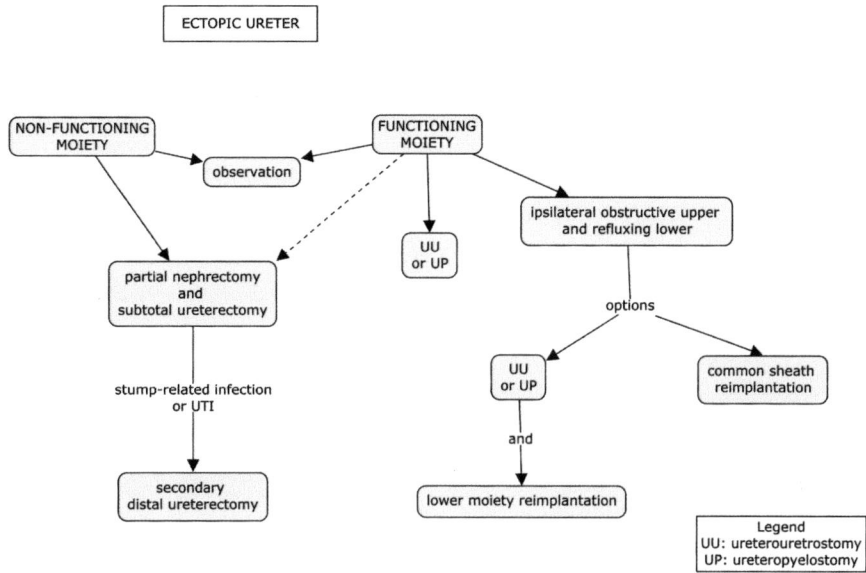

Fig. 8.11 Ectopic ureter management algorithm

partial nephrectomy alone [22, 52]. Scherz et al. reported 47 % of patients require a second bladder level surgery for UTI and VUR [53]. Thus, some believe in a combined primary repair including partial nephrectomy, ureterocelectomy and reimplantation. A 94 % success rate has been reported without the need for a second surgery [54, 55]. Husmann et al. clarified how to select patients who would most benefit from an initial combined surgery, sparing unnecessary morbidity in others. They reported a 62 % overall rate of reflux-correcting surgery in patients undergoing partial nephrectomy and subtotal ureterectomy alone in the context of a ureterocele and a nonfunctioning moiety. In patients with no initial VUR present, no one required a second surgery. If low-grade VUR was present in one ureter of the duplex system, 40 % required that second procedure. When low-grade VUR was present in more than one ureter or high-grade VUR was present, 96 % of patients required a second surgery. Indications for surgery were either the presence of VUR or UTIs [56]. The occurrence of ureterocele prolapse is another situation where bladder reconstruction is needed [57].

Cystoscopic unroofing of ureteroceles described by Tank remains an option for acute decompression in the septic patient when additional surgery is suspected [58]. Alternatively, endoscopic puncture of the ureterocele in the noninfected child can be a definitive procedure if it does not result in VUR [59].

Expectant management is being practiced in some with a nonfunctioning upper moiety and low-grade VUR in the lower moiety and no history of UTI. A cohort was kept on prophylactic antibiotics and 27 % have been successfully observed for 8 years [60]. Coplen and Austin describe successful expectant management with prophylactic antibiotics in children with a prenatal diagnosis of ureterocele associated with multicystic dysplasia of that renal moiety. Key features were absence of hydroureter, at most low-grade VUR in the ipsilateral renal moiety and absence of detectable function of the dysplastic moiety. All patients benefitted from involution of the affected moiety by 18 months of age, and none required surgical intervention over 36 months follow-up [61].

Ureterocele in Duplex System: Functioning Moiety

For a functioning moiety, one can decide to remove it if associated with a massively dilated ureter, as it maximally contributes only 10–15 % to the total renal function. This would preclude the morbidity from bladder surgery and risks to the good ureter.

Alternatively, in cases with no preoperative ipsilateral or contralateral reflux, UU or UP with subtotal ureterectomy can be performed. With the advent of injectable bulking agents such as Deflux, a noninvasive outpatient procedure can repair the secondary VUR in the non-ureterocele ureter, if the anatomy is favorable. However, when an upper moiety ureterocele is associated with lower moiety ipsilateral VUR, bladder reconstruction is more likely to be curative. DeFoor et al. applied Churchill's ectopic ureterocele classification to their patient series and concluded similarly that most grade I ectopic ureteroceles are successfully managed by an upper tract procedure, such as partial nephrectomy or UU/UP. Meanwhile, grade II–III ectopic ureteroceles more often require a second procedure, due to a persistent large ureterocele and UTI. A primary lower tract approach, such as ureterocelectomy and common sheath reimplantation, can circumvent the need for subsequent procedures. An upper tract approach successfully treated 85 % of grade I ectopic ureteroceles, whereas a lower tract approach was definitive in the treatment of 80 % of grade II and 100 % of grade III ureteroceles [62].

Obviously the child must be old enough with a bladder of adequate size to allow this reconstruction. To temporize, endoscopic puncture or incision can be performed while the infant is maintained on prophylactic antibiotics, decreasing the infection risk and ultimately simplifying the upcoming surgery. Increased interest in puncture has been peaked from Blyth et al. where he used a low transverse endoscopic incision to create a flap valve, with a 73 % definitive treatment rate. This approach is most successful in intravesical ureteroceles, with limited success in ectopic ones. Although an incision will successfully relieve obstruction, it only provides 50 % definitive treatment, as the incidence of iatrogenic VUR approaches 50 %. A 70 % reoperation rate has been estimated [59]. Husmann et al. showed that incision was more likely than partial nephrectomy to result in VUR into a non-refluxing system (64 % vs. 15 %) [63]. Cutaneous ureterostomy can also serve as a temporizing measure for the massively dilated upper moiety ureter until the bladder is amenable to reconstruction [64].

For small intravesical ureteroceles, a limited intravesical marsupialization has been described, instead of the more extensive enucleation. This approach is best suited for cases where the ureterocele has not caused a significant defect in the

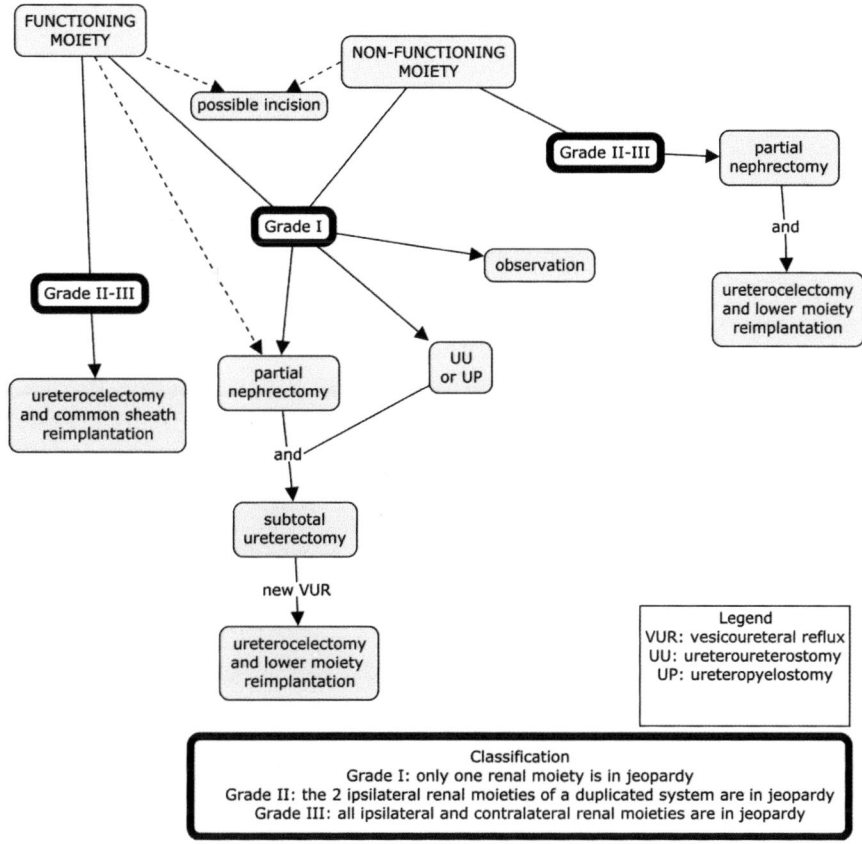

Fig. 8.12 Ureterocele management algorithm

bladder wall. In those situations a formal repair of the detrusor is required to avoid formation of a bladder diverticulum. An algorithm for the management of uretero-cele if is shown in Fig. 8.12.

Postoperative Follow-Up

An ultrasound to assess both kidneys and the bladder is routinely performed postop-eratively to image both the renal parenchyma and the presence or absence of hydro-nephrosis. VCUG will detect the persistence or appearance of VUR and depict the voiding pattern. Patients are often kept on prophylactic antibiotics until radiological evaluation is complete and satisfactory. It should be noted that 67% of patients complain of bladder dysfunction postoperatively following bladder reconstruction [65]. However, similar rates with upper tract surgery alone have been described [66], indicating a possible congenital component.

Conclusion

The presentation and management of duplication anomalies is obviously complex and best treated in centers with experienced clinicians who can best guide the family to the most ideal approach for their child's condition with the highest success rate, limited morbidity, and the lowest likelihood for requiring subsequent surgical intervention.

Acknowledgements We would like to acknowledge Nikta Khajeh, a UCI undergraduate student completing a urology clinical research internship, who has skillfully hand-drawn all the drawings included in this chapter. We are thankful for her contribution.

References

1. Spencer JR, Maizel M. Inhibition of protein glycosylation causes renal dysplasia in the chick embryo. J Urol. 1987;138:94.
2. Sariola H, Aufderheide E, Bernhardt H, Henke-Fahle S. Antibodies to cell surface ganglioside GD3 perturb inductive epithelial–mesenchymal interactions. Cell. 1988;54:235–45.
3. Hawthorne AB. The embryologicand clinical aspect of double ureter. JAMA. 1936;106:189.
4. Weigert C. Uebeteinige bil dunfehter der uretern. Virchows Arch. 1877;70:490–501.
5. Meyer R. Normal and abnormal development of the ureter in the human embryo: a mechanistic consideration. Anat Rec. 1946;96:355.
6. Fernbach SK, Feinstein KA, Spencer K, Lindstrom CA. Ureteral duplication and its complications. Radiographics. 1997;17:109–27.
7. Chwalla R. The process of formation of cystic dilation of the vesical end of the ureter and of diverticula at the ureteral ostium. Urol Cutan Ren. 1927;31:499–503.
8. Tokunaka S, Goth T, Koyanagi T, Tsuji I. The morphological study of ureterocele: a possible clue to its embryogenesis as evidenced by a locally arrested myogenesis. J Urol. 1981;126:726–9.
9. Mackie GG, Stephens FD. Duplex kidneys: a correlation of renal dysplasia with position of ureteral orifice. J Urol. 1975;114:274–80.
10. Stephens FD. Congenital malformations of the urinary tract. New York: Praeger; 1983. p. 320–2.
11. Churchill BM, Sheldon CA, McLorie GA. The ectopic ureterocele: a proposed classification based on renal unit jeopardy. J Pediatr Surg. 1992;27:497–500.
12. Ellsworth PI, Lim DJ, Walker RD, Stevens PS, Barraza MA, Mesrobian HG. Common sheath reimplantation yields excellent results in the treatment of vesicoureteral reflux in duplicated collecting systems. J Urol. 1996;155:1407–9.
13. Malek RS, Kelalis PP, Burke EC. Simple and ectopic ureterocele in infancy and childhood. Surg Gynecol Obstet. 1972;134:611–6.

14. Caldamone AA. Duplication anomalies of the upper urinary tract in infants and children. Urol Clin North Am. 1985;12:75–91.
15. Keating MA. Ureteral duplication anomalies: ectopic ureters and ureteroceles. In: Docimo SG, Canning DA, Khoury AE, editors. Clinical pediatric urology. 5th ed. 2007. Chap 40. p. 593–647.
16. Atwell JD, Cook PL, Howell CJ. Familial incidence of bifid and double ureters. Arch Dis Child. 1974;49:390–3.
17. Whitaker J, Danks DM. A study of the inheritance of duplication of the kidneys and ureters. J Urol. 1966;95:176–8.
18. Amitai M, Hertz M, Jonas P, Apter S, Heyman Z. Ectopic ureterocele in adults with a comparison of the anomaly in children. Urol Radiol. 1992;13:181–6.
19. Cronan JJ, Amis ES, Zeman RK, Dorfman GS. Obstruction of the upper-pole moiety in renal duplication in adults: CT evaluation. Radiology. 1986;161:17–21.
20. Ellerker AG. The extravesical ectopic ureter. Br J Surg. 1958;45:344–53.
21. Brock WA, Kaplan GW. Ectopic ureteroceles in children. J Urol. 1978;119:800–3.
22. Mandell J, Colodny A, Lebowitz RL, Bauer SB, Retik AB. Ureteroceles in infants and children. J Urol. 1980;123:921–6.
23. Uson AC, Lattimer JK, Melicow MM. Ureteroceles in infants and children: a report based on 44 cases. Pediatrics. 1961;27:971–83.
24. Barrett DM, Malek RS, Kelalis PP. Problems and solutions in surgical treatment of 100 consecutive ureteral duplications in children. J Urol. 1975;114:126–30.
25. Fernbach SK, Zawin JK, Lebowitz RL. Complete duplication of the ureter with ureteropelvic junction obstruction of the lower pole of the kidney: imaging findings. Am J Roentgenol. 1995;164:701–4.
26. Kaplan WE, Nasrallah P, King LR. Reflux in complete duplication in children. J Urol. 1978;120:220–2.
27. Afshar K, Papanikolaou F, Malek R, Bagli D, Pippi-Salle JL, Khoury A. Vesicoureteral reflux and complete ureteral duplication: conservative or surgical management? J Urol. 2005;173:1725–7.
28. Caldamone AA, Snyder 3rd HM, Duckett JW. Ureteroceles in children: follow-up of management with upper tract approach. J Urol. 1984;131:1130–2.
29. Finan BF, Mollitt DL, Golladay ES, Redman JF. Giant ectopic ureter presenting as abdominal mass in infant. Urology. 1987;30:246–7.
30. Williams DI. The ectopic ureter: diagnostic problems. Br J Urol. 1980;52:257–63.
31. Belarmino JM, Kogan BA. Management of neonatal hydronephrosis. Early Hum Dev. 2006;82:9–14.
32. Psooy K, Pike J. Investigation and management of antenatally detected hydronephrosis. Can Urol Assoc J. 2009;3:69–72.
33. Kaplan N, Elkin M. Bifid renal pelves and ureters. Radiographic and cinefluorographic observations. Br J Urol. 1968;40:235–44.
34. Senn S, Beasley SW, Ahmed S, et al. Renal function and vesicoureteral reflux in children with ureteroceles. J Pediatr Surg. 1992;27:192.
35. Bozorgi F, Connolly LP, Bauer SB, Neish AS, Tan PE, Schofield D, et al. Hypoplastic dysplastic kidney with a vaginal ectopic ureter identified by technetium-99 m-DMSA scintigraphy. J Nucl Med. 1998;39:113–5.
36. Pattaras JG, Rushton HG, Majd M. The role of 99mtechnetium dimercaptosuccinic acid renal scans in the evaluation of occult ectopic ureters in girls with paradoxical incontinence. J Urol. 1999;162:821–5.
37. Connolly LP, Connolly SA, Drubach LA, Zurakowski D, Ted Trevers S. Ectopic ureteroceles in infants with prenatal hydronephrosis: use of renal cortical scintigraphy. Clin Nucl Med. 2002;27:169–75.
38. Ritchie G, Wilkinson AG, Prescott RJ. Comparison of differential renal function using technetium-99 m MAG3 and technetium-99 m DMSA in a paediatric population. Pediatr Radiol. 2008;38:857–62.

39. Othman S, Al-Hawas A, Al-Maqtari R. Renal cortical imaging in children: 99mTc MAG3 versus 99mTc DMSA. Clin Nucl Med. 2012;37:351–5.
40. Wu F, Snow B, Taylor A. Potential pitfall of DMSA scintigraphy in patients with ureteral duplication. J Nucl Med. 1986;27:1154–6.
41. Matsuki M, Matsuo M, Kaji Y, Okada N. Ectopic ureter draining into seminal vesical cyst: usefulness of MRI. Radiat Med. 1998;16:309–11.
42. Gylys-Morin VM, Minevich E, Tackett LD, Reichard E, Wacksman J, Sheldon CA, et al. Magnetic resonance imaging of the dysplastic renal moiety and ectopic ureter. J Urol. 2000;164:2034–9.
43. Boss A, Martirosian P, Fuchs J, Obermayer F, Tsiflikas I, Schick F, et al. Dynamic MR urography in children with uropathic disease with a combined 2D and 3D acquisition protocol-comparison with MAG3 scintigraphy. Br J Radiol. 2014;87:20140426.
44. Plaire JC, Pope 4th JC, Kropp BP, Adams MC, Keating MA, Rink RC, et al. Management of ectopic ureters: experience with the upper tract approach. J Urol. 1997;158:1245–7.
45. Huisman TK, Kaplan GW, Brock WA, Packer MG. Ipsilateral ureteroureterostomy and pyelo-ureterostomy: a review of 15 years of experience with 25 patients. J Urol. 1987;138:1207–10.
46. Bochrath JM, Maizels M, Firlit CF. The use of ipsilateral ureteroureterostomy to treat vesico-ureteral reflux or obstruction in children with duplex ureters. J Urol. 1983;129:543–4.
47. Bieri M, Smith CK, Smith AY, Borden TA. Ipsilateral ureteroureterostomy for single ureteral reflux or obstruction in a duplicate system. J Urol. 1998;159:1016–8.
48. Lashley DB, McAleer IM, Kaplan GW. Ipsilateral uretero-ureterostomy for the treatment of vesicoureteral reflux or obstruction associated with complete ureteral duplication. J Urol. 2001;165:552–4.
49. el Ghoneimi A, Miranda J, Truong T, Monfort G. Ectopic ureter with complete ureteric duplication: conservative surgical management. J Pediatr Surg. 1996;31:467–72.
50. Smith FL, Ritchie EL, Maizels M, Zaontz MR, Hsueh W, Kaplan WE. Surgery for duplex kidneys with ectopic ureters: ipsilateral uretero-ureterostomy versus polar nephrectomy. J Urol. 1989;142:532–4.
51. Monfort G, Guys JM, Coquet M, Roth K, Louis C, Bocciardi A. Surgical management of duplex ureteroceles. J Pediatr Surg. 1992;27:634–8.
52. Mor Y, Goldwasser B, Ben-Chaim J, et al. Upper pole heminephrectomy for duplex systems in children: a modified technical approach. Br J Urol. 1994;73:584–5.
53. Scherz HC, Kaplan GW, Packer MG, Brock WA. Renal function and vesicoureteral reflux in children with ureteroceles. J Urol. 1989;142:538–43.
54. Decter RM, Sprunger JK, Holland RJ. Can a single individualized procedure predictably resolve all the problematic aspects of the pediatric ureterocele? J Urol. 2001;165:2308–10.
55. Beganovic A, Klijn AJ, Dik P, De Jong TP. Ectopic ureterocele: long-term results of open surgical therapy in 54 patients. J Urol. 2007;178:251–4.
56. Husmann DA, Ewalt DH, Glenski WJ, Bernier PA. Ureterocele associated with ureteral duplication and a nonfunctioning upper pole segment: management by partial nephroureterectomy alone. J Urol. 1995;154:723–6.
57. Gotoh T, Koyanagi T, Matsuno T. Surgical management of ureteroceles in children: strategy based on the classification of the ureteral hiatus and the eversion of ureteroceles. J Pediatr Surg. 1988;23:159–65.
58. Tank ES. Experience with endoscopic incisions and open unroofing of ureteroceles. J Urol. 1986;136:241–2.
59. Blyth B, Passerini-Glazel G, Camuffo C, Snyder HM. Endoscopic incision of ureteroceles: intravesical versus ectopic. J Urol. 1993;149:556–60.
60. Shankar KR, Vishwanath N, Rickwood AM. Outcome of patients with prenatally detected duplex system ureterocele; natural history of those managed expectantly. J Urol. 2001;165:1226–8.
61. Coplen DE, Austin PF. Outcome analysis of prenatally detected ureteroceles associated with multicystic dysplasia. J Urol. 2004;172:1637–9.
62. DeFoor W, Minevich E, Tackett L, Yasar U, Wacksman J, Sheldon C. Ectopic ureterocele: clinical application of classification based on renal unit jeopardy. J Urol. 2003;169:1092–4.

63. Husmann D, Strand B, Ewalt D, Clement M, Kramer S, Allen T. Management of ectopic ure-
    terocele associated with renal duplication: a comparison of partial nephrectomy and endo-
    scopic decompression. J Urol. 1999;162:1406–9.
64. Johnston JH. Urinary tract duplication in childhood. Arch Disease Child. 1960;180–9.
65. Abrahamsson K, Hansson E, Sillen U, Hermansson G, Hjalmas U. Bladder dysfunction: an
    integral part of the ectopic ureterocele complex. J Urol. 1998;160:1468–70.
66. Holmes NM, Coplen DE, Strand W, Husmann D, Baskin LS. Is bladder dysfunction and incon-
    tinence associated with ureteroceles congenital or acquired? J Urol. 2002;168:718–9.

Chapter 9
Congenital Anomalies of the Urinary Bladder

Patrick C. Cartwright

Abbreviations

CMMS   Congenital megacystis-megaureter syndrome
MMIHS Megacystis–microcolon–intestinal hypoperistalsis syndrome
UTI   Urinary tract infection
VCUG   Voiding cystourethrogram
VUR   Vesicoureteral reflux

Introduction

While congenital anomalies of the urinary tract are relatively common, the rate of those principally involving the bladder is low. This chapter will address anomalies of the bladder and associated problems with the urachus and proximal urethra. It does not cover bladder abnormalities or changes that develop secondary to bladder outlet or urethral obstruction.

Bladder anomalies can be identified by prenatal sonography but many are still discovered either at birth or due to later clinical concerns. This chapter reviews the basics of development of the bladder, urachus, and proximal urethra and the resultant disorders associated with maldevelopment. This includes a review of initial presentation, diagnosis, treatment options, potential complications, and clinical concerns as the child grows.

P.C. Cartwright, M.D. (✉)
Division of Urology, University of Utah, Primary Children's Hospital,
100 N. Mario Capecchi Dr. # 2200, Salt Lake City, UT 84113, USA
e-mail: patrick.cartwright@hsc.Utah.edu

© Springer International Publishing Switzerland 2016
A.J. Barakat, H. Gil Rushton (eds.), *Congenital Anomalies of the Kidney and Urinary Tract*, DOI 10.1007/978-3-319-29219-9_9

Development of the Bladder and Urachus

During the first few weeks of gestation, the cloaca develops on the ventral and caudal portion of the developing embryo. The cloacal membrane is a two-layered structure covering the cloacal channel on the surface of the developing fetus. The cloacal membrane serves as a central structure involved in understanding both bladder and cloacal exstrophy. Normally, the cloacal channel is partitioned in weeks 5-6 by descending growth of the urorectal septum, which fuses with lateral folds growing inward and separates the cloaca into the anterior urogenital sinus and the posterior anorectal canal. The cranial portion of the urogenital sinus connects with the allantois which extends into the umbilical cord. This superior portion of the urogenital sinus will eventually form the bladder and proximal urethra. The caudal portion of the urogenital sinus (below where the Wolffian duct enters) will form the phallic urethra in the male and distal vestibular structures in the female. Around midgestation the allantois begins to involute and elongate until it obliterates into a thick, fibrous cord referred to as the urachus or, anatomically, as the median umbilical ligament. It courses from the dome of the bladder to the base of the umbilicus.

Prenatal Sonography of the Bladder

Some anomalies of both bladder and urachal development may be noted prenatally. Urachal anomalies are detected as an abnormal fluid-filled structure noted somewhere between dome of bladder and base of umbilicus. Bladder anomalies largely fall into two categories prenatally: those causing persistent distention of the bladder and those leading to a poorly or non-visualized bladder. Causes of a persistently distended fetal bladder include a number of diagnoses secondary to bladder outlet obstruction. Included in this group would be posterior and anterior urethral valve, ureterocele at the bladder neck, urethral atresia, congenital urethral stenosis, and pelvic masses that compress the bladder neck and proximal urethra, such as sacrococcygeal teratoma and hydrocolpos. Those causes of a persistently dilated fetal bladder without bladder outlet obstruction include: prune belly syndrome, neurogenic bladder, megacystis–microcolon–intestinal hypoperistalsis syndrome (MMIHS) and megacystis–megaureter syndrome.

Megacystis–Megaureter Syndrome

Congenital megacystis–megaureter syndrome is noted in patients with very high volume vesicoureteral reflux (VUR) [1]. These patients will reflux such large volumes of urine into the upper tracts that even after voiding, the fetal bladder will promptly refill as urine recycles down from the capacious upper tracts. This leaves the prenatal sonographer to see a persistently dilated bladder on each spot check. There will also be associated dilated ureter and possibly mild-to-moderate hydronephrosis seen.

If patients with this problem are noted prenatally, they should be referred for a pediatric urologic evaluation shortly after birth. They should be placed on amoxicillin (20 mg/kg once daily) at birth with postnatal voiding cystourethrogram (VCUG) being diagnostic [2]. If not suspected prenatally, these patients will be normal at birth but prone to urinary tract infection. If ultrasound after UTI shows ureteral dilation or hydronephrosis, this should lead to VCUG for the purpose of finding patients with megacystis–megaureter syndrome and other patients with a high-grade VUR, both of who are at high risk for recurring UTI.

If diagnosed at birth, these patients can generally be kept infection free on anti-biotic prophylaxis generally using amoxicillin until 8 weeks of age and Septra suspension (0.25 ml/kg) after 6 weeks of age. At 6–9 months of age, bilateral ureteral reimplantation is the general course of management. If ureters are dilated above 1 cm distally, then tapering may be required for successful ureteral reimplantation. This generally lengthens the operative time and potentially, hospital stay slightly and these patients will require either internal or external ureteral stenting for a period of 10–21 days to allow healing of the tapered segment of the ureter.

These patients have normal bladder function and emptying once the reflux is corrected with successful reimplant surgery and they can be expected to develop normal continence and likely have a low risk for any progressive urologic issues.

Megacystis–Microcolon–Intestinal Hypoperistalsis Syndrome (MMIHS)

Another rare but devastating problem associated with prenatally detected persistent bladder distention is the megacystis–microcolon–intestinal hypoperistalsis syndrome (MMIHS). This is a rare disorder characterized by a grossly distended but non-obstructed bladder and profound hypoperistalsis of the bladder and portions of the gastrointestinal tract. It appears that a systemic smooth muscle myopathy underlies this disorder [3]. Patients with MMIHS are profoundly affected and most patients do not survive past the first year of life. Total parenteral nutrition is required for any even short-term survival and the urinary tract often requires intervention for drainage by means of intermittent catheterization or cutaneous vesicostomy. If not diagnosed antenatally, these infants quickly become apparent with extreme failure to thrive, inability to feed, or obvious distended bladder [4].

Non-distended or Non-visualized Fetal Bladder

Bladder Hypoplasia

The urinary bladder may be hypoplastic due to lack of filling and emptying with urine during fetal life. Conditions causing inadequate or no cyclic filling of the bladder during fetal life and, thus, predisposing to bladder hypoplasia include:

1. Urine bypassing the bladder, as will be found in ureteral ectopia with orifices located beyond the bladder neck.
2. Renal parenchymal disorders causing very low urine output.
3. Bladder outlet conditions causing incompetent bladder outlet such as epispadias and urogenital sinus.

All of these lead to incomplete bladder filling and cycling and hypoplasia of the bladder wall. Prenatally, this will lead to a poorly or non-visualized bladder. With surgical reconstruction, some hypoplastic bladders may be rehabilitated once they cycle urine, but most are persistently small and will require enterocystoplasty for continence [5].

Bladder Agenesis

The embryologic cause of true bladder agenesis is poorly understood. This rare anomaly is only compatible with life if the ureters enter and drain into müllerian structures in the female or into the anorectum in the male. Females tend to predominate among those cases noted. The distal urethra appears normal in these cases but urine drains from either vagina or rectum. Management would be with diversion of the ureters initially and then determined on an individual basis related to specific anatomy found.

Cloacal and Bladder Exstrophy—Prenatal Recognition

Both bladder and cloacal exstrophy result in an open and flattened bladder plate on the anterior abdominal wall with no retention of urine possible. Thus, prenatal ultrasound reveals no bladder-like structure in the pelvis but often irregular surface of the lower abdominal wall consistent with the exstrophied bladder plate. In addition, cloacal exstrophy will demonstrate prolapsing ileum within this plate creating a very distinct appearance on prenatal sonography [6].

Urachal Anomalies

The urachus represents the regressed and usually obliterated allantois. It extends in the midline from the bladder dome to the base of the umbilicus and is up to 10 cm in length and between 0.5 and 1 cm wide. It courses in a preperitoneal location with the posterior rectus and sheath on its anterior surface. It is flanked on each side by the obliterated umbilical arteries, also referred to as the medial umbilical ligaments. The common anatomic reference for urachus is also the median umbilical ligament.

Failure of the allantois to completely obliterate directly lends to a spectrum of abnormalities of the urachus including: patent urachus, urachal sinus, urachal cyst, and vesicourachal diverticulum (Fig. 9.1).

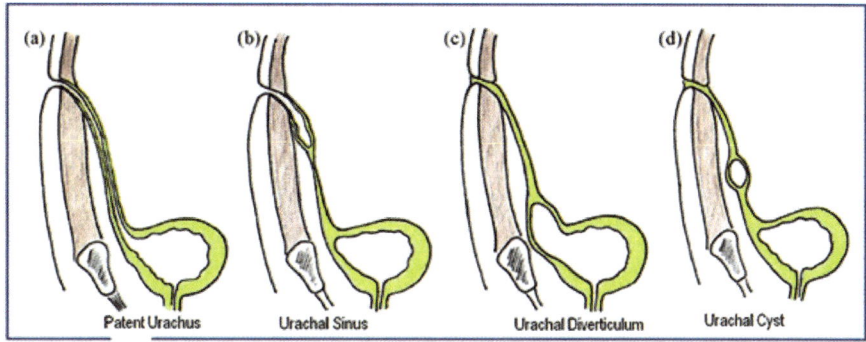

Fig. 9.1 Diagram of the variants of persistent urachus: (**a**) patent urachus, (**b**) urachal sinus, (**c**) vesicourachal diverticulum, (**d**) urachal cyst. With permission from Tazi F, Ahsaini M, Khalouk A, Mellas S, Stuurman-Wieringa RE, Elfassi MJ, Farih MH. Abscess of urachal remnants presenting with acute abdomen: a case series. J Med Case Rep 2012 30;6:226 [23]. Copyright ©2012 Tazi et al; licensee BioMed Central Ltd. This is an Open Access article distributed under the terms of the Creative Commons Attribution License (http://creativecommons.org/licenses/by/2.0), which permits unrestricted use, distribution, and reproduction in any medium, provided the original work is properly cited

Patent Urachus

Patent urachus represents a continuous internal lumen from the dome of the bladder to a location on the inferior edge of the umbilicus. This is rarely detected prenatally but becomes apparent in the infant due to persistent drainage at the umbilicus. There is some relationship between severe urethral obstruction and maintained patency of the urachus, but the majority of patients with posterior urethral valve and other outlet obstructions do not have associated urachal patency.

When persistent or intermittent umbilical drainage is noted early in infancy, patent urachus is on the differential diagnosis list along with omphalitis, urachal sinus, patent omphalomesenteric (vitelline) duct and granuloma. Umbilical granuloma occurs after the umbilical stump becomes disconnected and is characterized by a small, reddish lump of granulation within the base of the umbilicus causing intermittent bleeding or discharge. This can be topically treated with silver nitrate and generally resolves. Persistent omphalomesenteric duct is a result of failure of Meckel's diverticulum to disconnect from the base of the umbilicus during fetal development. Small bowel contents may be noted within the umbilicus along with severe skin irritation due to the alkaline nature of this fluid. Omphalitis can be life-threatening and is to be suspected with a swollen, infected and weeping umbilical stump associated with surrounding erythema. Patent urachus generally is characterized by slightly irritated umbilicus with watery drainage and sometimes persistence of the umbilical stump or failure to detach. Finally, urachal sinus is characterized most commonly by small volume, intermittent mucous drainage.

If patent urachus is suspected based upon persistent fluid drainage, then diagnosis should first be pursued by analyzing any collectible fluid for creatinine.

Fluid creatinine concentration higher than what would be expected in this serum is diagnostic for patency. Also, if inspection of the base of the umbilicus reveals an inferior pit or channel, then a small feeding tube may be placed and a contrast study via the tube may prove helpful diagnostically. In many cases, this cannot be achieved and ultrasound with specific emphasis from the dome of the bladder to the umbilicus is the most helpful first diagnostic step. A fluid-filled urachus is a diagnostic sonographic finding (Fig. 9.2). Rarely, VCUG may be needed if other modalities fail to demonstrate findings consistent with the clinical picture.

If patent urachus is suspected or diagnosed in early infancy, the option exists for early surgical excision or in asymptomatic patients, continued observation with hopes for spontaneous resolution in the first 3–6 months of life [7]. Some data suggests up 50 % of observed patients will resolve the various urachal abnormalities and avoid intervention. Repair of true patent urachus involves a small infraumbilical incision that can often be curvilinear and hidden on the inferior edge of the umbilicus. The urachus

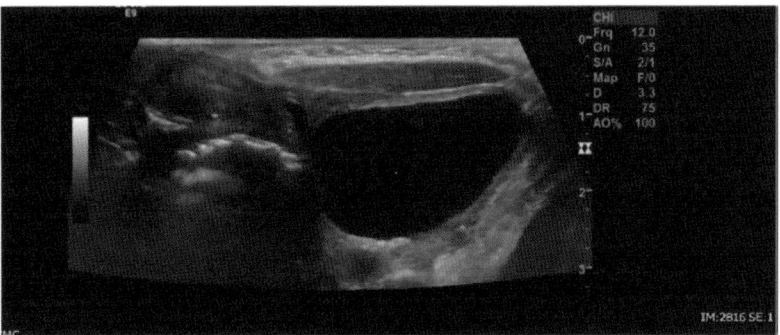

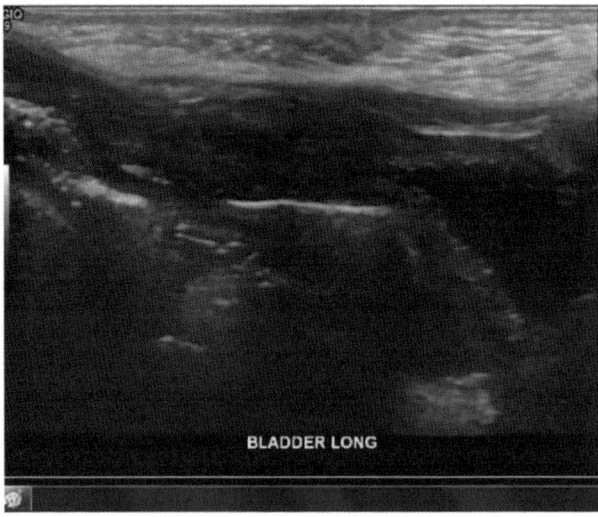

Fig. 9.2 Ultrasound of the bladder showing a fluid filled channel heading superiorly in the midline, indicating patent urachus

should be excised from the internal base of the umbilicus to the dome of bladder with simple repair of the dome using absorbable sutures. If the problem does not present until the patient is older, then laparoscopic excision is also a reasonable option.

Urachal Sinus

Urachal sinus represents patency of only a variable length of the urachus beginning at the base of the umbilicus and stopping somewhere along the course of the urachus toward the bladder. This results in intermittent umbilical discharge of epithelial debris, mucus or infected fluid. In some patients, this will be daily discharge and others will have discharge only every few days or weeks. At times, the urachal sinus may become infected and require oral antibiotic therapy. Involved organisms are most commonly staphylococcus aureus and various gram-negative organisms. Augmentin is a commonly chosen oral antibiotic based on this microbial spectrum.

Persistent concern of intermittent umbilical drainage warrants sonographic evaluation of the space between umbilicus and bladder. If a urachal remnant is suspected sonographically, then excision is required with an incision similar to that used for excising patent urachus. As with all surgery for umbilical remnants, the surgeon must take care dissecting the base of the umbilicus not to misidentify an omphalomesenteric duct and unknowingly detach this. Surgically, the entire urachus should be excised to avoid any persistent discharge.

Urachal cyst represents a patency in the midportion of the urachus with obliteration of the lumen at each end. This results in a cyst of variable size, which can range in position from near the bladder towards closer to the umbilicus. Urachal cyst may present as a palpable mass if large or as an abscess if it becomes infected [8]. Infected urachal cyst often requires initial drainage either percutaneously or open with appropriate antibiotics until the infection is resolved and later staged excision of the urachal cyst to prevent recurrence. It should be noted that low-grade inflammation of the urachus associated with either urachal sinus or urachal cyst may cause pain with voiding in a suprapubic or periumbilical area due to tension on the inflamed urachal remnant. Ultrasound is warranted in patients with this specific symptom even with lack of any concerning physical examination finding. Urachal excision may prove warranted.

Vesicourachal Diverticulum

In this situation, the urachus obliterates all but its most inferior portion, which appears as a diverticulum off of the dome of the bladder. This is generally asymptomatic and often only found incidentally when imaging is performed for other purposes. The diverticulum tends to be wide-mouthed and due to its superior location drains easily and does not predispose to infection or other concerns. Of note, patients with prune belly syndrome commonly have a vesicourachal remnant noted. Intervention is not generally required.

Bladder Diverticulum

Bladder diverticula may have three different etiologies:

1. Secondary due to bladder outlet obstruction or high intravesical pressures.
2. Iatrogenic after bladder surgery.
3. Congenital defects.

Bladder diverticulum is characterized by outpouching of bladder mucosa between defects in the detrusor. Bladder diverticula will vary in terms of size of the mouth of diverticulum, with small-mouthed diverticuli generally being more concerning as they may not drain easily with bladder emptying. The overall instance of bladder diverticuli in children is low.

The most common diverticulum noted is a paraureteral (Hutch) diverticulum [9]. A Hutch diverticulum may be primary, which is the result of incomplete muscular support around the entry point of the ureter into the bladder. This parameatal area will then result in mucosa bulging outward just around the ureteral orifice (Fig. 9.3). This will be seen incidentally on ultrasound or VCUG and often has no clinical significance. A secondary paraureteral diverticulum will occur due to a predisposition to weak muscular support in this area which

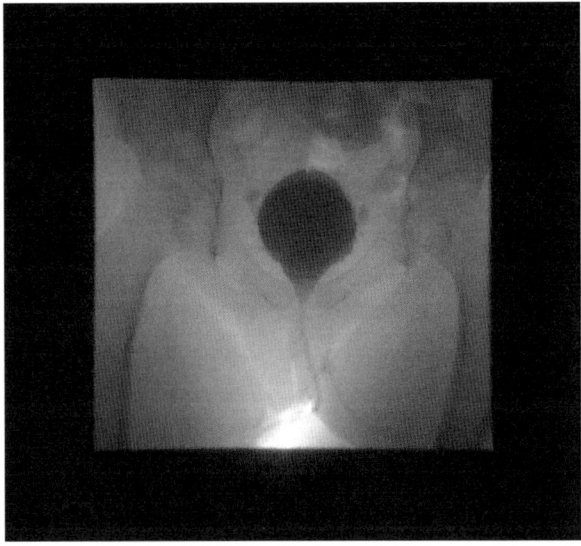

Fig. 9.3 VCUG showing modest paraureteral (Hutch) diverticulae of the bladder

is then accentuated by increased intravesical pressures from either bladder outlet obstruction or dysfunctional voiding and the resultant high intravesical pressures.

Most paraureteral diverticuli are small, asymptomatic and require no intervention. On occasion, they will become large and can be seen to empty poorly with voiding. This predisposes to UTI based on urinary stasis and in such cases excision of the diverticulum with reimplantation of the juxtaposed ureter will be required.

There are primary bladder diverticuli which may arise at other locations in the bladder and are often secondary to congenital connective tissue diseases such as Ehlers–Danlos, Williams syndrome, or Menkes syndrome. These diverticuli may be multiple and impressive in size in individual patients. They may be resected if symptomatic with UTI or urinary retention but these patients are prone to impaired healing and wound complications. Undertaking resection of multiple bladder diverticuli in such patients should be pursued with great caution.

Bladder Duplication

Duplication of the bladder and urethra is rare and can be seen in partial or complete forms. The duplication may occur in either the coronal or sagittal plane. Of all of the variants of bladder duplication, the most common seems to be complete duplication in the sagittal plane with duplication of each urethra. In this case, there is one ureter entering each bladder and a separate bladder neck and urethra involved. The majority of these patients will be diagnosed as newborns, as they have duplicate genital anatomy [10]. It should be noted that around 50 % of these patients will also have duplicate lower GI tract. The most likely embryologic explanation for this is partial twinning of the tail portion of the embryo.

Patients with partial bladder duplication may have a prominent septum either coronally or sagittally within the bladder but the two chambers will communicate at some point. There is great variation in potential anatomic structure of the urethra with some having duplex bladder neck but a fused common distal urethra and others having a single bladder neck at the base of the duplicated chambers.

Patients with complete duplication are often diagnosed in infancy due to the external abnormalities of the genitalia. Ultrasound and VCUG will be required at a minimum and often fully sorting out their anatomy requires endoscopic inspection. Surgical management will be highly individualized based on the anatomy noted.

Patients with partial bladder and urethral duplication may not present until later in life with a UTI, incontinence or other voiding issues. Standard evaluation for UTI will often show abnormalities by ultrasound or VCUG, which will lead to further evaluation with endoscopy and urodynamic studies to determine best management. In partial duplication, often the septum between the two chambers may be excised and a single bladder created surgically.

In all of these circumstances, the initial emphasis will be on relieving any obstruction and preserving optimal renal function with secondary consideration for achieving continence and reconstructing genitalia cosmetically. Complete evaluation of each patient and a decision on individualized care is appropriate, as there are many variations within this diagnosis.

Exstrophy and Epispadias

The congenital anomalies associated with exstrophy, referred to collectively as the exstrophy–epispadias complex are considered related by embryology and some of their anatomic features. Included within this spectrum are:

1. Epispadias: the urethra is partially or completely open on the dorsal surface of the penis (Fig. 9.4).
2. Bladder exstrophy: the bladder is an open plate and the urethra is open as complete epispadias (Figs. 9.5 and 9.6).
3. Cloacal exstrophy: the ileocecal segment of the bowel and bladder are exstrophied together (Fig. 9.7).
4. Exstrophy variants involving alternative or partial manifestations of the classic phenotypes.

Fig. 9.4 Penopubic epispadias. This is the most common form of epispadias and is associated with maldevelopment of the bladder neck and associated sphincteric musculature. Patients with this anomaly will almost uniformly have urinary incontinence and require bladder neck reconstruction as part of their eventual management

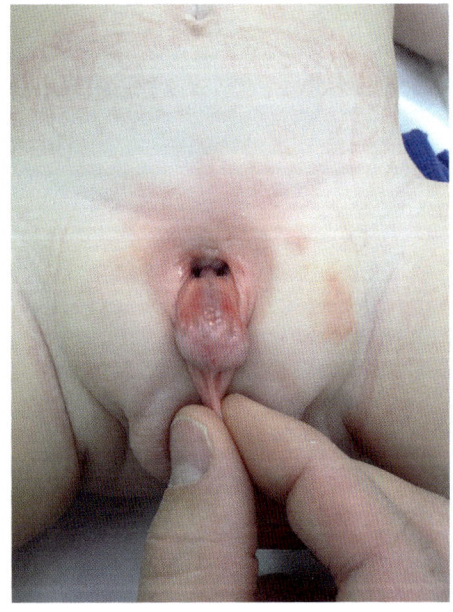

Fig. 9.5 Classic bladder exstrophy—male. The bladder plate is bulging outward and the open epispadiac urethra and open glans groove is visible on the dorsum of the penis. On the bladder plate, the ureteral orifices may be seen directly upon close inspection

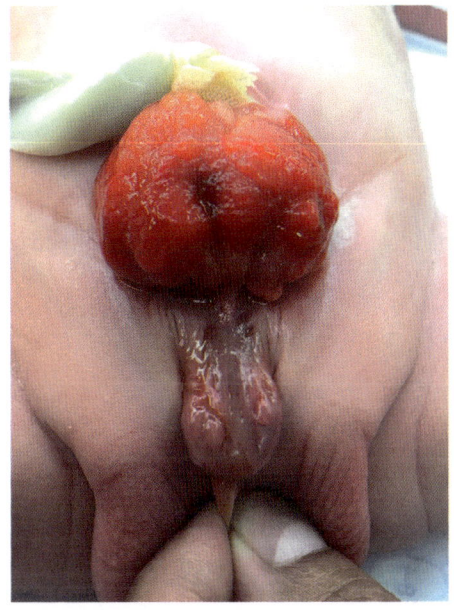

Fig. 9.6 Classic bladder exstrophy—female. Note the separation of the two bodies of the clitoris and open urethral plate between them. At time of bladder closure, the urethra is tubularized and the clitoral bodies may be joined in the midline just anterior to the urethra

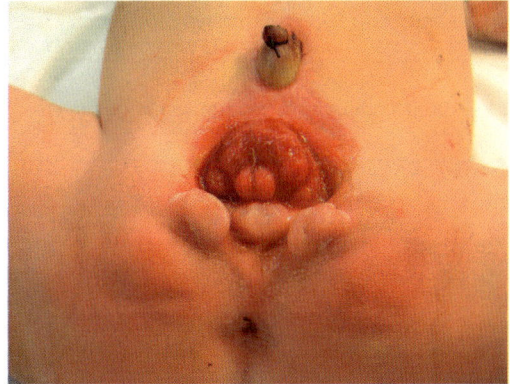

Classic Bladder Exstrophy

Bladder exstrophy occurs in around 1/30,000 live births and has preponderance in males with a ratio of 2.3–6:1. The risk of subsequent siblings being affected is roughly 1 % and the progeny risk from a parent with bladder exstrophy is 1.4 %.

Antenatal Findings

Sonographic findings during pregnancy that may lead to a high suspicion for bladder exstrophy include: non-visualization of the bladder, lower abdominal wall defect and irregularity, anteriorly placed scrotum, small phallus, and low-lying

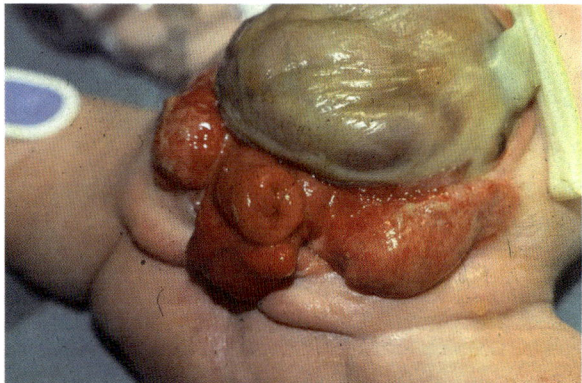

Fig. 9.7 Cloacal exstrophy—female. The bladder is in two "hemibladders" separated by an exstrophied portion of the cecum. The open cecum allows the terminal ileum to prolapse outward giving the typical "elephant trunk" appearance. There is almost always an associated omphalocele superiorly and the halves of the clitoris are separated by a large distance as they follow the pubic rami

umbilicus. A rapid screening sonography will often not recognize these findings and exstrophy is still most commonly diagnosed at the time of delivery. If exstrophy is suspected from sonography, fetal MRI can be quite accurate at confirming the associated anatomy and diagnosis [6].

Basic Anatomic Findings

The lower abdomen of a child born with bladder exstrophy will demonstrate an open bladder plate and epispadiac urethra. If male, the epispadiac urethra will be completely open from the glans back to the bladder neck. The verumontanum of the prostatic urethra and the ureteral orifices are visible directly from the surface. Bladder mucosa will often be hyperplastic with polypoid surface irregularities. In females, the epispadiac urethral plate will be associated with separation of the clitoral halves.

In association with the obvious bladder, urethral, and genital anomalies, exstrophy patients will also have a low-lying umbilicus attached to the superior edge of the exstrophic bladder plate. If a gloved finger is placed on the bladder plate and pushed gently in a posterior direction, the bladder will invert as there is a large fascial defect. This allows the examiner to easily feel the edges of the defect and judge its extent. The defect results from both inferior rectus fascia and muscles being located in an abnormally lateral fashion position as they extend inferiorly and insert into the widely separated halves of the pubis. There is no symphysis pubis but rather a wide and dense intersymphyseal band stretching transversely better the halves.

The scrotum in boys is often in an anteriorly located position, but both testes are generally descended. Hernia is a commonly associated finding (80 %) and should be repaired at the time of initial exstrophy closure. There is often a transverse area of non-rugated skin found between the penis and scrotum in boys with exstrophy, giving the appearance of slight separation of ventral penis from the scrotum itself. In girls, the entire vaginal canal and vestibule is anteriorly displaced with a large perineal body noted between anus and posterior forchette. VUR is commonly found once the exstrophic bladder is repaired but generally, the kidneys are healthy without hydronephrosis or other upper tract anomalies.

The exstrophied bladder may vary greatly in size and elasticity between patients. The smallest bladder plates create a clinical challenge in terms of posing a higher risk of complications at the time of early closure, in addition to more issues with poor bladder capacity increase over time. Studies of bladder wall composition and neural innervation in exstrophy have suggested some risk of both inelasticity due to high collagen–muscle ratio and altered innervation, which may affect contractility. As well, the muscular sphincters of the bladder neck are incompletely developed making complete, dribbling incontinence the norm after initial closure.

Other Defects Associated with Bladder Exstrophy

All patients with exstrophy have skeletal abnormalities [11]. Principal among these is diastasis of the symphysis pubis and external rotation of the anterior pelvis. These rotational deformities of the pelvis result in a short penile shaft noted in many males, as the corpora attach proximally to the inferior pubis ramus and follow the pubes as they rotate laterally, thus decreasing the length of corpora available to contribute to penile length. Substantial research has been done assessing angles of the pelvic bony malformation and its implications for repair and musculoskeletal function. These patients have a gait that shows some outward rotation at the hip but seems to cause little disability or athletic limitation. There may be a predisposition to osteoarthritis with aging.

Abdominal wall defects are also found in all patients with bladder exstrophy. The superior end of the triangular shaped musculofascial defect is the umbilicus with the bases of the triangle being the medial edge of the separated pubis on each side. These defects are closed at the time of early repair, but the pubes always drift apart again to some degree. Even with this, scarring of the fascia and midline repair keep the abdominal wall competent. As well, these patients will often lack a definitive umbilicus as they grow, since the malpositioned umbilical stump must be resected as part of the initial bladder closure.

The anus is generally displaced in an anterior location but has an intact and functioning sphincter mechanism able to achieve normal bowel continence over time. Untreated exstrophy patients are prone to rectal prolapse but after successful exstrophy closure this is rare to see. Rectal prolapse after closure suggests bladder outlet obstruction which must be evaluated carefully.

The male with bladder exstrophy demonstrates penile length around 50 % shorter than a mean for age. There is commonly dorsal chordee involved but the width of the corpora themselves is close to normal. The base of the corpora attaches to the inferior rami of the separated pubes, and this results in the shortness noted. Neural innervation is normal and the neurovascular bundles are typically located laterally on the corpora instead of the usually more dorsal position [12]. In young men born with exstrophy, the prostate appears to develop appropriately over time, although it has a predominantly posterior location relative to the urethra. In girls, the vagina is normal in caliber but shorter than usual with an orifice frequently narrowed and displaced anteriorly. The clitoris is bifid on each side of the epispadiac urethra. There are several variants of exstrophy, which have been given the terms: pseudoexstrophy, superior vesical fissure, duplicate exstrophy and covered exstrophy. All generally involve a less severe defect that classic bladder exstrophy but will present with genital and prepubic anatomy suggesting incomplete embryologic fusion and development.

Evaluation and Management of Bladder Exstrophy in the Newborn

If not suspected prenatally, bladder exstrophy becomes readily apparent at birth. The umbilical cord may be divided as usual, but it is preferable to ligate with suture rather than using the standard plastic cord clamp, in order to avoid the clamp traumatizing the bladder plate early on. The mucosa of the exstrophied bladder appears reddish-pink and is best protected by a simply placing non-adherent plastic wrap over it to avoid abrasion of the sensitive, exposed urothelium. Uncomplicated vaginal delivery is the norm for these children and there is no increased risk for peri-delivery respiratory or other complications. It is important to support the parents' needs after delivery; the support team should include social work and an experienced surgical team that may include a NICU nurse, pediatric urologist, orthopedic surgeon, neonatologist and anesthesiologist. If the child is delivered at a center without capacity for a full assessment, then timely transfer over the first day or two of life is appropriate to a children's hospital equipped for early surgical repair and post-op care.

If the child is well on general exam, then the only imaging needed prior to surgical repair is a renal ultrasound to assess for unanticipated upper tract issues and have a baseline study to assess against over time. Repair within the first week of life has traditionally been seen as optimal since the pelvic bones are maximally malleable at this point due to residual response to maternal relaxin around the time of delivery. This allows for repositioning of the pubic rami to the midline without osteotomy.

Occasionally, a patient will demonstrate such a small and poorly compliant exstrophied bladder plate that it will not allow for early reconstruction with an acceptable chance of success and delayed closure and management should be chosen [5]. Additionally, some centers have more recently chosen to electively delay early closure and wait until a few months of age when the closure may be carried out in a more elective fashion [13]. This choice involves mandated osteotomies to achieve appropriate repositioning of pubes in the midline. If osteotomy is required, it may be performed in several fashions including a posterior ileac osteotomy, opening of the innominate bone in a more lateral location or even cutting the anterior ramus of the pubis in a more lateral location to allow reapposition in the midline.

Traditional staged repair of bladder exstrophy involves three steps (boys): (1) initial bladder closure as newborn, leaving penopubic epispadias, (2) 6–12 months, repair of epispadias, (3) bladder neck reconstruction and ureteral reimplantation. The first stage involves extensive mobilization of the flat bladder plate in order to "sphericalize" it and allow placement back into the pelvis. The proximal urethra is reconstructed out to the base of the penis but the epispadias beyond this is left unrepaired. Once the bladder and proximal urethra are tucked into a more posterior position, the pubic rami are brought together anteriorly and sutured in place. This largely closes the triangular musculofascial defect in the midline. This traditional first-stage closure is completed by removal of the umbilical stump, closure of the anterior fascia and midline skin closure. More recently, some surgeons have chosen to create a needle umbilicus with small skin flaps at the superior end of this midline incision. Finally, some form of lower extremity and hip immobilization is required to keep the knees and hips from rotating outward and causing pubic separation before the wounds are well healed.

The alternative to this traditional first stage closure is to extend the closure through the entire epispadiac urethra to its distal most extent. As well, for complete initial closure of exstrophy, the corpora cavernosa are separated fully and the urethra is transposed to a ventral position before the corpora are reapproximated. This will often leave the shortened urethral plate in a hypospadiac position which will require later surgical repair. Dorsal chordee of the penis can also be corrected at this juncture. This procedure is advocated by some as improving bladder growth due to early bladder cycling, but it is a more extensive reconstruction with some risks associated [14].

With either traditional first stage repair or complete repair of exstrophy, attention to inguinal hernia should be made as 80 % of boys and 10 % of girls are affected. This warrants exploration and repair of hernia in both sexes at the time of initial bladder closure as it may be accomplished through the same midline incision with simple pre-fascial dissection gaining access to the inguinal canals.

If osteotomy is required with closure then bony fixation, in order to keep pubis together during healing, may be accomplished in several ways. Standard external fixators may be placed with pins into the anterior iliac crest, modified Buck's traction may be used, casting with lower extremity spica approach can be considered, and an alternative padded Velcro strapping method has been described, as well (Fig. 9.8) [15].

Most newborns remain in the NICU for a few days after surgery but can often be moved to the infant ward and then discharged by 7–10 days postop. Lower extremity mobilization to maintain medial rotation at the hips should be continued for 4–6 weeks postoperatively. The first stage in traditional exstrophy closure essentially converts the full bladder exstrophy into a penopubic epispadias with and incompetent bladder neck. Thus, urine is expected to drain principally through the suprapubic tube for the first few days, but then progressively more may be seen to exit the epispadiac urethra as surgical edema diminishes. The tube will remain in place for at least 3 weeks after closure. It is important to clamp the suprapubic tube and assure good drainage through the urethra before the tube is removed. Checking wound healing weekly is appropriate. Repeating the renal ultrasound at basic metabolic panel at 6–8 weeks post-op is wise to assure no new upper tract issues.

Fig. 9.8 Exstrophy patient immediately after closure with the legs restrained against outward rotation by the use of padded Velcro straps. These allow for cleaning and diaper changes, but remain in place for 4 weeks post-op

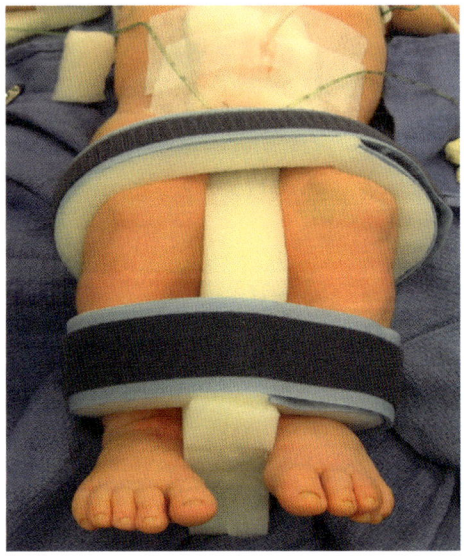

Following closure, all patients will have VUR and are should be maintained on antibiotic prophylaxis for (at least) the first 6 months of life. Continued surveillance is with ultrasound every 3–4 months for the first year of life and a VCUG at 1 year of age. If desired, VCUG may be done with a Foley balloon snugged down to occlude the bladder neck in order to estimate bladder capacity. If healing results in a scarred or overly tight bladder neck, then urinary retention, UTI and upper tract deterioration may be seen. If this occurs, then either dilatation of the bladder neck or intermittent catheterization may be required. Some patients in this circumstance will also require reimplantation of the ureters at an early age to avoid issues related to recurrent pyelonephritis.

In patients undergoing staged repair, the repair of the epispadias is carried out around 6–12 months of age. This involves one of several techniques for tubularization of the urethral plate and reconstruction of the shaft skin along with correction of dorsal chordee [16]. There is a paucity of normal dorsal penile skin and coverage of this area is achieved with skin flaps mobilized from later penile skin or ventral prepuce. A urethral stent is generally left in place for at least 10 days postoperatively. It should be noted that the risk of urethrocutaneous fistula and skin separation is substantially higher in epispadias repair than with hypospadias procedures, occurring in around 25 % of cases. One of the benefits of undertaking the epispadias repair at this age is the increased urethral resistance it creates; this leads to increased bladder filling, cycling and growth in capacity. If urethral fistula or skin separation does occur after epispadias repair, it is best to wait 4–6 months before undertaking revision.

In closing female exstrophy, the urethra is tubularized to the new meatus during the initial repair and the entire distal vagina is mobilized, as well. The perineal body is incised in the midline posterior to the vagina, and the vaginal vault is repositioned to this more posterior position, allowing adequate space for both urethra and vagina once the pubis is closed. Pubic closure brings the upper portion of the labia majora together along with the two halves of the clitoris. The medial sides of clitoral corpora and glans are de-epithelialized and brought together with a series of small absorbable sutures.

The third stage of bladder exstrophy repair is generally undertaken between 3 and 6 years of age. This involves reconstruction and tightening of the bladder neck to increase the potential for continence along with ureteral reimplantation. Prior to initiating this, bladder capacity must be estimated by either VCUG, cystometrogram, or via direct instillation during cystoscopy. If bladder capacity is less than 3–4 ounces, then reconstruction is likely to be unsuccessful at achieving improved continence [17]. Such patients should be considered for more extensive reconstruction including enterocystoplasty and creation of a catheterizable stoma in addition to bladder neck tightening and reimplant.

Bladder neck reconstruction may involve a fairly challenging and prolonged recovery with substantial discomfort and the need for a suprapubic tube drainage for around 3 weeks. At that point, clamping and voiding trails may be initiated. It is important to follow these children closely as this procedure may lead to elevated intravesical pressure and an increased risk of UTI and the development of hydronephrosis if the bladder is not being well emptied with each void. Until it is determined that all is going well, these patients are maintained on antibiotic prophylaxis and renal and bladder assessment with ultrasound is carried out periodically based on their clinical status. Post-void ultrasound images can be very helpful to assure good emptying once the suprapubic tube is gone.

Some patients with exstrophy will have a wide and depressed scar at the site of bladder repair and may need later revision that will include scar excision, rotational flap monsplasty and creation of neoumbilicus (Fig. 9.9a, b). Other long-term issues will be discussed, along with those for cloacal exstrophy patients, in the next section.

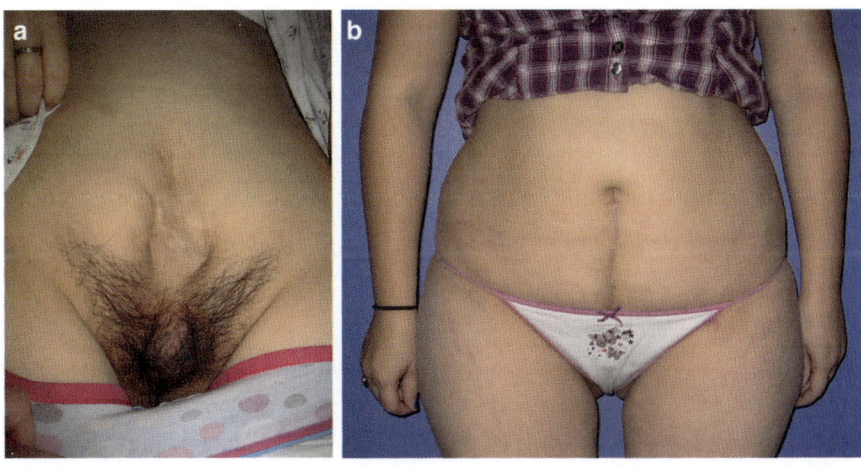

Fig. 9.9 (**a**) Adolescent female with disfiguring scar after childhood exstrophy repair and subsequent procedures. (**b**) After scar revision with rotational flap monsplasty and creation of neoumbilicus

Cloacal Exstrophy

The usual constellation of anomalies found in children with cloacal exstrophy includes: exstrophy of the bladder in two segments, complete separation of phallic corpora, very wide pubic diastasis, exstrophied cecum (with ileal prolapse) located between two bladder halves, rudimentary hindgut and absence of an anus. Virtually all affected children also have an omphalocele present just superior to the exstrophied cloaca. As opposed to patients with bladder exstrophy, who have few associated major defects, children with cloacal exstrophy routinely have multiple significant anomalies. Primary among these is a high instance of spina bifida and other vertebral anomalies at higher levels. Many of these patients will have associated peripheral skeletal anomalies such as club foot or a congenital hip dislocation, as well [18]. In terms of the intestinal tract, the omphalocele may involve liver and other portions of a small and large intestine. The exstrophied cecal segment often has the tiny appendix and hindgut traveling in a blind-ending fashion off its posterior wall. Many of these patients will develop short gut syndrome despite a relatively normal link of small bowel suggesting absorptive abnormalities. During repair, this makes it imperative to save the small segment of hindgut, especially for its water absorptive properties.

Patients with cloacal exstrophy commonly have müllerian abnormalities with uterine and vaginal duplication seen in over 90 %. As well, upper urinary tract anomalies occur in around 50 % of patients which includes UPJ obstruction, megaureter, multicystic dysplastic kidney and renal ectopy [19].

Prenatal Diagnosis of Cloacal Exstrophy

The large number of structural abnormalities in fetuses affected by cloacal exstrophy makes in utero diagnosis much more common than would be seen in bladder exstrophy. Specifically, the large abdominal wall defect with protruding ileum, omphalocele and myelomeningocele are rarely recognized sonographically [20]. When recognized, delivery certainly needs to be performed in a location with ready access to pediatric surgical and urologic expertise in addition to NICU care.

Early Care of the Infant with Cloacal Exstrophy

After birth, the patient should be cared for in an appropriate NICU setting. Patients should be monitored closely and stabilized early on with sonography to assess the upper urinary tracts being performed once possible. The exstrophied cloaca is again, protected with plastic wrap to avoid abrasion of the surface. Neurosurgical consultation is required due to the commonly present myelomeningocele and other vertebral anomalies.

The patient is thoroughly assessed and an individualized approach to repair is planned with all involved and the child's parents. The neurosurgical team will first close the myelomeningocele once the child is stable for transport to the operating room. Once the child has healed well in terms of myelomeningocele closure, the patient is returned to the operating room for dressing the omphalocele and exstrophied defects. It is most important at this point to close the omphalocele to prevent rupture. Simultaneously, the exstrophied bowel segment is detached centrally from the two halves of the bladder. Due to the concerning overall metabolic status of patients with ileostomy, it is always advantageous to tubularize the exstrophed cecum and mobilize the small rudimentary hindgut and create an end colostomy utilizing the entire hindgut in the process. This shortened section of hindgut may substantially change the patient's clinical status due to its role in fluid absorption [21]. Once this bowel segment has been tubularized and end colostomy is created, an assessment is made about the remaining halves of the bladder. Often, it is not possible to mobilize bladder halves and close the bladder exstrophy simultaneously due to the size of the abdominal wall defect. If this is the case, the bladder walls are brought together and sewn in the midline and the omphalocele defect repaired. This is thus converted omphalocele with cloacal exstrophy to an anatomic appearance more similar to a classic bladder exstrophy. The closure of the exstrophied bladder may be undertaken at any time in the future based on the patient's progress and healing.

An additional major issue in cloacal exstrophy involves the genitalia and their reconstruction along with gender assignment. In males, the corpora may often be unbalanced and diminutive. In the past, many XY patients with diminutive corporal development underwent removal of testes and gender conversion, psychosexual evaluation over time and determination of gender identity. Currently, most surgeons and physicians involved in the management of such patients recommend assigning gender that is consistent with karyotypic makeup of the individual, if this is at all possible given anatomic considerations [22]. Patients with cloacal exstrophy routinely require pelvic osteotomy at the time of bladder closure to allow the very wide pubic diastasis to be brought into a reasonable apposition.

Long-Term Issues in Cloacal Exstrophy

Long-term bladder function and potential for urinary continence is affected not only by the exstrophied bladder segment and its limited growth but also by innervation abnormalities associated with spina bifida. It is highly likely that in order to achieve urinary continence, these patients will need extensive urinary reconstruction at an older age. This will likely involve bladder neck tightening or closure to increase bladder outlet, augmentation of bladder volume with intestine, and creation of catheterizable stoma for the urinary reservoir. This is all complicated by the already existing short gut and these patients may be one of the only subgroups in whom gastric augmentation remains a viable alternative, as they are often insensate due to the neurologic defect associated with spina bifida and small bowel is in somewhat short supply.

In terms of bowel continence, these patients often have a permanent end colostomy and manage this with an external collection device. Long-term survival in patients with cloacal exstrophy has greatly improved over the past 30 years. Phallic reconstruction remains an issue for boys with particularly diminutive natural corpora and sometimes full neophallus construction from free flaps may be required. Boys with cloacal exstrophy generally have very limited fertility and while girls appear to be much more fertile overall, while they do suffer from higher rates of cervical and uterine prolapse.

References

1. Harrow BR. The myth of the megacystis syndrome. J Urol. 1967;98:205.
2. Mandell J, Lebowitz RL, Peters CA, Estroff JA, Retik AB, Benacerraf BR. Prenatal diagnosis of the megacystis-megaureter association. J Urol. 1992;148:1487–9.
3. Lashley DB, Masliah E, Kaplan GW, McAleer IM. Megacystis microcolon intestinal hypoperistalsis syndrome: bladder distension and pyelectasis in the fetus without anatomic outflow obstruction. Urol. 2000;55:774.
4. Mc Laughlin D, Puri P. Familial megacystis microcolon intestinal hypoperistalsis syndrome: a systematic review. Pediatr Surg Int. 2013;29:947–51.
5. Gearhart JP. Exstrophy, epispadias, and other bladder anomalies. In: Walsh PC, Retik AB, Vaughan ED, et al., editors. Campbell's urology. 8th ed. Philadelphia: WB Saunders; 2002.
6. Gearhart JP, Ben-Chaim J, Jeffs RD, Sanders RC. Criteria for the prenatal diagnosis of classic bladder exstrophy. Obstet Gynecol. 1995;85:961–4.
7. Galati V, Donovan B, Ramji F. Management of urachal remnants in early childhood. J Urol. 2008;180:1824–6.
8. Berrocal T, Lopez-Pereira P, Arjonilla A, Gutierrez J. Anomalies of the distal ureter, bladder and urethra in children: embryologic, radiologic and pathologic features. Radiographics. 2002;22:1139–64.
9. Hutch JA. Saccule formation at the ureterovesical junction in smooth walled bladders. J Urol. 1961;86:390–9.
10. Abrahamson J. Double bladder and related anomalies: clinical and embryological aspects and a case report. Br J Urol. 1961;33:195–212.
11. Sponseller PD, Bisson LJ, Gearhart JP, Jeffs RD, Magid D, Fishman E. The anatomy of the pelvis in the exstrophy complex. J Bone Joint Surg Am. 1995;77:177–89.
12. Perovic SV, Djinovic RP. New insight into surgical anatomy of epispadiac penis and its impact on repair. J Urol. 2007;179:689–95.
13. Canning DA. Re: Delayed primary closure of bladder exstrophy: immediate postoperative management leading to successful outcomes. J Urol. 2012;188:959.
14. Grady RW, Mitchell ME. Complete primary repair of exstrophy. J Urol. 1999;162:1415–20.
15. Wallis MC, Oottamasathien S, Wicher C, Hadley D, Snow BW, Cartwright PC. Padded self-adhesive strap immobilization following newborn bladder exstrophy closure: the Utah straps. J Urol. 2013;190:2216–20.
16. Baird AD, Gearhart JP, Mathews RI. Applications of the modified Cantwell-Ransley epispadias repair in the exstrophy-epispadias complex. J Pediatr Urol. 2005;1:331–6.
17. Purves JT, Baird AD, Gearhart JP. The modern staged repair of bladder exstrophy in the female: a contemporary series. J Pediatr Urol. 2008;4:150–3.
18. Jain M, Weaver DD. Severe lower limb defects in exstrophy of the cloaca. Am J Med Genet. 2004;128:320–4.
19. Diamond DA. Management of cloacal exstrophy. Dial Pediatr Urol. 1990;13:2.

20. Austin P, Holmsy YL, Gearhart JP, Porter K, Guidi C, Madsen K, et al. Prenatal diagnosis of cloacal exstrophy. J Urol. 1998;160:1179–81.
21. Husmann DA, McLorie GA, Churchill BM. Closure of the exstrophic bladder: an evaluation of the factors leading to its success and its importance on urinary continence. J Urol. 1989;142:522–4.
22. Reiner WG. Psychosexual development in genetic males assigned female: the cloacal exstrophy experience. Child Adolesc Psychiatr Clin North Am. 2004;13:657–74.
23. Tazi F, Ahsaini M, Khalouk A, Mellas S, Stuurman-Wieringa RE, Elfassi MJ, et al. Abscess of urachal remnants presenting with acute abdomen: a case series. J Med Case Rep. 2012;30(6):226.

Chapter 10
Prune Belly Syndrome

David B. Joseph

Abbreviations

PBS Prune belly syndrome
UTI Urinary tract infection

Introduction

A 6-year-old child's appearance was described as that of "a wrinkled prune" by William Osler in 1901 [1]. Since that report, prune belly syndrome (PBS) became synonymous with Triad Syndrome originally reported by Parker in 1895 [2]; the clinical association of a thin flaccid, wrinkled, abdominal wall; undescended, intraabdominal testicles; and bladder enlargement with hydroureters (Fig. 10.1) [2]. Over the years, PBS has also become known as the Eagle–Barrett syndrome and the abdominal muscular deficiency syndrome. Classically PBS occurs in boys; however, 5 % are girls presenting with similar physical and urinary tract findings, with the exception of the gonadal abnormality. The incidence of PBS in the United States has remained stable and approximates 1/26,000 live births; 50 % Caucasian, 31 % African-American and 10 % Hispanic [3, 4]. Most cases are sporadic, although a familial occurrence has been described and associated with trisomies 13, 18, 21, and possibly influenced by the HNF1ß gene [5, 6].

D.B. Joseph, M.D., F.A.C.S., F.A.A.P. (✉)
Department of Urology, The University of Alabama at Birmingham,
1600 7th Ave South, Birmingham, AL, USA
e-mail: david.joseph@childrensal.org

© Springer International Publishing Switzerland 2016   197
A.J. Barakat, H. Gil Rushton (eds.), *Congenital Anomalies of the Kidney and Urinary Tract*, DOI 10.1007/978-3-319-29219-9_10

Fig. 10.1 Newborn with
PBS and associated patent
urachus (*arrow*). With
permission from Gonzales
ET, Bauer SB (eds).
Pediatric urology practice.
Philadelphia, PA:
Lippincott, 1999

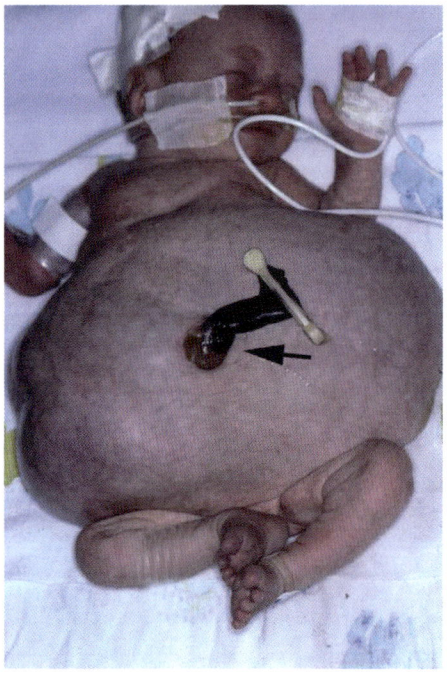

Pathogenesis

There is no single theory, which incorporates all aspects of PBS. The two most appealing are based on the primary abnormality resulting from either urethral obstruction, or a mesenchymal defect [7, 8].

Urethral Obstruction

The theory of obstruction is based on a blockage at the junction of the prostatic and membranous urethra; a location similar to that of a posterior urethral valve [8]. This temporary obstruction causes compression of the prostate resulting in posterior urethral dilatation. Distention of the bladder occurs resulting in urinary ascites and degeneration of the abdominal wall muscle. Elevated bladder pressure leads to upper urinary tract ectasia and renal dysplasia. The massive distention of the bladder mechanically prevents the testicle from entering the internal ring and descending. Later in fetal development the posterior urethral lesion ruptures eliminating identifiable obstruction in neonates with PBS.

An alternative obstructive theory has been proposed with the pathology occurring at the distal urethra during weeks 11–16 of gestation resulting in a delay of canalization of the spongy glanular urethra [9]. The timing of this defect helps to explain the poor prostatic development which occurs during the 11th week and the persistence of a patent urachus which typically closes by week 15. Urinary tract distension during week 13–15 could account for the degenerative changes of the abdominal wall and contribute to malrotation of the gastrointestinal tract.

The clinical absence of abdominal wall changes and intrabdominal testes in patients with documented urethral obstruction from a posterior urethral valve combined with postmortem comparison of patients with PBS to that of posterior urethral valves has placed an obstructive etiology in doubt, supported by abnormal development of the seminal duct vesicles and prostatic glands noted only in children with PBS [10].

Mesodermal Defect

The theory of a mesodermal defect is based on abnormal development during the third week of gestation affecting the medial somites and the lateral plate contributing to maldevelopment of the mesonephros, mesonephric duct (Wolffian), and metanephros [8]. Smooth muscle of the genitourinary and gastrointestinal tract derives from the visceral layer of the lateral plate, with a deficiency in equal distribution of mesoderm resulting in the occurrence of PBS [11].

Post mortem findings in children with PBS reveals the terminal portion of the Wolffian duct appropriates into the prostatic and membranous urethra; overexpansion of the Wolffian duct and ureteric bud enhances dilatation of the prostatic urethra and prostatic hypoplasia and residual membranous leaflets supporting the appearance of an obstruction [10]. Dilatation of the ureteric bud results in megaureters and ectopic insertion into the metanephric blastema induces renal dysplasia [12, 13]. Simultaneous failure of myoblasts to migrate from the thoracic somites results in laxity of the abdominal wall [8].

Although the mesodermal defect theory explains most of the features of PBS, it does not explain the significant male predominance that appears with PBS. It has been proposed that there is a greater demand on the mesoderm for differentiation of the Wolffian versus Müllerian system accounting for the male predominance [11, 14].

Features of the Prune Belly Syndrome (PBS)

Abdominal Wall

Classic description of PBS is based on the wrinkled, lax appearance of the abdominal wall ranging from variable, patchy, asymmetric muscular deficiency limited to the lower abdomen to an extensive asymmetric deficiency throughout. Asymmetric bulging of the abdominal wall can be visualized when the child stands and strains. The rectus abdominous is often poorly developed in the caudal portion and results in a cephalic displacement of the umbilicus. The blood supply and segmental nerve distribution remains normal [15–17]. The abdominal wall abnormality can result in functional consequences. Some children have difficulty changing from a supine to sitting position and delaying ambulation [18]. Deficiency in abdominal musculature also inhibits productive coughing resulting in a higher incidence of upper respiratory infections in a pulmonary compromised patient [19].

Kidneys

Renal development in PBS covers a spectrum from a normal kidney to one that is small, hypoplastic, cystic dysplastic, and/or hydronephrotic. The degree of hydronephrosis may not be proportional to the degree of hydroureter or megacystis. Renal function can be preserved supporting a mesenchymal defect as the etiology. Renal abnormalities have been broadly categorized into one of three groups [20]. The first group consists of severely affected dysplastic kidneys characterized by gross parenchymal disorganization with few nephrons, primitive tubules, embryonic mesodermal cysts, and metaplastic cartilage [21]. The second group is characterized by smaller kidneys with cystic dysplasia, consisting of subcortical, glomerular, and tubular cysts within fibrous tissue surrounding medullary collecting ducts [8, 14]. The third group consists of a combination of cystic dysplasia explained by the Mackie-Stephens theory of renal development with dysplasia due to abnormal induction of nephrogenic mesenchyme by a defective ureteral bud or vascular ischemia [8, 12].

Ureters

The ureters are grossly elongated, tortuous and dilated. The distal ureter is often asymmetrically more involved with significant ectasia. Secondary obstruction may result from kinking and folding of the redundant ureter. Primary obstruction has been reported at the ureteropelvic and ureterovesical junctions, but obstruction is not synonymous with hydroureters [16, 17, 22]. The ureteral orifices are lateral, often golf hole in appearance, and associated with a diverticulum and vesicoureteral reflux in 75 % of children [23, 24].

Microscopically, there is an increase in fibrous tissue at the expense of normally developed ureteric muscle, the suggestion of degeneration of non-myelinated Schwann fibers, and decreased number of nerve plexus [8]. These findings may help explain the poor dynamic characteristics of the ureter resulting in ineffective peristalsis and stagnant urine [15, 16, 25, 26]. Ureteral pathology tends to predominate in the distal portion of the ureter which must be considered when urinary reconstruction is undertaken (Fig. 10.2).

Fig. 10.2 Upper tract specimen of cystic dysplastic kidneys with tortuous asymmetrically dilated megaureters. With permission from Gonzales ET, Bauer SB (eds). Pediatric urology practice. Philadelphia, PA: Lippincott, 1999

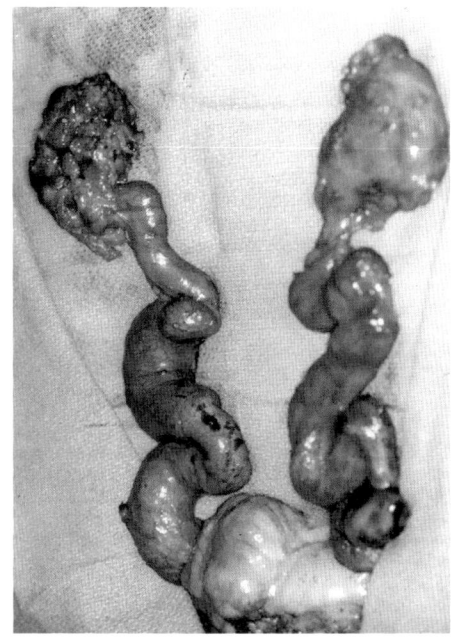

Bladder

The bladder is often massively enlarged with a pseudo diverticulum in the bladder dome, representing a remnant of the urachus (Fig. 10.3). A patent urachus or urachal cyst has been reported in 25–50 % of children [10, 16, 27]. Histologically the bladder wall is thickened due to increased collagen deposits. When true obstruction is present, muscular hypertrophy may account for some detrusor thickening. However, without obstruction there is an increase in the ratio of collagen to muscle fibers [28]. There is no apparent neurological deficit of the bladder with normal distribution of ganglion cells [15].

Typically, the PBS bladder is highly compliant, allowing for an excessive volume of urine stored at low pressure. Decreased effective detrusor contractility is associated with the increased capacity leading to urinary stasis in the lower and upper urinary tract and a tendency for subsequent sepsis. Spontaneous voiding can be achieved but usually at the expense of significant residual urine. The residual urine rarely leads to upper tract deterioration because of the highly compliant bladder. Urodynamic assessment has been described as three distinct voiding patterns; normal with modest post-void residual, prolonged voiding with low leak point pressure, and an intermittent pattern. Voiding is often accomplished by increasing intra-abdominal pressure via diaphragmatic contraction or manual suprapubic compression. Voiding efficiency has marginal benefits following urinary reconstruction, which may include a reduction cystoplasty; the initial post operative improvement in voiding after reduction cystoplasty is not long lasting.

Fig. 10.3 Bladder with
pseudo diverticulum
(*double arrows*) and
bilateral intra-abdominal
testicles (*single arrow*).
With permission from
Gonzales ET, Bauer SB
(eds). Pediatric urology
practice. Philadelphia, PA:
Lippincott, 1999

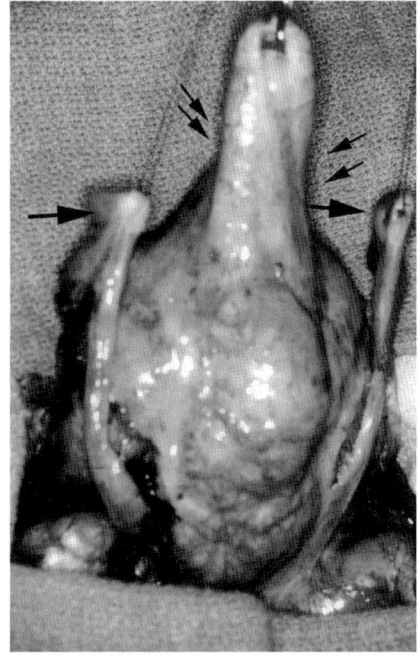

Prostate and Prostatic Urethra

The prostate is hypoplastic with tubuloalveolar glands present in very sparse populations [10, 29]. As with other components of the urinary system there is an increase in the ratio of fibrous tissue and collagen fibers to smooth muscle. The verumontanum is poorly developed and reported as flat, absent, or replaced by a small rounded utriculus [10]. The prostatic urethra is typically an expanded pouch with an abrupt junction between the prostatic and membranous urethra often giving the false appearance of an obstruction (Fig. 10.4) [8].

Genital Tract

The vas deferens is narrow and convoluted from the prostate gland to the testicle; with attachment of the epididymis to the testicle tenuous or nonexistent [10]. The seminal ducts may be poorly developed with mid-line fusion and the seminal vesicles can be very rudimentary or absent.

Anterior Urethra

Anatomic abnormalities of the penile urethra span a spectrum from normal to bulbous or atretic and are not a requirement for the diagnosis of PBS. Measurements of urethral caliber are distinctly abnormal in boys with PBS compared to boys with

Fig. 10.4 Voiding
cystourethrogram, *arrows*
indicate bladder neck. The
prostatic urethra is
patulous. With permission
from Gonzales ET, Bauer
SB (eds). Pediatric urology
practice. Philadelphia, PA:
Lippincott, 1999

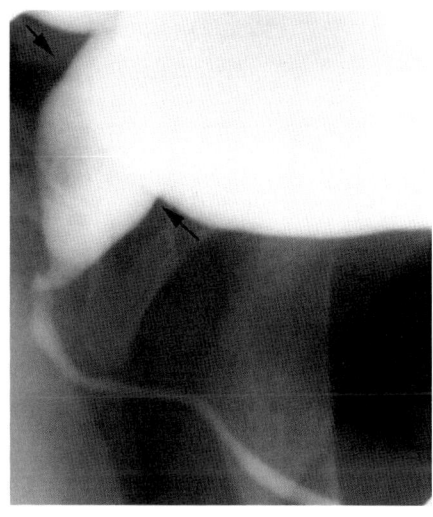

posterior urethral valves and normal controls [9]. Megalourethra, often seen in PBS, represents a continuation of the mesodermal theory of maldevelopment. Megalourethra is classified as scaphoid or fusiform. The scaphoid defect is more common with deficiency of the corpus spongiosum confined to the penile portion of the urethra, resulting in a variable length of massively enlarged ventral, anterior urethra similar in appearance to a saccular diverticulum. The fusiform variety encompasses a defect of the corpus spongiosum in association with a deficiency of one or both corpora cavernosum, resulting in circumferential ballooning of the urethra and generalized penile flaccidity. Urethral atresia is usually associated with a patent urachus.

Testicles

By definition, the testicles in patients with PBS are intra-abdominal and usually located overlying the ventral aspect of the distal ureter. Gubernacular attachment to the testis occurs proximally at the tail of the epididymis and distally at the pubic tubercle. The gubernaculum itself is histologically normal with a normal neuronal input [30]. The histological pattern of PBS testicle shows absence of spermatogenesis, decreased number of spermatogonium and Sertoli cells, and Leydig cell hyperplasia [31, 32]. With the lack of spermatogonia, the risk of a germ cell tumor has been considered minimal [32]. However, the histological similarities with intratubular germ cell neoplasia have been noted reinforcing the importance of long term follow-up [33]. To date, reports of paternity with PBS are rare, likely due to histological abnormalities of the testicle and structural abnormalities of the genital ductal system. Intracytoplasmic sperm injection may be a feasible alternative [34, 35].

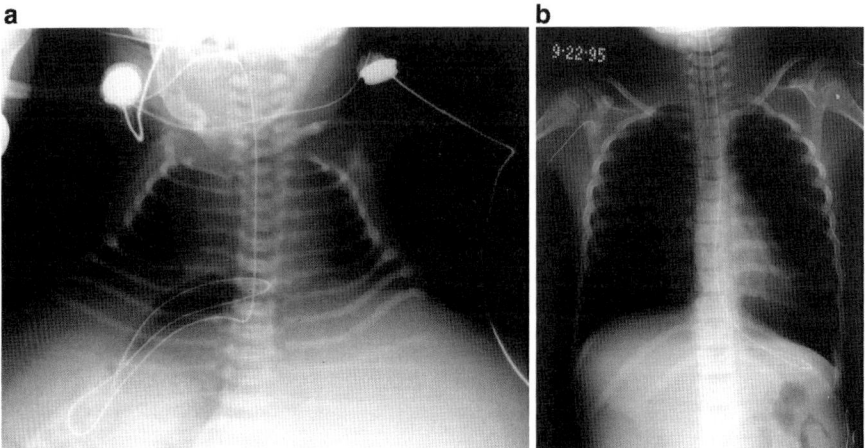

Fig. 10.5 (**a**) Newborn chest X-ray with splayed appearance of lower ribs due to severe abdominal distention. (**b**) Seven year follow-up of the same child showing normalization of chest after urinary diversion. With permission from Gonzales ET, Bauer SB (eds). Pediatric urology practice. Philadelphia, PA: Lippincott, 1999

Associated Organ System Anomalies

PBS is associated with other anomalies in 75 % of patients. Thoracic skeletal deformity is common resulting in a protruded upper sternum, depressed lower sternum, and splayed ribs (Fig. 10.5). Other skeletal deformities include talipes equinovarus, congenital hip dislocation, calcaneus valgus, polydactyly, syndactyly, arthrogryposis, scoliosis, and lordosis. Intestinal malformations are noted in over 30 % of affected children; most due to defective fixation or malrotation of the midgut. Cardiac atrial or ventricular septal defects, patent ductus arteriosus, and teratology of Fallot have been reported in 15 % of these children [5]. Oral manifestations of enamel hypoplasia and jaw bone abnormalities have recently been described, possibly due to chronic renal insufficiency [36]. Perinatal mortality is high and influenced by prematurity and pulmonary complications.

Diagnosis

The diagnosis of PBS can be established in utero with fetal sonography. However, the findings and appearance are similar to, and often confused with obstruction from a posterior urethral valve or the megacystis–megaureter syndrome. The clinical manifestations of those diagnoses and potential for in utero treatment requires very close inspection for a thinned, deficient or absent abdominal wall musculature that supports the diagnosis of PBS. In utero diagnosis allows for planned neonatal support at a high-risk maternal–fetal center. PBS should be obvious at birth with the pathogno-monic physical findings of a loose, lax, wrinkled abdominal wall; flared chest; and undescended testicles. The diagnosis is further supported with renal/bladder sonog-raphy revealing a large bladder and significant hydroureteronephrosis.

PBS has several classifications most based on clinical presentation and morbidity of the neonate. For practical purposes, neonates can be classified as mild, moderate, or severe based on their clinical status. Neonates classified as mild do not suffer from respiratory or renal compromise. While long-term follow-up is necessary within the mild group, operative intervention is often limited to orchiopexy and pos-sibly abdominal wall reconstruction.

Moderate PBS has features of combined renal and respiratory insufficiency, man-dating close observation. Early intervention in neonates within the moderate group is necessary to minimize the sequelae of pulmonary and renal compromise. The combina-tion of increased bilateral renal sonographic echogenicity, chronic urinary tract infec-tions (UTIs), and a nadir serum creatine of >0.7 mg/dL are prognostic for eventual renal failure as the child ages [37]. Monitoring the urinary system and referral to pediatric nephrology and urology is mandatory to minimize progressive renal deterioration due to stagnation of urinary flow, UTIs, and possible urinary tract obstruction. Urinary tract reconstruction may play an important role in limiting long-term morbidity, but should be limited to children who do not respond to medical management. Reconstruction should not be based on the dramatic abnormal appearance of imaging studies.

Severe PBS relates to significant respiratory compromise due to pulmonary immaturity and dysplasia and extensive renal dysplasia, resulting in a Potter-like syndrome. Survival in the severe form is limited.

Evaluation

A team approach to care is required; in addition to the pediatric nephrologist and urologist, consultation may be required from a neonatologist, pulmonologist, cardi-ologist, and orthopedic surgeon in order to maximize patient outcome. It is impor-tant to quickly establish the cardiorespiratory status of the neonate. The baby should undergo a chest X-ray and if indicated, echocardiography. Urological evaluation commences with an abdominal (renal/bladder) sonogram and baseline serum chem-istries. The upper and lower urinary tract requires assessment, placing attention on the volume and echogenicity of the renal parenchyma and degree of hydronephro-sis. Disproportionate distal hydroureter compared to the proximal ureter and renal pelvis may be impressive. On occasion, a marked transition of ureteral dilation is noted with the lower ureter being more involved than the upper ureter and kidney. A patent urachus may be present promoting passive drainage of urine from the blad-der. There should be no rush to close a draining urachal remnant.

When the infant is clinically stable with normal renal function and voiding per urethra, further diagnostic testing can be placed on hold. Neonates with renal insufficiency, however, require diagnostic testing to differentiate renal dysplasia and stagnant urine flow within a dilated system from true obstruction. The MAG-3 renal scan remains an objective diagnostic tool but it has limitations in the newborn period particularly in the face of renal insufficiency. A voiding cystourethrogram can assess vesicoureteral reflux and the effectiveness of bladder emptying. However, the neonate with PBS is susceptible to bacteriuria and can quickly become symptomatic and septic. When present, bacteriuria often persists and is difficult to clear. Therefore, it cannot be overemphasized that any invasive lower urinary tract imaging is undertaken in a sterile environment, with the child receiving pre- and postprocedural antibiotics.

Indications for Surgery

PBS requires individualized care as each neonate presents with a unique constellation of problems resulting in its own set of considerations [38]. No single treatment plan is appropriate for all children making an algorithm for care difficult. In general, operative management is organized into three broad areas: the need for reconstruction of the urinary tract, the appearance of the abdominal wall, and transfer of the intra-abdominal testicle to the scrotum.

Urinary Tract Reconstruction

The need for aggressive urinary tract reconstruction should be tempered and based on the clinical status of the child, not their physical appearance or imagining abnormality. Early aggressive operative intervention for all children is countered by the fact that renal dysplasia may be inherent preventing any intervention from improving the functional status. In addition, imaging studies revealing significant hydroureteronephrosis do not correlate with obstruction or subsequent symptoms; hydroureteronephrosis by itself does not mandate reconstruction. Urinary tract reconstruction should be reserved for the child who has obstructive uropathy and has shown improved renal function with decompression of the urinary system; the child who has progressive hydroureteronephrosis associated with increasing renal compromise; or the child who has recurrent symptomatic UTIs due to significant stagnant urine flow.

Temporary Diversion of the Upper Tract

Urinary diversion plays an initial temporary role in the management of acute renal failure or sepsis. Upper urinary tract decompression via nephrostomy tube drainage stabilizes an acute problem but with limited long-term effectiveness as a more formal upper urinary tract diversion is ultimately needed. There is a theoretical advantage of performing proximal upper tract diversion (renal pelvis or proximal ureter) in an effort to maximally relieve stress on the kidney and improve the egress of stagnant urine within a dilated tortuous ureter. However, there is often a disproportionate degree of distal versus proximal ureteral dilation that can prevent easy access of a minimally dilated proximal ureter. A low distal cutaneous ureterostomy can adequately decompress stagnant urine flow and stabilize renal function. Low distal diversion has the advantage of leaving the proximal upper tract uncompromised an important factor when it comes time for "undiversion."

Temporary Diversion of the Lower Tract

Children with urethral atresia or obstruction will often present with a patent urachus, effectively emptying their lower tract. Neonates with associated posterior urethral abnormalities resulting in poor bladder emptying, who are not candidates for intermittent catheterization, benefit from a vesicostomy. A vesicostomy, while draining the bladder, may not adequately drain the upper urinary tract due to an obstruction of the ureter at the level of the bladder or poor urinary transport due to a highly compliant, adynamic ureter. Vesicostomy should be considered only after bladder catheterization has shown effective decompression of the upper urinary tract. Otherwise, temporary diversion of the upper urinary tract will be required.

Reconstruction or Undiversion of the Upper Tract

When definitive upper urinary reconstruction is necessary, the initial approach to the ureter can be an extravesical reimplant. If an obvious transition is noted on imaging between the dilated distal ureter and a more normal proximal ureter, consideration should be given to removing as much distal ureter as possible, limiting the need for aggressive tapering of the ureter. During dissection, the adventitial tissue surrounding the ureter must be preserved to prevent devascularization. The ureter is reimplanted in the bladder in a standard fashion or with the assistance of a psoas hitch.

   If total proximal and distal ureteral tailoring is necessary due to massive dilation, redundancy, and tortuosity, complete mobilization of the ureter will most likely require transperitoneal exposure. The dynamic capability of the ureter to transmit urine into the bladder parallels the degree of hydroureter. Therefore, ureteral tapering may enhance urinary flow into the bladder. Multiple techniques exist for ureteral tailoring and include ureteral imbrication and formal ureteral excision. The technique selected will be determined by the bulk of ureter present. If a large, redundant renal pelvis is present in association with a dilated proximal ureter, a reduction pyeloplasty should be performed in line with the proximal ureteral excision taking great care to preserve the proximal ureteral blood supply.

Reconstruction or Undiversion of the Lower Tract

It is compelling to perform a reduction cystoplasty during urinary reconstruction in a child with PBS. However, long-term follow-up has been mixed regarding identifiable objective advantages [39–41]. With time, the bladder often returns to its preoperative state and regains its large size, loses its tone, and results in inadequate emptying. For these reasons, it is not practical to routinely proceed with reductive cystoplasty as the primary indication for urinary reconstruction. Intermittent catheterization is a more appropriate form of initial management for the large, poorly contracting bladder. However, when undertaking formal urinary reconstruction with upper tract ureteral tailoring, reductive cystoplasty is practical and may provide limited improved bladder emptying [41].

Reconstruction of the Abdominal Wall

Abdominal wall reconstruction allows for an improvement in cosmetic and functional outcome. It should be individualized based on the degree of abdominal wall laxity [42–45]. Timing for this procedure is based on the need for other operative intervention. If the child does not need upper urinary tract reconstruction, abdominal wall reconstruction can be undertaken at any time. If, however, there is the potential for upper urinary tract intervention, abdominal wall reconstruction should be deferred until the time of that procedure or thereafter.

Several techniques have been developed to maximize the cosmetic benefits of abdominal wall reconstruction in children with PBS. There is evidence indicating that the muscular defect is more pronounced centrally and caudally. Early reconstructive efforts were based on removal of this abnormal tissue. While the appearance of the abdomen was improved, it was not ideal and resulted in a transverse incision and loss of the umbilicus. Monfort subsequently described preservation of the umbilicus, and others have added various modifications [42–44, 46–48]. The Monfort approach begins with a midline incision from the tip of the xiphoid process carried inferiorly, circumscribing the umbilicus, leaving an adequate umbilical island of tissue, and ending at the symphysis pubis (Fig. 10.6). Full-thickness skin flaps are created laterally. The peritoneum is entered lateral to the superior epigastric artery from the costal margin to the symphysis pubis on each side. The central fascial bridge with the umbilical island is now supported by both sets of epigastric arteries. The two lateral incisions provide excellent exposure for orchiopexy and major urinary tract reconstruction when required. During closure, the lateral abdominal fascia wall is secured to the central fascial strip in a pants-over-vest technique providing additional ventral support. The skin flaps are tailored, with the excess dermis removed, allowing for a midline and periumbilical closure. A laparoscopic-assisted approach has been described that may be helpful with simultaneous orchiopexy; however, this can be easily completed via the open abdominal exposure at the time of abdominoplasty [49].

Fig. 10.6 Abdominal exposure with reflected skin flaps. *Large arrow* indicates retained umbilicus. *Small arrows* entrance into the peritoneum lateral to the superior upper epigastric artery. With permission from Gonzales ET, Bauer SB (eds). Pediatric urology practice. Philadelphia, PA: Lippincott, 1999

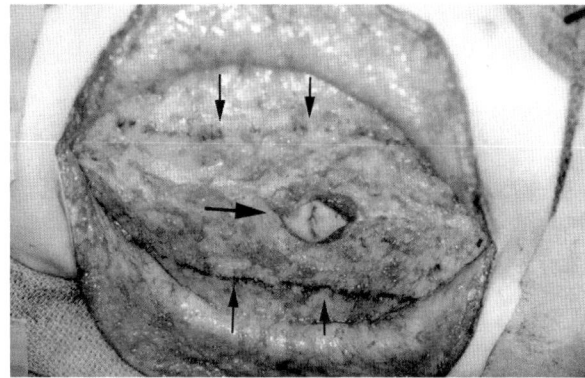

Orchiopexy

The age for orchiopexy is individualized to the child's need for urinary reconstructive surgery. If early urinary reconstructive surgery is required, orchiopexy can be performed simultaneously. If urinary reconstructive surgery is not required, the timing and approach are variable. Placement of the testicle within the scrotum is important for maintaining hormone function, allowing for pubertal development and sexuality, but fertility is not improved [50].

The testicle is often closely adherent to a dilated distal ureter and should be released from the ureter initially without sacrifice of the gonadal artery in order to determine whether the testicle can be delivered into the scrotum. This is often possible when undertaken within the first 6 months of life [38]. After the testicle is separated from the ureter, an incision is made in the peritoneum lateral to the gonadal artery and directed to the internal ring. A second incision medial to the gonadal vessels is made in the peritoneum and continued caudally along the course of the vessels and vas deferens. It is important not to disrupt the vascular supply of the peritoneal pedicle running on both sides of the vas deferens. If it becomes apparent that the testicle will not reach the scrotum after mobilization, the gonadal vessels are sacrificed, as described by Fowler and Stephens [51]. The blood supply to the testicle is maintained by the vasal artery and small anastomotic channels within the peritoneal flap. A tunnel is then made into the scrotum and an incision placed inferiorly in the scrotum to create a dartos pouch for testicular placement. Care must be taken not to twist or place the peritoneal pedicle on tension. A laparoscopic primary or staged approach works well when the orchiopexy is an independent procedure [52].

Urethral Reconstruction

Correction of the megalourethra is dependent on presenting symptoms of urinary dribbling and/or urinary infections. Most often operative correction is undertaken because of the unusual appearance of the megalourethra. Urethral tapering is an appropriate treatment.

Operative Results

The results of urologic reconstruction can be very gratifying in the initial postoperative period, in particular the cosmetic appearance of the abdomen and the improvement in upper urinary tract drainage. Voiding function may become more effective due to the benefits of abdominal wall reconstruction and reduction cystoplasty [44, 45]. However, with time there can be an increase in both bladder size and ureteral dilation. This is often due to ineffective voiding and is independent of bladder reduction. For those reasons, long-term follow-up of the urinary tract is required. Patients should be prepared for the potential need for intermittent catheterization. Because of normal sensation, children are often unwilling to cooperate with urethral catheterization. Placement of an appendicovesicostomy should be considered at the time of urinary reconstruction if catheterization appears to be a realistic future possibility. An appendicovesicostomy provides excellent access to the bladder in a normally sensate child. Long-term antibiotic prophylaxis is indicated in these high risk children with dilated collecting systems and large bladders usually associated with vesicoureteral reflux.

Sexual Function

Preservation of the upper urinary tract in children with PBS has lead to increased survival through puberty and into adulthood. A small survey of adults with PBS found all able to achieve normal erections and orgasm. However, most reported retrograde ejaculation. Serum testosterone levels were normal in 66 % along with elevated levels of luteinizing hormone and follicle stimulating hormone. All men were infertile [53]. Paternity is limited but it must be kept in mind that the adult population includes men who had orchidopexy at a late age. The current philosophy of early orchidopexy may improve chances for paternity but it is not expected based on underlying histologic and anatomic abnormality. Rare success with ICSI has been reported.

Conclusion

Children with PBS present a complex set of problems. The outlook remains poor for those neonates born with severe pulmonary and renal dysplasia resulting in early end-stage renal disease and renal transplantation in 15 % [54]. Children with minimal to marginal pulmonary dysplasia can do quite well regardless of renal dysplasia provided appropriate nephrologic and urologic care is undertaken. Nutrition, prophylactic antibiotics, and intermittent catheterization play a critical role in the management of these children. A small, select group of children benefit from aggressive urinary reconstruction. Current techniques for abdominal wall reconstruction provide satisfactory cosmetic results with preservation of the umbilicus. All boys benefit from bilateral orchidopexy either from open or laparoscopic exposure. Early intervention might allow the testicles to be brought into the scrotum without transection of the spermatic vessels.

References

1. Osler W. Congenital absence of the abdominal muscles with distended and hypertrophied urinary bladder. Bull Johns Hopkins Hosp. 1901;12:331–3.
2. Parker RW. Absence of abdominal muscles in an infant. Lancet. 1895;23:1252.
3. Routh JC, Huang L, Retik AB, Nelson CP. Contemporary epidemiology and characterization of newborn males with prune belly syndrome. Urology. 2010;76:44–8.
4. Lloyd JC, Wiener JS, Gargollo PC, Inman BA, Ross SS, Routh JC. Contemporary epidemiological trends in complex congenital genitourinary anomalies. J Urol. 2013;190:1590–5.
5. Strand WR. Initial management of complex pediatric disorders: prunebelly syndrome, posterior urethral valves. Urol Clin North Am. 2004;31:399–415.
6. Granberg CF, Harrison SM, Dajusta D, Zhang S, Hajarnis S, Igarashi P, et al. Genetic basis of prune belly syndrome: screening for HNF1β gene. J Urol. 2012;187:272–8.
7. Stumme EG. Ueber die symmetrischen kongenitalen Bauchmuskeldefekte und uber die Kombination derselben mit anderen Bildungsanomalien des Rumpfes. Mitt Grenzgebiete Med Chir. 1903;11:548–90.
8. Wheatley JM, Stephens FD, Hutson JM. Prune belly syndrome: ongoing controversies regarding pathogenesis and management. Semin Pediatr Surg. 1996;5:95–106.
9. Beasley SW, Bettenay F, Hutson JM. The anterior urethra provides clues to the etiology of prune-belly syndrome. Pediatr Surg Int. 1988;3:169–72.
10. Stephens FD, Gupta D. Pathogenesis of the prune belly syndrome. J Urol. 1994;152:2328–31.
11. Ives EJ. The abdominal muscle deficiency triad syndrome—experience with 10 cases. Birth Defects. 1974;10:127–35.
12. Mackie GG, Stephens FD. Duplex kidneys: a correlation of renal dysplasia with position of the ureteral orifice. J Urol. 1975;114:274–80.
13. Stephens FD. Morphology and embryogenesis of the triad. In: Stephens FD, editor. Congenital malformation of the urinary tract (chap 32). New York, NY: Praeger; 1983. p. 485–91.
14. Greskovich FJ, Nyberg LM. The prune belly syndrome: a review of its etiology, defects, treatment and prognosis. J Urol. 1988;140:707–12.
15. Nunn N, Stephens FD. The triad syndrome: a composite anomaly of the abdominal wall, urinary system and testes. J Urol. 1961;86:782–94.
16. Wigger HJ, Blanc WA. The prune-belly syndrome. Pathol Annu. 1977;12:17–39.
17. Moerman P, Fryns J-P, Goddeeris P, Lauweryns JM. Pathogenesis of the prune-belly syndrome: a functional urethral obstruction caused by prostatic hypoplasia. Pediatrics. 1984;73:470–5.
18. Duckett Jr JW. Prune belly syndrome. In: Welch KJ, Randolph JG, Ravitch MM, et al., editors. Pediatric surgery. Chicago: Year Book Medical Publishers; 1986. p. 1193–203.
19. Panitch HB. Pulmonary complications of abdominal wall defects. Paediatr Respir Rev. 2015;16:11–7.
20. Skoog SJ. Prune belly syndrome. In: Kelalis PP, King LR, Belman AB, editors. Clinical pediatric urology. Philadelphia: WB Saunders; 1992. p. 943–76.
21. Osathanondh V, Potter EL. Pathogenesis of polycystic kidneys. Arch Pathol. 1964;77:510–3.
22. Manivel JC, Pettinato G, Reinberg Y, Gonzalez R, Burke B, Dehner LP. Prune-belly syndrome: clinicopathologic study of 29 cases. Pediatr Pathol. 1989;9:691–711.
23. Berdon WE, Baker DH, Wigger HJ, Blanc WA. The radiologic and pathologic spectrum of the prune-belly syndrome. The importance of urethral obstruction in prognosis. Radiol Clin North Am. 1977;15:83–92.

24. Fallat ME, Skoog SJ, Belman AB, Eng G, Randolph JG. The prune belly syndrome: a comprehensive approach to management. J Urol. 1989;142:802–5.
25. Gearhart JP, Lee BR, Partin AW, Epstein JI, Gosling JA, Kogan BA. Quantitative histological evaluation of the dilated ureter of childhood, II: Ectopia, posterior urethral valves and the prune belly syndrome. J Urol. 1995;153:172–6.
26. Ehrlich RM, Brown WJ. Ultrastructural anatomic observations of the ureter in the prune belly syndrome. Birth Defects. 1977;13:101–3.
27. Lattimer JK. Congenital deficiency of the abdominal musculature and associated genitourinary anomalies: a report of 22 cases. J Urol. 1958;79:343–52.
28. Workman SJ, Kogan BA. Fetal bladder histology in posterior urethral valves and the prune-belly syndrome. J Urol. 1990;144:337–9.
29. Deklerk DP, Scott WW. Prostatic maldevelopment in the prune belly syndrome: a defect in prostatic stromal–epithelial interaction. J Urol. 1978;120:341–4.
30. Tayakkanonta K. The gubernaculum and its nerve supply. Aust N Z J Surg. 1963;33:61–7.
31. Orvis BR, Bottles K, Kogan BA. Testicular histology in fetuses with prune belly syndrome and posterior urethral valves. J Urol. 1988;139:335–7.
32. Uehling DT, Zadina SP, Gilbert E. Testicular histology in triad syndrome. Urology. 1984;23:364–6.
33. Massad CA, Cohen MB, Kogan BA, Beckstead JH. Morphology and histochemistry of the infant testis in the prune belly syndrome. J Urol. 1991;146:1598–600.
34. Kolettis PN, Ross JH, Kay R, Thomas AJ. Sperm retrieval and intracytoplasmic sperm injection in patients with prune-belly syndrome. Fertil Steril. 1999;72:948–50.
35. Fleming SD, Varughese E, Hua V, Robertson A, Dalzell F, Boothroyd CV. Normal live births after intracytoplasmic sperm injection in a man with the rare condition of Eagle-Barrett syndrome (prune-belly syndrome). Fertil Steril. 2013;100:1532–5.
36. Pessoa L, Galvao V. Oral manifestations associated with systemic complications of prune belly syndrome. Oral Surg Oral Med Oral Pathol Oral Radiol. 2013;115:e37–40.
37. Noh PH, Cooper CS, Winkler AC, Zderic SA, Snyder 3rd HM, Canning DA. Prognostic factors for long-term renal function in boys with the prune-belly syndrome. J Urol. 1999;162:1399–401.
38. Woodard JR. Prune-belly syndrome: a personal learning experience. BJUI. 2003;92:10–1.
39. Bukowski TM, Perlmutter AD. Reduction cystoplasty in the prune-belly syndrome: a long-term follow-up. J Urol. 1994;152:2113–6.
40. Kinahan TJ, Churchill BM, McLorie GA, Gilmour RF, Khoury AE. The efficiency of bladder emptying in the prune-belly syndrome. J Urol. 1992;148:600–3.
41. Denes FT, Arap MA, Giron AM, Silva FA, Arap S. Comprehensive surgical treatment of prune belly syndrome: 17 years' experience with 32 patients. Urology. 2004;64:789–93.
42. Denes FT, Lopes RI, Oliveira LM, Tavares A, Srougi M. Modified abdominoplasty for patients with the prune belly syndrome. Urology. 2014;83:251–4.
43. Lesavoy MA, Chang EI, Suliman A, Taylor J, Kim SE, Ehrlich RM. Long-term follow-up of total abdominal wall reconstruction for prune belly syndrome. Plast Reconstr Surg. 2012;129:104e–9.
44. Fearon JA, Varkarakis G. Dynamic abdominoplasty for the treatment of prune belly syndrome. Plast Reconstr Surg. 2012;130:648–57.
45. Smith CA, Smith EA, Parrott TS, Broecker BH, Woodard JR. Voiding function in patients with the prune-belly syndrome after Monfort abdominoplasty. J Urol. 1998;159:1675–9.
46. Bukowski TM, Smith CA. Monfort abdominoplasty with neoumbilical modification. J Urol. 2000;164:1711–3.
47. Ehrlich RM, Lesavoy MA, Fine RN. Total abdominal wall reconstruction in the prune-belly syndrome. J Urol. 1986;136:282–5.
48. Montfort G, Guys JM, Boccoardo A, Coquet M, Chevallier D. A novel technique for reconstruction of the abdominal wall in the prune belly syndrome. J Urol. 1991;146:639–40.
49. Fishman AI, Franco I. Laparoscopic-assisted surgical reconstruction of a rare congenital abdominal wall defect in two children misdiagnosed with prune-belly syndrome. J Pediatr Urol. 2013;9:448–52.

50. Patil KK, Duffy PG, Woodhouse RJ, Ransley PG. Long-term outcome of Fowler-Stephens orchiopexy in boys with prune-belly syndrome. J Urol. 2004;171:1666–9.
51. Fowler R, Stephens FD. The role of testicular vascular anatomy in the salvage of high undescended testis. Aust NZ J Surg. 1959;29:92–106.
52. Philip J, Mullassery D, Craigie RJ, Manikandan R, Kenny SE. Laparoscopic orchidopexy in boys with prune belly syndrome—outcome and technical considerations. J Endourol. 2011;25:1115–7.
53. Woodhouse CRJ, Synder H. Testicular and sexual function in adults with prune belly syndrome. J Urol. 1985;133:607–9.
54. Seidel NE, Arlen AM, Smith EA, Kirsch AJ. Clinical manifestations and management of prune-belly syndrome in a large contemporary pediatric population. Urology. 2015;85:211–5.

Chapter 11
Congenital Neuropathic Bladder

Stuart B. Bauer

Abbreviations

CIC   Clean intermittent catheterization
DSD   Dyssynergy
UTI   Urinary tract infection
VUR   Vesicoureteral reflux

First Impressions

Since the mid-portion of the 2nd decade of the twentieth century, there has been a paradigm shift in the evaluation and management of newborns with myelodysplasia due to the successful development of prenatal closure of the spinal defect [1]. The improved cognitive ability with the apparent reduced need for shunting the cerebrospinal fluid in these infants is driving families and practitioners to seek prenatal treatment of the defect at an expanding number of locations around the USA. Although definitive urologic findings from the largest series of prenatal closures (the MOMS trial) have not been published yet, several reports involving small groups of these children have shown that the neuro-urologic findings may differ in these infants from newborns closed postnatally [2, 3]. It is imperative, therefore, that newborns who have had prenatal closure undergo lower urinary tract assessment as soon as feasible after delivery to characterize its function and then apply treatment based on the algorithm outlined in this chapter.

S.B. Bauer, M.D. (✉)
Department of Urology (Surgery), Harvard Medical School, Boston Children's Hospital,
300 Longwood Avenue, Hunnewell 3rd Floor, Boston, MA 02115, USA
e-mail: stuart.bauer@childrens.harvard.edu

© Springer International Publishing Switzerland 2016   215
A.J. Barakat, H. Gil Rushton (eds.), *Congenital Anomalies of the Kidney and Urinary Tract*, DOI 10.1007/978-3-319-29219-9_11

For most practitioners, however, the urologic management of the newborn with myelodysplasia begins shortly after birth. Evaluating neonates this early provides clinicians with information about bladder compliance, presence of detrusor overactivity, bladder contractility at capacity, ability to empty at acceptable pressures and presence of detrusor sphincter dyssynergia. Although it would be helpful to know what effect postnatal closure has on lower urinary tract function, only one center has been able to accomplish that with pre- and post-closure urodynamic testing. Only 3.2 % of these babies incurred a change in function from the closure [4]. As the study involved only 23 infants, it is not known if this low rate of change is universal or not. Spinal shock with paralysis of the bladder for several days to weeks or even a month or two, occurs in about 10 % of these children [5]. The most important concern following initial closure is "can the child empty his or her bladder and at what pressure to insure a normal upper urinary tract?"

Answering these questions involves obtaining a post-void residual urine measurement by catheterizing the bladder immediately after the infant has leaked urine or voided spontaneously. If the residual is above 5 ml repeating the measurement following a Credé maneuver aids in determining if clean intermittent catheterization (CIC) or continuous Foley catheter drainage should be instituted. CIC is performed every 4 h during the day. If the child fails to empty after the postoperative catheter is removed, presumably secondary to spinal shock (10 %), either CIC is begun then or the Foley catheter is replaced and removed periodically to see if bladder function has returned [5]. Adequate bladder drainage is the mainstay of treatment to prevent urinary tract infection (UTI) during this time before the second portion of the question can be answered.

Initial Comprehensive Assessment

The initial comprehensive assessment (Table 11.1) begins with an examination of the lower extremities, checking muscle mass, spontaneous movements, deep tendon reflexes, sensation (both lower extremity and perineal areas), and anal tone in order to determine what are the child's sensory and motor neurological levels. Despite a comprehensive examination, little predictability has been noted between the neurological level and UTI [6]. However, some clues do exist that can suggest what type of bladder and sphincter behavior is present, i.e., a patulous anus is often seen in children with complete lower motor neuron lesions involving the external urethral sphincter, whereas an anal wink (anal muscle reactivity to gentle scratching the pigmented, ruggated skin adjacent to the anus) implies intact sacral spinal cord function and reflexes. This creates the potentiality that detrusor-sphincter dyssynergia is present that must be investigated when urodynamic testing is undertaken.

Urodynamic evaluation is performed within the first several weeks but no later than 3 months after birth [7, 8]. It includes slow fill cystometrography (≤5 ml per minute) using saline warmed to 37 °C [9], looking at detrusor compliance, contractility, leak-point pressure, and the ability to void and empty at capacity with

Table 11.1 Initial workup and noteworthy parameters

Postvoid residual
• After a spontaneous void or Credé maneuver
Renal and bladder ultrasound
• Kidney size, appearance, parenchymal thickness, collecting system dilation
• Ureteral dilation—proximal and distal
• Bladder wall thickness and residual urine volume
Urodynamic study
• Cystometrogram (compliance, contractility, detrusor overactivity, leak-point pressure)
• Voiding pressure studies and ability to empty at specific pressures
• External urethral sphincter electromyography (baseline potentials, sacral reflex responses, response to voiding, or maneuvers to empty)
Neurologic examination
• Lower extremity strength, tone, reflexes, sensation, spontaneous movements
• Perineal tone and sensation
• Spine examination
Laboratory values
• Urine culture
• Serum creatinine after 5–7 days of life
Voiding cystourethrogram
• Bladder wall characteristics (trabeculation)
• Bladder neck appearance and pelvic floor position
• Vesicoureteral reflux—when during filling, grade and laterality
• Ability to empty
Nuclear scintigraphy
• DMSA scan if reflux is present
• Mag3 lasix renogram if hydronephrosis or hydroureteronephrosis is present

acceptable pressures. The normal bladder capacity at this age varies between 10 and 15 ml. Simultaneously, external sphincter electromyography is done using a 24 gauge concentric needle electrode placed in the external urethral sphincter to evaluate individual motor unit action potentials at rest, in response to various sacral stimuli, bladder filling, and emptying [10]. This is preferable to patch EMG electrodes placed perineally, as the latter only records the overall activity to filling and emptying of the bladder and does not provide any data about the characteristics of the bioelectric activity, which could be important in neurosurgical management of these patients. The most important findings include: end detrusor filling pressure that provides a measure of compliance, leak or voiding pressure, the presence of detrusor overactivity, and reactivity of the external urethral sphincter to a bladder contraction. This test answers the 2nd part of the question posed earlier and helps determine what type of treatment or further assessment, if any, should be instituted at this time.

Although still somewhat controversial [11–17] urodynamic testing in the newborn period provides important knowledge that includes: (1) an understanding of current knowledge of the lower urinary tract physiology; (2) a baseline assessment allowing for comparisons to be made if changes occur in either neurological or urologic function over time; (3) a degree of predictability for urinary tract deterioration if the child is managed expectantly; (4) a reason to initiate prophylactic therapy in infants who have a normal appearing upper urinary tract in order to prevent deterioration; and (5) an accurate picture to counsel parents about future bladder and sexual function [18].

Renal ultrasonography, often performed prior to urodynamic testing, is needed to determine size, position, and appearance of the kidneys, the collecting system, the distal ureters and bladder wall thickness to corroborate urodynamic findings and the need for early intervention. The kidneys are normal in 98 % of cases. Of all the potential anomalies, horseshoe kidneys have been the only reported abnormality with any consistency in the newborn period, but even that is rare. Historically, voiding cystography is undertaken only when renal ultrasonography suggests reflux or another abnormality, or the urodynamic study indicates the possibility of dyssynergy and/or vesicoureteral reflux (VUR) (Table 11.2) [19].

Although some clinicians rely solely on ultrasound and radiologic imaging to determine whether or not intervention should be undertaken [16], most centers now obtain urodynamic testing at this age and base management on the combination of findings from these studies [13, 18, 20, 21]. Two philosophies of management have emerged—expectant versus prophylactic therapy. The "observers" cite: (1) the incidence of deterioration is low; (2) any abnormality can be reversed if treatment is instituted after it occurs; (3) overall renal function is not impaired when comparing expectant to prophylactic treatment; (4) why subject the child and family to risks that might be unfounded; and (5) why subject parents to undertake CIC and be even more burdened when caring for their children than they truly need to be [15, 16, 22, 23]. "Interventionists" report, however, that prophylactic therapy begun in the newborn period has not been shown to harm any infant, does not place significant hardships on parents, and rarely leads to repeated UTI or other complications from catheterization or injury to the urethra [21, 24]. In fact, several bene-

Table 11.2 Indications for cystography (conventional/nuclear)	*Ultrasound*
	• Hydronephrosis-either static or changing throughout the exam
	• Discrepancy in kidney size or segmental parenchymal thinning
	• Increased bladder wall thickness
	Urodynamic studies
	• Poor compliance during filling (maximum detrusor pressure >25 cm H_2O)
	• High-pressure detrusor overactivity (>25 cm H2O)
	• High voiding pressure (>75 cm H_2O)
	• Dyssynergic sphincter activity at capacity or during voiding
	• Leak-point pressure (>75 cm H_2O) with/without complete sphincter denervation
	• Post-void residual >10 % of bladder capacity

fits are evident following initiation of CIC: ease in which children adjust to accepting it as they grow; ability to attain continence with less adjunctive medical and surgical measures; an earlier goal for achieving independence and self-management of the lower urinary tract; and reduced risk of renal function deterioration [25]. In addition, early intervention has resulted in a reduced need for augmentation cystoplasty that is now well documented [20, 26, 27].

Newborn Urodynamic Findings

Urodynamic studies in newborns have demonstrated unexpected results when compared to findings in older children, reflecting the dynamic nature of the neurological lesion in myelodysplasia. Bladder function classified using current International Children's Continence Society terminology [28] refers to "contractile" which denotes a voiding contraction occurring at capacity "during a cystometrogram, whereas "acontractile" implies no bladder contraction at all.

Of 225 newborns (Table 11.3) 63 % demonstrated a contractile bladder and 37 % did not. Of the latter, 20 % had good and 17 % poor compliance (end filling pressure at capacity of <40 cm H_2O) [29]. Electromyographic (EMG) assessment of the external urethral sphincter revealed intact sacral cord function with normal motor unit potentials and normal responses to sacral stimuli in 40 %, partial denervation of

Table 11.3 Urodynamic studies in 225 myelodysplastic newborns

Bladder function	
Contractile	63 %
Acontractile-poor compliance	17 %
Acontractile-good compliance	20 %
Sphincter innervation:	
Intact sacral reflex arc	40 %
Partial denervation	24 %
Complete denervation	36 %
Lower urinary tract function:	
Dyssynergy	37 %
Synergy	26 %
Complete denervation	36 %

The types of bladder function and sphincter innervation noted in 225 newborns with myelodysplasia who underwent urodynamic testing within the first month of life over the last 25 years at our institution. Combined lower urinary tract function refers to the response of the sphincter to bladder filling at the time capacity was reached. Complete denervation is applied to those infants with no bioelectric activity in the sphincter during needle electromyography the sphincter with variable sacral reflex responses in 24 %, and complete denervation with no electrical activity and no responses to sacral stimulation in 36 %.

Detrusor and urethral sphincter function can be integrated to denote reactivity of the latter in response to the contractility of the former. Synergy means quieting of the sphincter when the bladder contracts at capacity, whereas dyssynergy (DSD) implies the urethral sphincter activity increases in response to a bladder contraction or fails to relax as the bladder is filled to capacity or when leakage occurs. The incidence of synergy in our newborn series was 26 %, DSD occurred in 37 %, and complete denervation was seen in 36 % [29].

Initial Treatment

Initial management is predicated by the urodynamic findings as well as the state of the upper urinary tract (Table 11.4) [30–34]. No intervention is necessary with a synergic sphincter, complete emptying and normal kidneys. Similarly, no treatment is needed in the child with complete denervation, a low leak-point pressure, and sporadic but complete emptying. However, CIC is considered mandatory when a child has DSD because experience has shown expectant therapy alone often leads to bladder decompensation with poor compliance, hydroureteronephrosis and VUR, that is not always reversible with aggressive subsequent management (Fig. 11.1). Additionally, augmentation cystoplasty is needed much more often if aggressive management is not undertaken early, as muscular thickening and inelasticity progress from continued high bladder outlet resistance associated with DSD [20, 26]. New renal damage demonstrated by dimercaptosuccinic acid (DMSA) renal scans has provided another paramount reason for intervening early, as reversibility of renal injury from high-pressure VUR and recurrent urinary UTI rarely occurs once it is established [5].

As noted earlier, spinal shock following meningocele repair occurs in up to 10 % of newborns [35, 36]. Its presence is denoted on urodynamic testing—an underactive detrusor (unsustained or acontractile bladder) and no reactivity of the urethral sphincter muscle to sacral stimuli despite normal potentials. In other instances, complete denervation of the urethral sphincter and an acontractile detrusor are present; this leads to poor bladder emptying. Despite low filling and leak point pressures, when emptying is incomplete, CIC is initiated but only continued until the bladder regains its contractility and complete emptying occurs. The time to resolution is

Table 11.4 Management based on urodynamic findings

No intervention (Observation)	Minimal intervention (CIC only)	More involved intervention (CIC + anticholinergic meds)
Synergic voiding with complete emptying	Dyssynergy	DSD + poor compliance
Low LPP 2° denervation fibrosis	Reflux ≤ grade 2	DSD + poor compliance + reflux ≥ grade 3

UDS Findings in
225 Myelodysplastic Newborns

- **Bladder function**

Contractile	63%
Acontractile - poor compliance	17%
Acontractile - good compliance	20%

- **Sphincter innervation**

Intact sacral reflex arc	40%
Partial denervation	24%
Complete denervation	36%

- **Lower urinary tract function**

Dyssynergy	37%
Synergy	26%
Complete denervation	36%

Fig. 11.1 Comparison made of the response in those 225 infants followed postnatally with either expectant (71) or prophylactic (122) therapy, excluding 32 children who already had deterioration of their urinary tract at the time of birth, presumably from the prenatal effects of increased bladder outlet resistance. With permission from: Corcos J, Ginsberg D, Karsenty G. Textbook of the Neurogenic Bladder, 3rd ed. Chapter 56: Initial Management of Meningomyelocele Children. CRC Press, 2015 © Taylor and Francis

variable, but spinal shock may last up to 2–4 weeks after surgery [36]. Prophylactic antibiotics are administered during the first few weeks after CIC is initiated so as to minimize the threat of UTI while parents are adjusting to catheterization.

When spinal shock is not the issue and DSD is noted, CIC is begun in earnest as a permanent means of emptying the bladder to avoid the potentially hazardous effects of high voiding or leak-point pressures that lead to upper urinary tract damage [25] and to the creation of an inelastic thick-walled bladder over time [26, 37].

If the initial urodynamic studyreveals poor detrusor compliance with end filling pressure exceeding 20 cm H_2O, detrusor overactivity with pressures exceeding 50 cm H_2O, or voiding pressures greater than 80 cm H_2O, anticholinergic medication is begun as an adjunct to CIC (Fig. 11.2) [23, 33, 38, 39]. Oxybutynin HCl available in liquid form allows easy titration based on the child's age and/or weight. Dosing is based on 1 mg/year of age bid or tid, proportioned for children under 1 year as 0.1 mg at birth, increased by 0.1 mg each 5 weeks thereafter until age 1 year and by 0.25 mg each 3 months after that (Fig. 11.3) [40]. Side effects from this dosage schedule have been minimal, with facial flushing as the most likely observed symptom; no long-term sequelae have been noted affecting the gastrointestinal tract or the cardiovascular system. The incidence of urinary tract deterioration is low (15 %) in these proactively treated children, and substantially lower than the 38 % of children treated expectantly during the same time period (Figs. 11.4 and 11.5) [31].

Credé voiding to empty the bladder is to be avoided on a routine basis. It may be effective in young babies when the bladder remains an abdominal organ, but as children age and the pelvis deepens, the bladder descends more into the pelvis, reducing this maneuver's effectiveness. More importantly, it should only be used

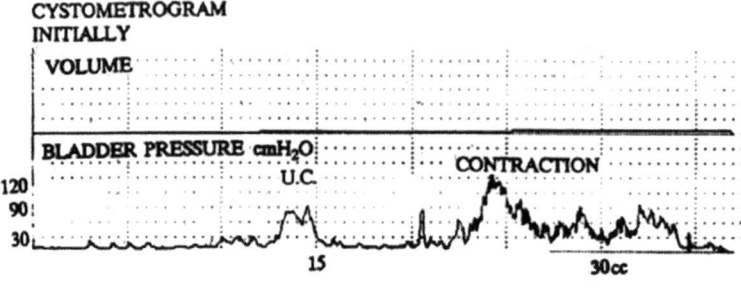

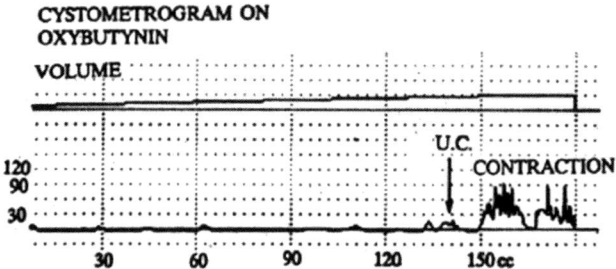

Fig. 11.2 Effect of oxybutynin HCl administered orally (according to dosing noted in the text) on bladder function for infants with increased bladder outlet resistance showing a reduction in uninhibited bladder activity at the time of birth, presumably from the prenatal effects of increased bladder outlet resistance. With permission from: Corcos J, Ginsberg D, Karsenty G. Textbook of the Neurogenic Bladder, 3rd ed. Chapter 56: Initial Management of Meningomyelocele Children. CRC Press, 2015 © Taylor and Francis

when the external urethral sphincter is not reactive to sacral stimuli [41], for under these conditions there is no corresponding increase in activity (nor any increase in urethral resistance) when the bladder is "emptied" in this manner. In contrast, a reactive sphincter muscle tightens in response to any increase in abdominal pressure causing bladder outlet resistance to rise, resulting in high pressure "voiding" as the bladder is emptied (Fig. 11.6).

Vesicoureteral Reflux

The incidence of vesicoureteral reflux (VUR) varies between 3 and 5 % in newborns with myelodysplasia, usually found in association with poor detrusor compliance, detrusor overactivity, and/or DSD [5, 42], the probable result of 2 or more months of in utero voiding against a tightening sphincter [31]. When VUR is detected, additional treatment measures are instituted based on the severity of the reflux. The higher the grade, the more that intervention is necessary. For grades I or II, just CIC is begun. Higher grades may require anticholinergic medication, based on urodynamic assessment. Prophylactic antibiotics are either initiated or

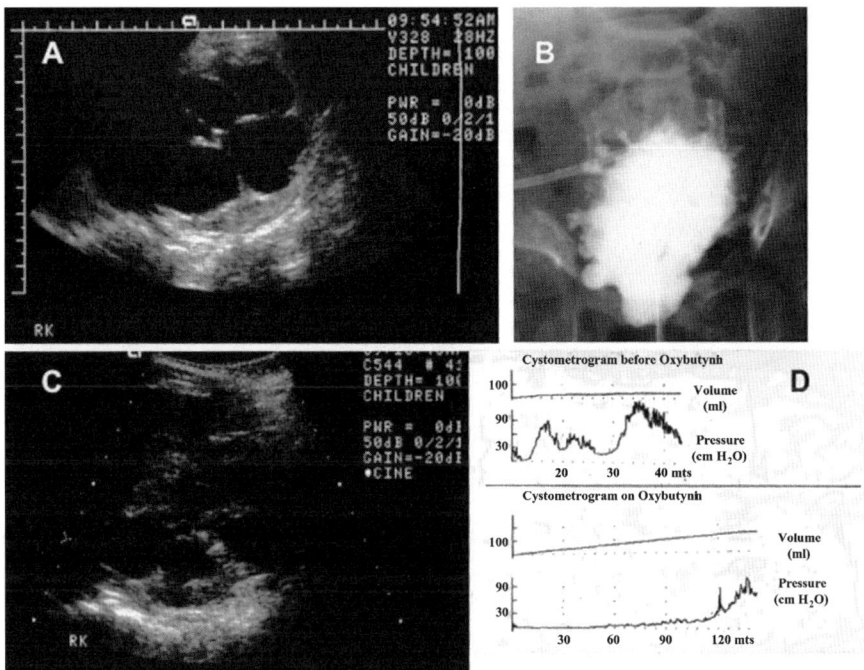

Fig. 11.3 Ultrasound of the right kidney (**A**), voiding cystogram (**B**), and urodynamic study (**D**) in a 1-year-old girl with detrusor-sphincter dyssynergy. Note severe right hydronephrosis caused by high filling pressures despite the absence of reflux. Once treatment with CIC and oxybutynin were begun the right kidney improved (**C**), but did not completely resolve its hydronephrosis at the time of birth, presumably from the prenatal effects of increased bladder outlet resistance. With permission from: Corcos J, Ginsberg D, Karsenty G. Textbook of the Neurogenic Bladder, 3rd ed. Chapter 56: Initial Management of Meningomyelocele Children. CRC Press, 2015 © Taylor and Francis

continued on a regular basis for all grades higher than grade I. A DMSA renal scan is advisable with grades ≥III reflux to determine the likely presence and extent of parenchymal damage secondary to the VUR [43]. Knowing whether or not renal damage has occurred as a result of in utero high pressure voiding associated with bladder-sphincter dyssynergy during this critical time in development of the kidney is paramount to insuring that no further injury takes place.

If the initial cystometrogram demonstrates poor compliance, high-pressure overactive contractions (>25 cm H$_2$O), or high voiding pressures (>75 cm H$_2$O), anticholinergic medication is begun, if not started already, so as to lower intravesical pressure and minimize the VUR [25, 32, 38, 42, 44]. Dosing of oxybutynin (as noted earlier) is administered thrice daily to maximize its effectiveness in these conditions.

For those children receiving expectant therapy (based on our criteria) urine cultures are obtained twice a year, whereas those on CIC with or without VUR, cultures are necessary every 4 months, or when symptoms suggesting an infection are

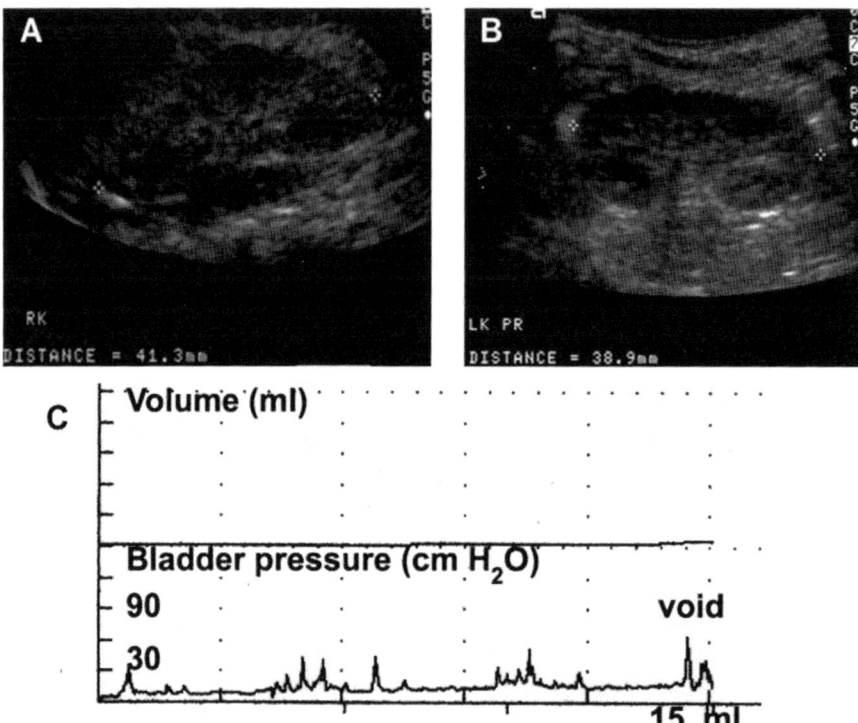

Fig. 11.4 This newborn boy with a lumbar level myelodysplasia had normal kidneys (**A**, **B**) and a benign urodynamic study initially (**C**) with low filling and voiding pressures and complete denervation in the sphincter (not shown) at the time of birth, presumably from the prenatal effects of increased bladder outlet resistance. With permission from: Corcos J, Ginsberg D, Karsenty G. Textbook of the Neurogenic Bladder, 3rd ed. Chapter 56: Initial Management of Meningomyelocele Children. CRC Press, 2015 © Taylor and Francis

present. If hydroureteronephrosis is evident on ultrasonography, it should be repeated 6 months later to determine resolution. Otherwise, sonography is repeated at age 1 and yearly thereafter. Urodynamic testing is repeated at 6 months if the child has been given anticholinergic medication due to poor compliance with or without VUR, and yearly thereafter. For those with VUR, video urodynamics or simultaneous nuclear cystography/cystometrography is performed to denote (1) the continued presence of VUR and its grade, and (2) the efficacy of anticholinergic medication in lowering detrusor pressure and improving the grade of reflux.

The indications for antireflux surgery are similar to those in normal children: recurrent breakthrough febrile UTI despite continuous antibiotics; persistent high-grade reflux (>III) despite improvement in detrusor compliance and/or overactivity with anticholinergic medication; failure of renal growth on serial ultrasounds; development or progression of renal scarring on subsequent DMSA studies; and the need to perform bladder outlet surgery to improve urinary continence [45, 46]. Excellent success rates for reflux resolution have been achieved when surgery is

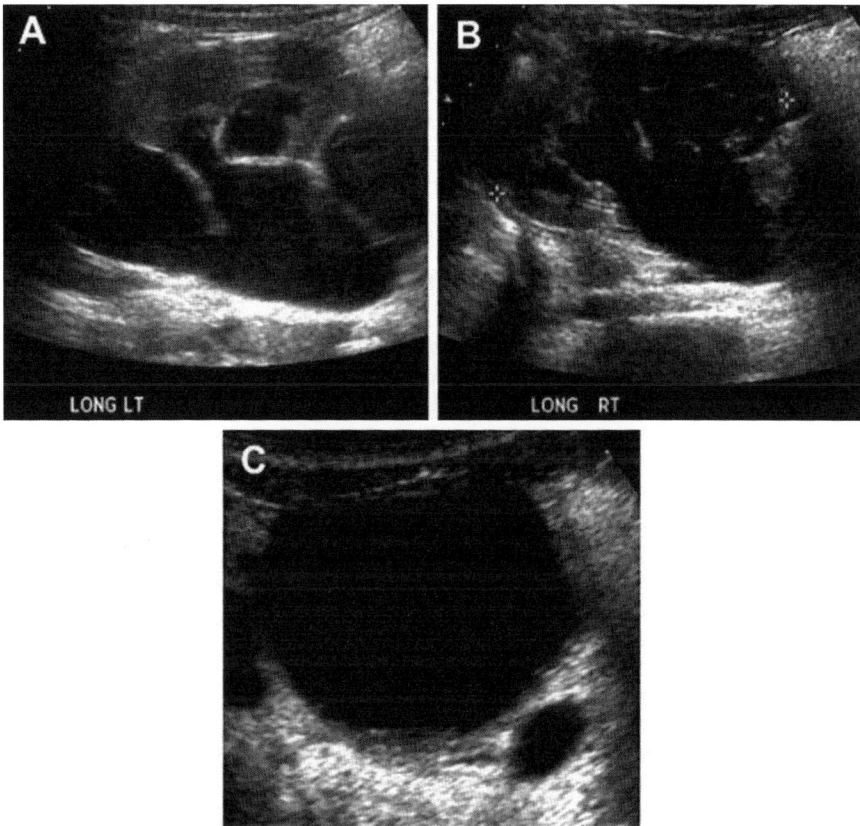

Fig. 11.5 At 1 year of age this same boy had a urinary tract infection and his ultrasound now reveal bilateral hydronephrosis (**A, B**) with a dilated right ureter extending down to the bladder (**C**). A voiding cystogram demonstrated grade 5/5 reflux bilaterally (**D**), narrowing in the region of the external urethral sphincter (**E**), and a markedly hypertonic bladder (**F**). His EMG revealed reinnervation of the sphincter with concomitant dyssynergy at capacity (not shown) at the time of birth, presumably from the prenatal effects of increased bladder outlet resistance. With permission from: Corcos J, Ginsberg D, Karsenty G. Textbook of the Neurogenic Bladder, 3rd ed. Chapter 56: Initial Management of Meningomyelocele Children. CRC Press, 2015 © Taylor and Francis

combined with anticholinergic medication and CIC to insure low detrusor filling pressure and complete emptying [47, 48]. Cross-trigonal versus ureteral advancement or extravesical techniques is probably preferable as some of these children may eventually need bladder outlet surgery to achieve dryness later in life.

Endoscopic management of VUR has become increasingly popular in recent years, thus lowering the threshold for correcting reflux in these children (Fig. 11.7). However, long-term efficacy of bulking agents has not been clearly established [49, 50]. The risk of recurrence of reflux, especially when the disease process is dynamic,

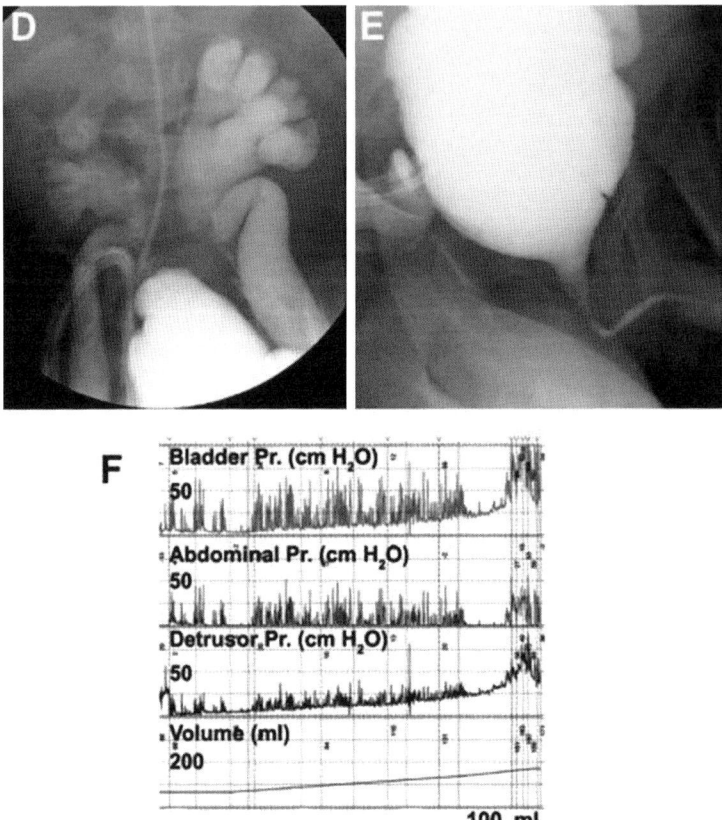

Fig. 11.5 (continued)

is unknown. Therefore, caution regarding its use in patients with neuropathic bladders is advised.

Again, Credé voiding to empty the bladder should be avoided in babies who have a reactive external urethral sphincter as the increased "voiding" pressure generated by a reactive sphincter may lead to more injury from the reflux [41].

Vesicostomy Drainage

Before CIC was considered a safe undertaking in early infancy, vesicostomy drainage was frequently employed to drain the bladder, especially in those with VUR and/or hydronephrosis [51, 52]. In recent times, fewer vesicostomies have been performed, mostly in children whose parents are unable to adhere to a regular catheterization

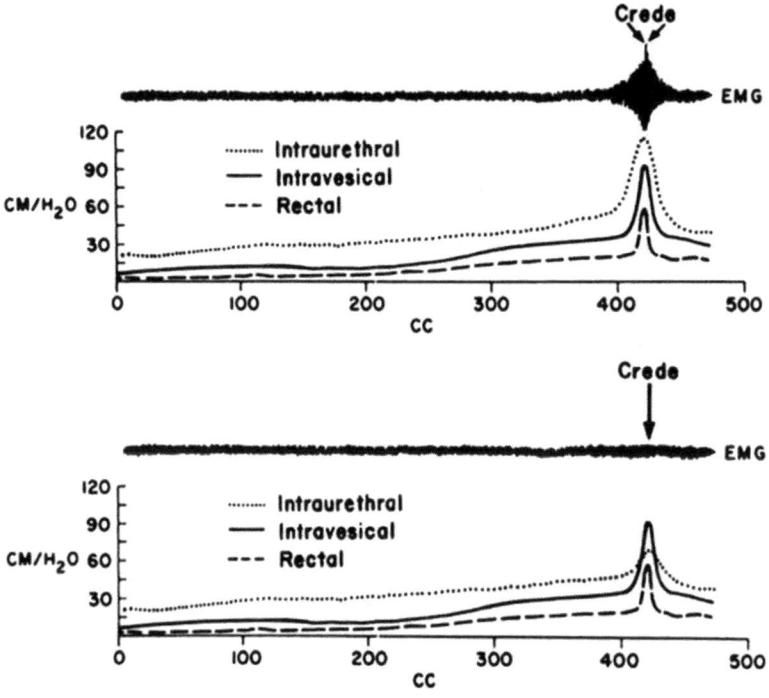

Fig. 11.6 When the urethral sphincter is reactive to sacral reflexes a Credé maneuver can lead to increases in abdominal pressure and high pressure "voiding" (upper tracing). When the sphincter is extensively denervated, however, there is no corresponding reaction to a Credé maneuver so bladder outlet resistance does not change (lower tracing). Thus, it is relatively safe to perform, at the time of birth, presumably from the prenatal effects of increased bladder outlet resistance. With permission from: Corcos J, Ginsberg D, Karsenty G. Textbook of the Neurogenic Bladder, 3rd ed. Chapter 56: Initial Management of Meningomyelocele Children. CRC Press, 2015 © Taylor and Francis

schedule, or who experience urethral injury, or for those who exhibit a poorly compliant or markedly overactive detrusor unresponsive to anticholinergic medication in the face of high-grade VUR and/or hydronephrosis [53]. It is applicable when there is no ureterovesical junction obstruction. Vesicostomy should be considered as only a temporary measure to drain the bladder due to the difficulty in maintaining a collecting bag over the ostomy site as the child grows too big for diapers. As the child approaches 3–4 years of age it should be reversed and CIC and drug therapy instituted. It is difficult to predict preoperatively the outcome from closing the vesicostomy, so repeat cystography and urodynamic study are necessary shortly after it is done. Definitive antireflux surgery and/or augmentation cystoplasty may be needed at some point after this "undiversion," as the vesicostomy rarely improves the underlying bladder dysfunction.

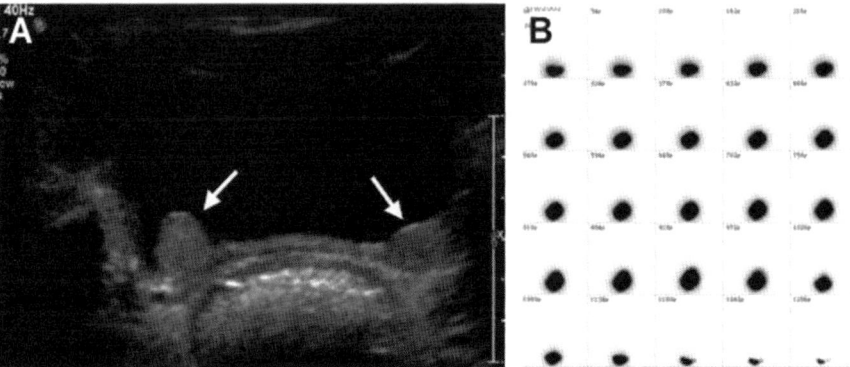

Fig. 11.7 Following Deflux injected into each ureteral orifice in the boy shown in Fig. 11.6 a mound can be seen (*arrows*) surrounding each intramural ureter (**A**), while no reflux is noted during a postinjection nuclear cystogram (**B**) at the time of birth, presumably from the prenatal effects of increased bladder outlet resistance. With permission from: Corcos J, Ginsberg D, Karsenty G. Textbook of the Neurogenic Bladder, 3rd ed. Chapter 56: Initial Management of Meningomyelocele Children. CRC Press, 2015 © Taylor and Francis

Neurological Changes

From longitudinal assessments of children with myelodysplasia over the last 20 years it is apparent that the neurological injury in myelodysplasia is not a static lesion but rather a dynamic disease process (Fig. 11.8) [54]. Comparing prenatal closure findings of sacral cord function with those of similar children whose spinal defects were closed after birth [2] and the finding that early infancy neuro-urologic function does not always correlate with what is seen in later life on X-ray imaging and urodynamic studies, there is strong evidence that as the fetus or infant grows, secondary injury to the spinal cord occurs over time. Sometimes a change in neuro-urologic function is the primary reason for failure of initial management. A 19 % incidence of change during the first several years of life has been noted, with most of the changes occurring in the first 2–3 years [55].

The change in neurological function is not confined to just one specific level of lesion [56, 57]. In addition, a 32 % risk for deterioration over several years was seen in newborns with normal urodynamic findings (Fig. 11.9) [58]. Therefore, vigilance is the key to following these children, noting any changes and referring them for neurosurgical assessment when the possibility of neuro-urologic function is suspected. Repeating urodynamic studies routinely in those children with normal or almost normal bladder and sphincter function and those who demonstrate either a change in urinary and/or fecal continence, upper urinary tract drainage, recurrent UTI or alterations in lower extremity neurological examinations, especially if there is no change in the degree of hydrocephalus or a malfunction of the shunt, is mandatory. Any urodynamic change that cannot be explained otherwise warrants referral to neurosurgery.

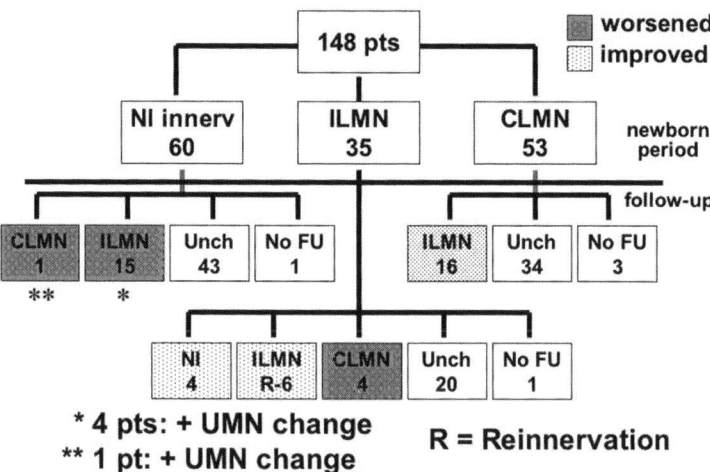

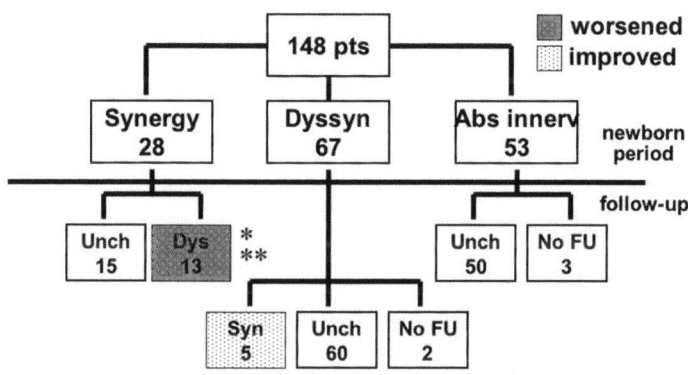

Fig. 11.8 The flowchart emphasizes the changing neurologic lesion involving (a) lower motor neuron (sacral reflex) and (b) upper motor neuron (spinal cord) function in newborns with myelodysplasia over time. *ILMN* incomplete lower motor neuron, *CLMN* complete lower neuron, *UMN* upper motor neuron, *Nl* normal, *innerv* innervation, *Unch* unchanged, *Abs innerv* absent sphincter activity (complete denervation), *FU* follow-up, *Dyssyn or Dys* dyssynergy, *Syn* synergy at the time of birth, presumably from the prenatal effects of increased bladder outlet resistance. With permission from: Corcos J, Ginsberg D, Karsenty G. Textbook of the Neurogenic Bladder, 3rd ed. Chapter 56: Initial Management of Meningomyelocele Children. CRC Press, 2015 © Taylor and Francis

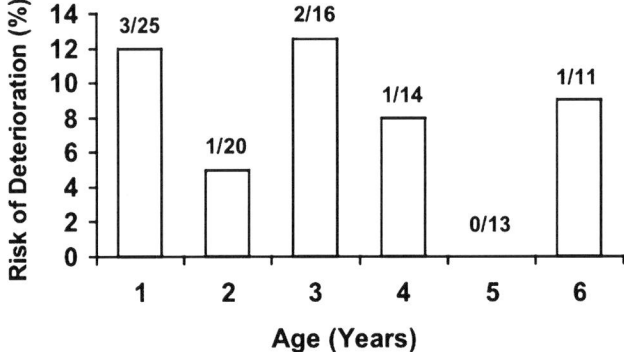

Fig. 11.9 Risk of deterioration with increasing age in 25 newborns with myelodysplasia who had normal urodynamic findings and normal neurologic exams at birth. The denominator above each column refers to the number of infants at risk while the numerator refers to those who actually changed at that particular age, at the time the analysis was undertaken. Once a child deteriorated he/she was not included in those at risk for neurologic deterioration the following year, at the time of birth, presumably from the prenatal effects of increased bladder outlet resistance. With permission from: Corcos J, Ginsberg D, Karsenty G. Textbook of the Neurogenic Bladder, 3rd ed. Chapter 56: Initial Management of Meningomyelocele Children. CRC Press, 2015 © Taylor and Francis

Table 11.5 Surveillance of measured parameters/tests after initial evaluation

Parameter/test	Type of urodynamic finding		
	Complete denervation	Normal bladder/ sphincter function	Dyssynergy ± detrusor overactivity
Residual urine	2–3×/year	2–3×/year	N/A
Urine C/S	2–3×/year	2–3×/year	2–3×/year
Renal ECHO	Yearly	Yearly	Yearly
Urodynamic study	Age 1	Yearly till 6 years	Only to evaluate effectiveness of therapy
Cystography (VCUG/ nuclear)	Only if UTI	Only if UTI	Yearly, to follow progression of reflux
DMSA (high grade reflux)	Biennial	Biennial	Biennial

Subsequent Surveillance

Surveillance depends on several factors: the neuro-urologic findings in the early newborn period, the type of intervention undertaken, if any, and the potential for neurological and/or urologic change over time (Table 11.5). If a child has a complete lower motor neuron lesion with no bioelectric activity in the sphincter, a good compliant bladder with low filling and leak-point pressure at capacity, little residual, and a normal renal ultrasound, he or she can be followed expectantly. Periodic residual urine measurements with urine cultures about 2–3 times a year and yearly renal ultrasounds for the first several years after birth are all that is necessary until it is time to attempt to achieve continence. When reinnervation of the external urethral sphincter does occur (25 %), it produces increased bladder outlet resistance in the form of DSD. Denervation fibrosis of the external sphincter can occur in 21 % resulting in increased urethral resistance leading to increased residual urine [59]. Any change in PVR, development of recurrent UTI, ureteral dilation and or hydronephrosis on ultrasonography warrants further investigation with repeat urodynamic studies to determine its cause, as well as voiding cystography or isotope renography, (depending on the new findings) to denote its consequence.

If the child has normal bladder and external urethral sphincter function with a good compliant bladder early in filling, a normal voiding contraction at capacity with normal pressure, normal or only partial denervation in the sphincter with normal sacral reflexes and detrusor-sphincter synergy, and normal kidneys on ultrasound, then a residual urine volume with urine cultures twice a year and a yearly renal ultrasound and urodynamic study are recommended to insure a stable neurological picture. Both upper (detrusor overactivity and/or DSD) as well as, lower (acontractility and/or sphincter denervation) motor neuron deterioration is possible. The earlier it is detected, the greater the likelihood that detrusor and external urethral sphincter function can be reversed or preserved with secondary spinal cord untethering [60].

A repeat urodynamic study is warranted if the clinician needs to know (1) the effectiveness of anticholinergic medication after it has been started, (2) why an increase in residual urine has occurred if the child has been voiding spontaneously to completion previously, (3) the reason for a change in the child's level of continence, (4) what effect recurrent UTI has had on detrusor muscle compliance and contractility, and (5) what may have caused an increase in collecting system dilation on radiological imaging. As noted, external urethral sphincter EMG should be repeated as part of the urodynamic study if there is any apparent change in lower extremity function, an increase in detrusor leak-point pressure and/or residual urine, a change in the level of urinary and/or fecal continence, or an increase in or new onset of upper urinary tract dilation, for these signs might suggest either reinnervation of the external urethral sphincter, with or without the development of detrusor sphincter dyssynergy or deterioration in sphincter function, which results in increasing wetness from loss of sphincter function [61].

Depending on the change that is noted, various treatment measures will need to be started [62]. If the child has new onset or worsening detrusor overactivity, a poorly compliant bladder with high leak-point pressure, detrusor-sphincter dyssynergy or a nonrelaxing sphincter at capacity, elevated residual urine after a spontaneous void, hydronephrosis and/or dilated ureter(s), more rigorous CIC and more aggressive medical therapy is undertaken. On the other hand, when further denervation occurs and bladder outlet resistance is lowered resulting in increased incontinence, more frequent catheterization along with alpha sympathomimetic agents may be attempted. However, it is likely that surgery will be required to achieve continence. When surgery is indicated (open or endoscopic treatment of VUR, vesicostomy, bladder outlet) follow-up is predicated on what has been instituted. Surveillance with urine cultures and residual urine measurements at least twice a year and renal ultrasonography yearly is usually the minimum standard of follow-up [62].

Nuclear or voiding cystography is indicated on a yearly basis to follow children with high grade VUR (just as one would do for children with normal lower urinary tract function) or if there is a change in function on the urodynamic study, dilation of the upper urinary tract on renal ultrasonography, or recurrent febrile UTI that warrants a repeat study. Renal scintigraphy with DMSA is helpful in detecting any upper urinary tract deterioration in those children with recurrent UTI, persistent high-grade VUR, new onset of hypertension or deterioration in lower urinary tract function on urodynamic studies that predisposes them to kidney damage. Currently, some clinicians are recommending baseline DMSA scanning in infancy for those with any upper urinary tract abnormality and periodically for the child with recurrent infection or stable but persistent hydronephrosis as a means to stave off progressive renal failure that is being seen with increasing regularity as more of these children survive and transition into adulthood [43].

Serum creatinine measurements have not been a useful tool for either the initial assessment or subsequent follow-up because these children have diminished muscle mass development compared to normally ambulatory children in addition to the test not being an accurate way to detect early changes in renal function. However, an initial serum creatinine level may be helpful when juxtaposed against later measurements in those children who have repeated UTI in the face of VUR, persistent hydronephrosis and/or kidneys that do not grow with advancing age [25]. Glomerular filtration rates are more apt to accurately show subtle changes in function much earlier than serum creatinine values would.

Conclusion

Advances in the evaluation and management of the child with myelodysplasia have been nothing short of miraculous during the last 35 years [61]. One could sum up the entire management philosophy of years ago into a couple of phrases—*watchful waiting*, or *urinary diversion* in those with any signs of deterioration or just the presence of myelodysplasia. The advent of CIC, the development of numerous drugs that modulate lower urinary tract function and minimally invasive therapies have profoundly altered the way these children are initially assessed and treated at the current time. There is still some controversy whether or not proactive treatment versus careful surveillance with rapid initiation of therapy when a change takes place is the correct method of treatment. The important outcome, however, is that the children are receiving a substantially higher level of urologic care that they did in the 1960s and 1970s. Their quality of life, their overall kidney health, and their ability to integrate into and become functional in society are clearly much better than they were in the past [5, 8].

References

1. Adzick NS, Thom EA, Spong CY, Brock III JW, Burrows PK, Johnson MP, et al. A randomized trial of prenatal versus postnatal repair of myelomeningocele. N Engl J Med. 2011;364:993–1004.
2. Koh CJ, DeFilippo RE, Borer JG, Khoshbin S, Bauer SB. Bladder and external urethral sphincter function after prenatal closure of myelomeningocele. J Urol. 2006;176:2232–6.
3. Lee NG, Gomez P, Uberoi V, Kokorowski PJ, Khoshbin S, Bauer SB, et al. In utero closure of myelomeningocele does not improve lower urinary tract function. J Urol. 2012;188:1567–71.
4. Kroovand RL, Bell W, Hart LJ, Benfeld KY. The effect of back closure on detrusor function in neonates with myelodysplasia. J Urol. 1990;144:423–5.
5. Chiaramonte RM, Horowitz EM, Kaplan GA, Brock WA. Implications of hydronephrosis in newborns with myelodysplasia. J Urol. 1986;136:427–9.
6. Bauer SB, Labib KB, Dieppa RA, Retik AB. Urodynamic evaluation in a boy with myelodysplasia and incontinence. Urology. 1977;10:354–62.
7. Bauer SB, Austin PF, Rawashdeh YF, de Jong TP, Franco I, Siggard C, et al. International Children's Continence Society's recommendations for initial diagnostic evaluation and follow-up in congenital neuropathic bladder and bowel dysfunction in children. Neurourol Urodyn. 2012;31:610–4.
8. Frimberger D, Cheng E, Kropp BP. The current management of the neurogenic bladder in children with spina bifida. Pediatr Clin North Am. 2012;59:757–67.
9. Joseph DB. The effect of medium-fill and slow-fill cystometry on bladder pressure in infants and children with myelodysplasia. J Urol. 1992;147:444–6.
10. Blaivas JG, Labib KB, Bauer SB, Retik AB. A new approach to elec-tromyography of the external urethral sphincter. J Urol. 1977;117:773–7.
11. McGuire EJ, Woodside. JR, Borden TA, Weiss RM. The prognostic value of urodynamic testing in myelodysplastic patients. J Urol. 1981;126:205–9.
12. Bauer SB, Hallet M, Khoshbin S, Lebowitz RL, Winston KR, Gibson S, et al. The predictive value of urodynamic evaluation in the newborn with myelodysplasia. JAMA. 1984;152:650–2.
13. Sidi AA, Dykstra DD, Gonzalez R. The value of urodynamic testing in the management of neonates with myelodysplasia: a prospective study. J Urol. 1986;135:90–3.
14. Perez LM, Khoury J, Webster GD. The value of urodynamic studies in infants less than one year old with congenital spinal dysraphism. J Urol. 1992;148:584–7.
15. Teichman JMH, Scherz HC, Kim KD, Cho DH, Packer MG, Kaplan GW. An alternative approach to myelodysplasia management: aggressive observation and prompt intervention. J Urol. 1994;152:807–11.
16. Hopps CV, Kropp KA. Preservation of renal function in children with myelomeningocele managed with basic newborn evaluation and close followup. J Urol. 2003;169:305–8.
17. Snodgrass WT, Gargollo PC. Urologic care of the neurogenic bladder in children. Urol Clin North Am. 2010;37:207–14.

18. Bauer SB. Myelodysplasia: newborn evaluation and management. In: McLaurin RL, editor. Spina bifida: a multidisciplinary approach. New York: Praeger; 1984. p. 262–7.
19. Kopp C, Greenfield SP. Effects of neurogenic bladder dysfunction in utero seen in neonates with myelodysplasia. Br J Urol. 1993;71:739–42.
20. Wu H-Y, Baskin LS, Kogan BA. Neurogenic bladder dysfunction due to myelomeningocele: neonatal versus childhood treatment. J Urol. 1997;157:2295–7.
21. Kurzrock EA, Polse S. Renal deterioration in myelodysplastic children: urodynamic evaluation and clinical correlates. J Urol. 1998;159:1657–61.
22. Klose AG, Sackett CK, Mesrobian H-GJ. Management of children with myelodysplasia. Urologic alternatives. J Urol. 1990;144:1446–9.
23. Tanaka H, Kakizaki H, Kobayashi S, Shibata T, Ameda K, Koyanagi T, et al. The relevance of urethral resistance in children with myelodysplasia: its impact on upper urinary tract deterioration and the outcome of conservative management. J Urol. 1999;161:929–32.
24. Joseph DB, Bauer SB, Colodny AH, Mandell J, Retik AB. Clean intermittent catheterization in infants with neurogenic bladder. Pediatrics. 1989;84:78–83.
25. Kari JA, Safdar O, Jamjoom R, Anshasi W. Renal involvement in children with spina bifida. Saudi J Kidney Dis Transpl. 2009;20:102–5.
26. Kaefer M, Pabby A, Kelly M, Darbey M, Bauer SB, et al. Improved bladder function after prophylactic treatment of the high risk neurogenic bladder in newborns with myelomeningocele. J Urol. 1999;162:1068–71.
27. Bauer SB. Early evaluation and management of children with spina bifida. In: King LR, editor. Urologic surgery in neonates and young infants. Philadelphia: WB Saunders; 1988. p. 252–64.
28. Austin PF, Bauer SB, Bower W, Chase J, Franco I, Hoebeke P, et al. The standardization of terminology of lower urinary tract function in children and adolescents: update report from the Standardization Committee of the International Children's Continence Society. J Urol. 2014;191:1863–5.
29. Bauer SB. Neuropathic dysfunction of the lower urinary tract. In: Wein AJ, Kavoussi LR, Novick AC, Partin AW, Peters CA, editors. Campbell-walsh urology. 9th ed. Philadelphia: Saunders Elsevier; 2006. p. 3625–55.
30. van Gool JD, Dik P, de Jong TP. Bladder-sphincter dysfunction in myelomeningocele. Eur J Pediatr. 2001;160:414–20.
31. Bauer SB. The management of spina bifida from birth onwards. In: Whitaker RH, Woodard JR, editors. Paediatric urology. London: Butterworths; 1985. p. 87–112.
32. Edelstein RA, Bauer SB, Kelly MD, Darbey MM, Peters CA, Atala A, et al. The long-term urologic response of neonates with myelodysplasia treated proactively with intermittent catheterization and anticholinergic therapy. J Urol. 1995;154:1500–4.
33. Dik P, van Gool JD, de Jong-de Vos van Steenwijk CC, de Jong TP. Early start therapy preserves kidney function in spina bifida patients. Eur Urol. 2006;49:908–13.
34. Seki N, Masuda K, Kinukawa N, Senoh K, Naito S. Risk factors for febrile urinary tract infection in children with myelodysplasia treated by clean intermittent catheterization. Int J Urol. 2004;11:973–7.
35. Van Gool JD, Juijten RH, Donckerwolcke RA, Kramer PP. Detrusor- sphincter dyssynergia in children with myelomeningocele: a prospective study. Z Kinderchir. 1982;37:148–51.
36. Stoneking BJ, Brock JW, Pope JC, Adams MC. Early evolution of bladder emptying after myelomeningocele closure. Urology. 2001;58:767–71.
37. Ghoniem GM, Roach MB, Lewis VH, Harmon EP. The value of leak point pressure and bladder compliance in the urodynamic evaluation of myelomeningocele patients. J Urol. 1990;144:1440–2.
38. Geranoitis E, Koff SA, Enrile B. Prophylactic use of clean intermittent catheterization in treatment of infants and young children with myelomeningocele and neurogenic bladder dysfunction. J Urol. 1988;139:85–6.
39. Landau EH, Churchill BM, Jayanthi VR, Gilmour RF, Steckler RE, McLorie GA, et al. The sensitivity of pressure specific bladder volume versus total bladder capacity as a measure of bladder storage dysfunction. J Urol. 1994;152:1578–81.

40. Kasabian NG, Bauer SB, Dyro FM, Colodny AH, Mandell J, Retik AB. The prophylactic value of clean intermittent catheterization and anticholinergic medication in newborns and infants with myelodysplasia at risk of developing urinary tract deterioration. Am J Dis Child. 1992;146:840–3.
41. Barbalais GA, Klauber GT, Blaivas JG. Critical evaluation of the Credé maneuver: a urodynamic study of 207 patients. J Urol. 1983;130:720–8.
42. Flood HD, Ritchey ML, Bloom DA, Huang C, McGuire EJ. Outcome of reflux in children with myelodysplasia managed by bladder pressure monitoring. J Urol. 1994;152:1574–7.
43. Stein DR, Gordon CM, Feldman HA, Hobbs NM, Bauer SB, Baum MB. Chronic kidney disease in children with myelodysplasia/spina bifida. Poster presentation, Pediatric Academic Societies; 2011. (Abstract # 752298).
44. Agarwal SK, McLorie GA, Grewal D, Joyner BD, Bägli DJ, Khoury AE, et al. Urodynamic correlates of resolution of reflux meningomyelocele patients. J Urol. 1997;158:580–2.
45. Bauer SB, Colodny AH, Retik AB. The management of vesico-ureteral reflux in children with myelodysplasia. J Urol. 1982;128:102–5.
46. Kaplan WE, Firlit CF. Management of reflux in myelodysplastic children. J Urol. 1983;129:1195–7.
47. Jeffs RD, Jones P, Schillinger JF. Surgical correction of vesico-ureteral reflux in children with neurogenic bladder. J Urol. 1976;115:449–55.
48. Kass EJ, Koff SA, Lapides J. Fate of vesico-ureteral reflux in children with neuropathic bladders managed by intermittent catheterization. J Urol. 1981;125:63–4.
49. Schlussel R. Cystoscopic correction of reflux. Curr Urol Rep. 2004;5:127–31.
50. Elder JS, Diaz M, Caldamone AA, Cendron M, Greenfield S, Hurwitz R. Endoscopic therapy for vesicoureteral reflux: meta-analysis. I. Reflux resolution and urinary tract infection. J Urol. 2006;175:716–22.
51. Duckett JW. Cutaneous vesicostomy in childhood. Urol Clin North Am. 1974;1:485–95.
52. Mandell J, Bauer SB, Colodny AH, Retik AB. Cutaneous vesicostomy in infancy. J Urol. 1981;126:92–3.
53. Morrisroe SN, O'Connor RC, Nanigian DK, Kurzrock EA, Stone AR. Vesicostomy revisited: the best treatment for the hostile bladder in myelodysplastic children? BJU Int. 2005;96:397–400.
54. Spindel MR, Bauer SB, Dyro FM, Krarup C, Khoshbin S, Winston KR, et al. The changing neuro-urologic lesion in myelodysplasia. JAMA. 1987;258:1630–3.
55. Lais A, Kasabian NG, Dyro FM, Scott RM, Kelly MD, Bauer SB. Neurosurgical implications of continuous neuro-urological surveillance of children with myelodysplasia. J Urol. 1993;150:1879–83.
56. Dator DP, Hatchett L, Dyro EM, Shefner JM, Bauer SB. Urodynamic dysfunction in walking myelodysplastic children. J Urol. 1992;148:362–5.
57. Pontari MA, Keating M, Kelly MD, Dyro F, Bauer SB. Retained sacral function in children with high level myelodysplasia. J Urol. 1995;154:775–7.
58. Tarcan T, Bauer S, Olmedo E, Koshbin S, Kelly M, Darbey M. Long-term follow-up of newborns with myelodysplasia and normal urodynamic findings: is it necessary? J Urol. 2001;165:564–7.
59. Mandell J, Lebowitz RL, Hallett M, Khoshbin S, Bauer SB. Urethral narrowing in region of external sphincter: radiologic urodynamic correlations in boys with myelodysplasia. Am J Roentgenol. 1980;134:731–5.
60. Bauer SB. The value of needle EMG in open and occult spinal dysraphisms. Vanderbilt Children's Hospital Lecture. Accessed 6 Mar 2015.
61. Bauer SB. The management of the myelodysplastic child: a paradigm shift. BJU Int. 2003;92:23–8.
62. Rawashdeh YF, Austin P, Siggaard C, Bauer SB, Franco I, de Jong TP, et al. International Children's Continence Society's recommendations for therapeutic intervention in congenital neuropathic bladder and bowel dysfunction in children. Neurourol Urodyn. 2012;31:615–20.

Chapter 12
Imaging of Congenital Anomalies of the Kidney and Urinary Tract

Nora G. Lee, Sherry S. Ross, and H. Gil Rushton

Abbreviations

ADPKD	Autosomal dominant polycystic kidney disease
APD	Anterior–posterior diameter
ARPKD	Autosomal recessive polycystic kidney disease
CT	Computerized tomography
DMSA	Dimercaptosuccinic acid
DRF	Differential renal function
IVP	Intravenous pyelography
KUB	Abdominal plain film of kidney ureter, bladder
MCDK	Multicystic dysplastic kidney
MRI	Magnetic resonance imaging
PUV	Posterior urethral valve
RNC	Radionuclide cystography
SFU	Society for fetal urology
UPJ	Ureteropelvic junction
UTI	Urinary tract infection
VCUG	Voiding cystourethrogram
VUR	Vesicoureteral reflux

N.G. Lee, M.D.
Department of Urology, University of Virginia Health System, Charlottesville, VA, USA

S.S. Ross, M.D.
Department of Urology, The University of North Carolina at Chapel Hill,
Chapel Hill, NC, USA

H. Gil Rushton, M.D. (✉)
Division of Pediatric Urology, Children's National Medical Center, Departments of Urology
and Pediatrics, The George Washington University School of Medicine,
Washington, DC, USA
e-mail: hrushton@cnmc.org

© Springer International Publishing Switzerland 2016
A.J. Barakat, H. Gil Rushton (eds.), *Congenital Anomalies of the Kidney
and Urinary Tract*, DOI 10.1007/978-3-319-29219-9_12

237

Introduction

With advances in technology and technique, radiographic imaging of the urinary tract for pediatric patients has become progressively sophisticated for diagnosis and evaluation of urologic conditions. Due to its non-invasive nature and lack of radiation, ultrasonography is often utilized as the initial diagnostic tool for evaluation of the urinary tract. Importantly this modality is the primary imaging modality in the prenatal detection of genitourinary anomalies. Voiding cystourethrography and nuclear scintigraphy are also important diagnostic studies used in the postnatal patient that further aid in diagnosis and management. Over the last decade, computerized tomography (CT) and magnetic resonance imaging (MRI) have become more refined in providing clearer imaging with additional benefits to ultrasonography. These imaging modalities are fundamental in the management and treatment of patients with congenital urologic anomalies and will be discussed in detail in this chapter.

Imaging Modalities

Ultrasonography

Ultrasonography utilizes high-frequency sound waves to image organs and structures. It is one of the most important imaging modalities in the pediatric population. This relatively inexpensive study is frequently used since it is noninvasive and has the unique capability of visualizing structures in real time without exposure to radiation or nephrotoxic contrast agents. However, ultrasound provides no functional data, and the quality and clarity of the study is operator and equipment-dependent. Additionally impediments such as bowel gas and body habitus in older or obese children may limit visualization of structures and impact the quality of the exam [1].

Gray-scale, two-dimensional ultrasonography is the most commonly utilized mode for ultrasound. This pulsed-wave technique produces real-time images consisting of shades of gray as determined by the amplitudes of echoes reflected from the tissue. By convention, the liver is used as a benchmark to measure echogenicity of an image. Structures similar in brightness are considered isoechoic. Tissues with high-signal intensity, such as the peripelvic fat adjacent to the normal renal pelvis, appear brighter than the liver and are described as hyperechoic (Fig. 12.1). Hypoechoic tissues have less-intense signals relative to the liver and are transmitted as darker shades of gray, while those with no internal echo such as fluid or urine are anechoic and appear black on images (Fig. 12.2). Images are oriented with the cranial aspect of a structure to the left and the caudal aspect to the right. Three-dimensional and four-dimensional scanning are highly sophisticated modes of ultrasound utilized most commonly in obstetrics and prenatal imaging but have limited application in the routine evaluation of urinary anomalies postnatally due to its complex and expensive computational infrastructure.

Fig. 12.1 Ultrasound of normal kidney. Hyperechoic peripelvic fat adjacent to the normal renal pelvis appears as white tissue in the central portion of the kidney as indicated by the *arrow*. Hypoechoic areas in the medulla of the kidney demonstrate normal corticomedullary differentiation and can be mistake for hydronephrosis (*asterisk*)

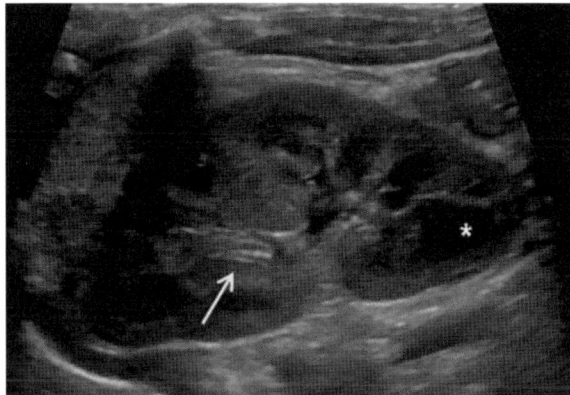

Fig. 12.2 Ultrasound of normal bladder. Urine within bladder appears black or anechoic

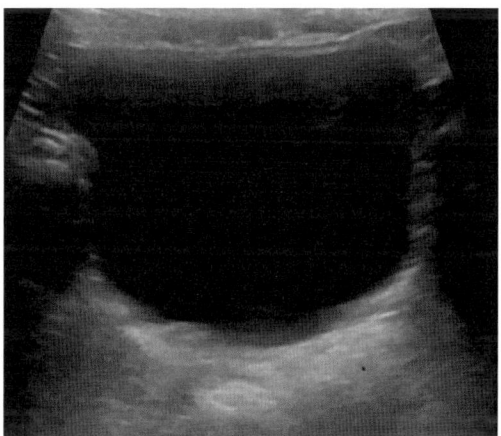

Doppler ultrasound mode is utilized for characterization of motion and is based on the principle of frequency shift when sound waves strike a moving target. Color Doppler is most commonly used to evaluate blood flow with the color blue indicating motion away from the transducer and the color red indicating motion toward the transducer. The velocity of motion is designated by the intensity of the color with higher speeds producing brighter hues.

Prenatal Ultrasonography

The number of routine prenatal ultrasounds performed in the United States has increased twofold between 1998 and 2005 [2]. Universally the sensitivity for detecting urologic anomalies before birth is high at 88 %. However, the overall sensitivity of the prenatal ultrasound varies for each disease process and is lower for congenital anomalies outside the genitourinary system [3].

By 16–17 weeks of gestation, the kidneys and bladder can be identified in 90 % of fetuses [4]. Bladder filling can be noted as early as 14–15 weeks which often

Fig. 12.3 Ultrasound of kidney from prenatal study. The kidney, surrounded by crosses, can be seen as hypoechoic paraspinal structure with a more echogenic renal pelvis. Pelviectasis is present as demonstrated by the central anechoic area (*arrow*)

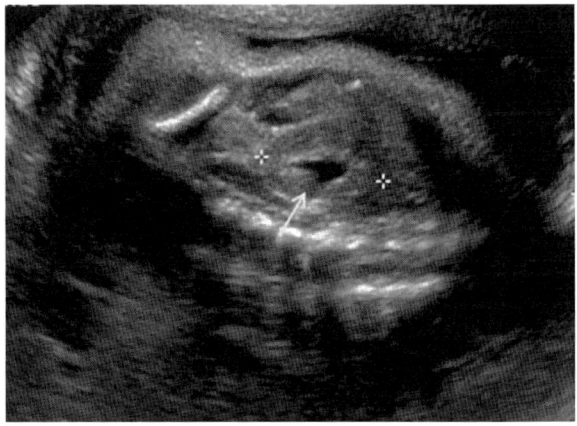

allows identification of abnormalities such as ureteroceles, diverticula, or poor bladder emptying [5]. The kidneys appear as hypoechoic paraspinal structures with an echogenic renal pelvis (Fig. 12.3). Kidney length is measured to ensure appropriate growth for gestational age [6] (Table 12.1), and the kidneys are examined for evidence of hydronephrosis or abnormal cystic or solid structures. When hydronephrosis is noted, the degree and progression of dilatation often correlates with persistent postnatal pathology [7]. In one study 12 % of mild, 45 % of moderate and 88 % of severe hydronephrosis were associated with postnatal pathology [8]. The most commonly used method for defining antenatal hydronephrosis is anterior–posterior diameter (APD) of the renal pelvis. APD is determined by measuring the transverse axial image of the renal pelvis at the approximate level of the renal hilum. The Society for Fetal Urology (SFU) classification system is based on renal APD measurements in the second and third trimesters (Table 12.2) [9].

Amniotic fluid levels should be assessed especially in cases of bilateral hydronephrosis or when there is suspicion of poorly functioning kidneys. Oligohydramnios (defined as amniotic fluid index <5) and polyhydramnios (defined as amniotic fluid index >24) can indicate significant problems with urinary function and can be associated with complex congenital anomalies. Fetal urine chemistry compositions are an adjunct to prenatal imaging and allow classification of fetal renal function into good and poor functioning groups. While fetal management is beyond the scope of this chapter, prenatal imaging plays an important role in perinatal management and offers some insight into postnatal renal function (Refer to Chap. 13).

Abdominal Plain Film of Kidney, Ureter, Bladder (KUB)

While a plain abdominal film is the simplest radiographic study, its utility in congenital urologic anomalies is limited. A KUB is most useful in evaluating spinal or skeletal abnormalities which may indicate pathology such as spinal dysraphisms. It

Table 12.1 Normal fetal renal length during development

Renal length during development	
Gestational age	Length (cm)
18	2.2
19	2.3
20	2.6
21	2.7
22	2.7
23	3
24	3.1
25	3.3
26	3.4
27	3.5
28	3.4
29	3.6
30	3.8
31	3.7
32	4.1
33	4.0
34	4.2
35	4.2
36	4.2
37	4.2
38	4.4
39	4.2
40	4.3
41	4.5

With permission from Cohen HL, Cooper J, Eisenberg P, et al. Normal length of fetal kidneys: sonographic study in 397 obstetric patients. AJR Am J Roentgenol. 1991;157:545–8 [6]

Table 12.2 Classification scheme for grading hydronephrosis based on society for fetal urology consensus statement

Degree	Second trimester (mm)	Third trimester (mm)
Mild	4–<7	7–<9
Moderate	7–<10	9–<15
Severe	>10	>15

Data from Nguyen HT, Herndon CD, Cooper C, et al. The Society for Fetal Urology consensus statement on the evaluation and management of antenatal hydronephrosis. J Pediatr Urol. 2010;6:212–31 [9]

is also useful in the evaluation of bowel gas patterns and constipation. When combined with renal ultrasound, KUB can play an important role in the diagnosis of nephrolithiasis in the pediatric patient.

Intravenous pyelogram (IVP) is an antiquated study which is rarely used at the present time in pediatric urology. This contrast study begins with a scout KUB followed by injection of an intravenous contrast. Images of the kidneys are then obtained during various stages of contrast uptake and drainage. IVP has ultimately been replaced by newer imaging techniques such as sonography and nuclear scintigraphy in the evaluation of hydronephrosis, and by CT scan in the evaluation of urolithiasis. One area where IVP may be useful is in acute trauma situations with an unstable patient and the need for evaluation of the renal collecting system. In this situation, 2 mL/kg of contrast is injected, and images are obtained approximately 10–20 min after contrast administration [10]. This may reveal renal pelvic or ureteral extravasation indicative of injury to the urinary tract and the need for surgical management.

Voiding Cystourethrography (VCUG)

The VCUG is a contrast imaging study which allows evaluation of the urinary bladder and urethra, and is the gold standard for the detection and grading of vesicoureteral reflux (VUR). A urethral catheter or feeding tube is placed in the bladder, and the bladder is filled to capacity with contrast medium. The study requires an initial scout KUB followed by fluoroscopic images of the bladder and upper urinary tract obtained during bladder filling and voiding.

During contrast instillation, filling detects are seen as darker areas surrounded by white contrast medium. The filling phase is important in identifying abnormalities such as ureteroceles since these structures may collapse and disappear as the bladder pressure increases with filling. Once the bladder is at full capacity, anteroposterior images and steep oblique images are obtained. This allows for identification of posterior bladder abnormalities including low grade reflux and bladder diverticula. Imaging during the voiding phase is important since 20 % of VUR may occur during the voiding phase and may be missed when these images are not included [11]. The voiding phase is also necessary for adequate visualization of the urethra. It is during this phase of the study that abnormalities such as a posterior urethral valve (PUV) and strictures are diagnosed. The voided volume is measured to determine actual bladder capacity in comparison to estimated bladder capacity (eBC): eBC (in ounces) = age (years) + 2 × 30) [10]. The efficiency of bladder emptying may also be determined.

When voiding is complete, the renal fossa should be examined as retained contrast from reflux may be visualized. With high grade reflux, a delayed abdominal film may be performed 15 min after voiding to differentiate simple reflux from reflux associated with ureteropelvic or ureterovesical junction obstruction [12]. Recent improvements to decrease radiation doses include low-dose fluoroscopy techniques and pulse fluoroscopy with digital enhancing modalities.

Nuclear Medicine Scintigraphy

Radionuclide Cystography (RNC)

Radionuclide cystography avoids the use of iodinated intravenous contrast agents, and is associated with lower radiation exposure as compared to contrast VCUG. Images are obtained from the patient's posterior position; therefore, right-sided structures are on the right side of the image and vice versa. It is ideal for patients requiring repeat imaging to evaluate resolution of VUR, for postoperative imaging after antireflux procedures, and/or sibling screening for reflux [10]. A dose of 0.5 mCi of Tc-99m-pertechnetate in isotonic saline is instilled into the bladder through a catheter. Continuous monitoring under a gamma camera provides a detailed cystogram and increases the sensitivity of the study without increasing ionizing radiation exposure to the patient. RNC offers limited detailed anatomic information of the bladder and urethra; however with continuous monitoring it is more sensitive than a VCUG for detection of VUR (Fig. 12.4) [10]. The determination of VUR grade is typically graded on a scale of 1–3 (Table 12.3) [13].

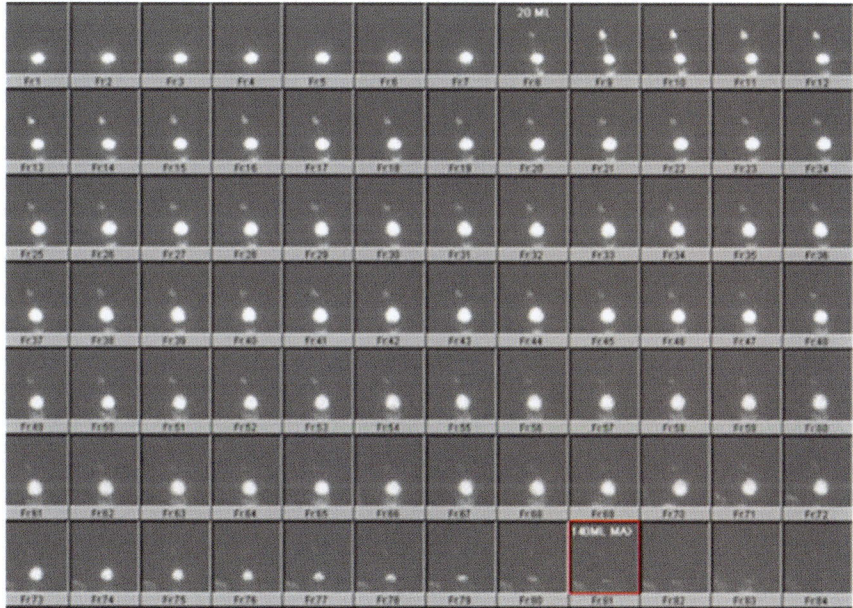

Fig. 12.4 Radionuclide cystogram. Mild left vesicoureteral reflux is first demonstrated at 20 mL of filling of the bladder and persists throughout filling and during voiding

Table 12.3 RNC grading system

RNC grade	International reflux grading system	Description
Grade 1	Grade 1	Activity limited to ureter
Grade 2	Grades 2–3	Activity reaching the collecting system with none or minimal activity in ureter
Grade 3	Grades 4–5	Dilatation of the collecting system and dilated tortuous ureter

Data from Willi U, Treves S. Radionuclide voiding cystography. Urol Radiol. 1983;5:161–73) [13]

Technetium-99m Dimercaptosuccinic Acid (DMSA)

Tc-99m-DMSA is a chelating agent taken up by and fixed to the proximal convoluted tubules in the renal cortex. There is little accumulation of the agent in the renal papilla and medulla with minimal excretion making it an excellent marker for renal cortical activity and function [12]. Renal scans are typically obtained 1.5–2 h after an intravenous injection of 0.05 mCi/kg of 99mTc-DMSA. Three techniques of imaging are performed: planar with parallel hole collimator, planar with parallel hole and pinhole collimator, and SPECT. Magnified posterior and posterior-oblique views are obtained using an ultrahigh resolution parallel collimator. DMSA scintigraphy is the gold standard for the diagnosis of acute pyelonephritis and is the best imaging modality to identify renal cortical scarring. It is also useful in the diagnosis of some congenital renal anomalies such as ectopic kidneys or ectopic ureters that may be associated with poorly functioning renal moieties or duplicated collecting systems. It provides accurate differential renal function of the kidneys and can even provide differential function between upper and lower pole moieties in a duplex system.

DMSA scan is the imaging modality of choice for diagnosing acute pyelonephritis which is demonstrated by decreased accumulation of the radiotracer in the affected area (Fig. 12.5) [14]. Decreased uptake of radioisotope by tubular cells due to ischemia, inflammation, and/or decreased cellular enzyme function results in areas of diminished uptake of isotope on the final image defined as photopenia [4]. These areas of photon deficiency are associated with preservation of the normal renal contour. Over time these areas may resolve, and follow-up DMSA imaging may reveal normal appearing parenchyma with retained renal function or, alternatively, the insult may progress resulting in an irreversible renal scar characterized by parenchymal volume loss or a wedge defect associated with contraction of the damaged renal cortex (Fig. 12.6).

SPECT imaging using multidetector cameras has been applied to DMSA scans to increase sensitivity for detection of "defects" when compared to pinhole imaging. In an experimental study comparing pinhole and SPECT imaging to histology in a refluxing piglet model, SPECT was more sensitive (91 %) than pinhole imaging (86 %), however its specificity was lower (82 % compared with 95 %). The overall accuracy was 88.5 % for both [15].

Fig. 12.5 DMSA scan showing acute pyelonephritis. Acute inflammation prevents normal radiotracer DMSA uptake and creates areas of photopenia as indicated by the *arrow*. However the normal renal contour is preserved

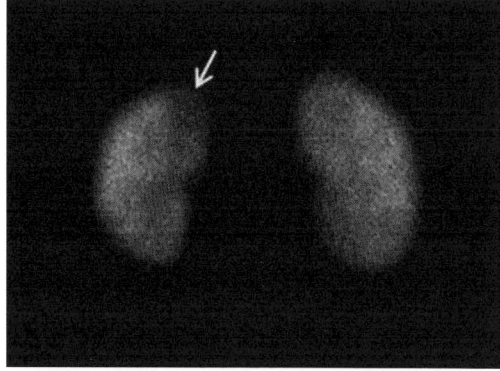

Fig. 12.6 DMSA scan showing renal scarring. Renal scarring results in photopenia associated with loss or contraction of the normal renal contour, as indicated by the *arrow*

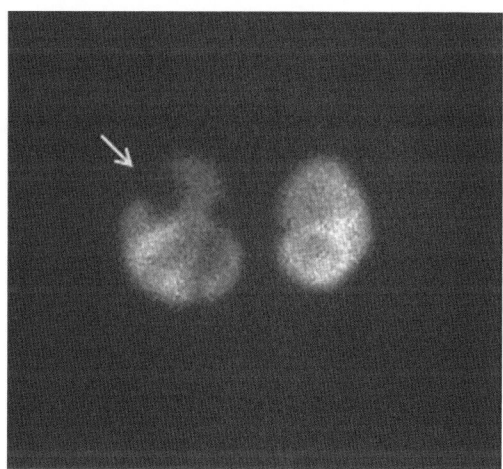

Technetium 99m-Mercaptoacetyl Triglycine (MAG-3)

MAG-3 renal scan is the study of choice when both differential renal function and drainage of the renal collecting system require evaluation. Consequently, it is used primarily in the evaluation of hydronephrosis that may be secondary to an obstructive uropathy. MAG-3 is taken up by the proximal tubule and is cleared mainly by tubular secretion, independent of glomerular filtration rate. Patients are hydrated intravenously (15–20 mL/kg over 30–60 min), and a urinary catheter or feeding tube is inserted into the bladder and left in place to allow maximal bladder draining during the study. Images of the kidneys and bladder are obtained for 30 min after injection of 0.05 mCi/kg of radioisotope. A diuretic (furosemide 1 mg/kg; max 40 mg) is administered intravenously, and additional images are obtained for an additional 15–30 min to evaluate drainage of the collecting system. Various protocols exist for the timing of diuretic administration. Some institutions administer the diuretic 20 min prior to injection of the radioisotope, while others routinely inject at 15–30 min after administration of the radioisotope. Since filling and drainage of the collecting system can be affected by the severity of hydronephrosis, the patient's

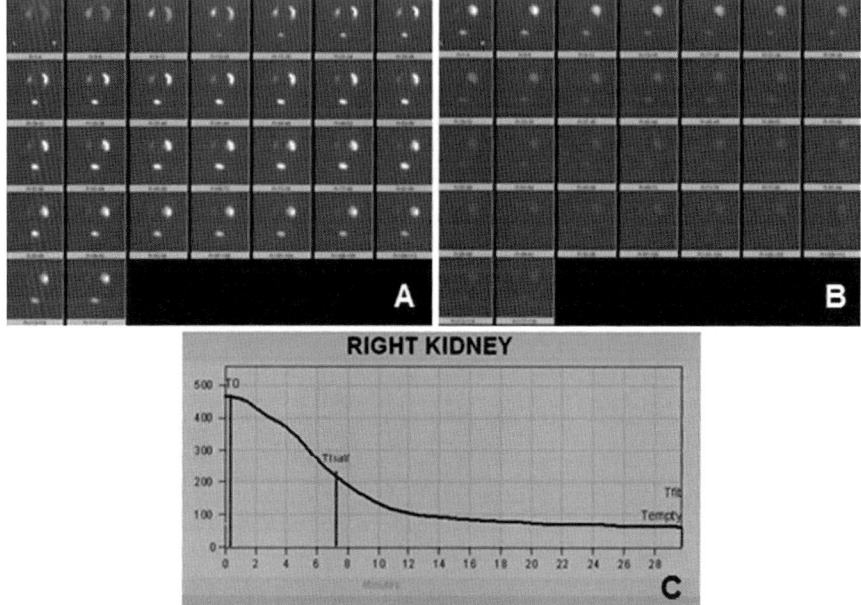

Fig. 12.7 MAG-3 scan demonstrating a non-obstructed kidney. Both kidneys demonstrate prompt uptake of radiotracer. (**a**) Pre-diuretic images reveal symmetric function determined in the first two images of uptake. There is prompt spontaneous drainage of radiotracer by the left system with retained radiotracer in the right system. (**b**) In post-diuretic images, the right kidney is cleared of radiotracer. (**c**) This is further depicted by the rapid downward slope of the drainage curve and a normal drainage T1/2 time of 7 min

hydration status, and the relative function of the involved kidney, we recommend that the collecting system should be maximally filled with radioisotope prior to administration of the diuretic. Additional images are obtained at 15–30 min after the administration of the diuretic to evaluate drainage of the collecting system. After 15 min of upright positioning, patients can be reimaged to assess for further clearance of the radioisotope resulting from gravity drainage.

Radiotracer counts are plotted on a time graph creating a three-phase curve [12]. The initial perfusion phase is characterized by a rapid rise in isotope counts reflecting blood flow to the kidneys. The renal phase follows and is used to assess differential renal function (DRF). In this phase, images are obtained 2–3 min following injection of the isotope before it gets excreted into the collecting system. In the final excretory phase, 1-min images are taken over a 30-min period and should demonstrate a gradual decline in radiotracer associated with drainage of urine from the kidney into the bladder. If retention of isotope is seen within a dilated renal pelvis or ureter, the diuretic is administered to increase urine flow in order to further assess drainage of the system. Drainage is determined by calculating the slope of the drainage curve in the excretory phase and the drainage half-time (T1/2). The T1/2 is defined as the time it takes for half of the isotope to clear from the collecting system. A non-obstructed kidney will demonstrate rapid washout of the radio-

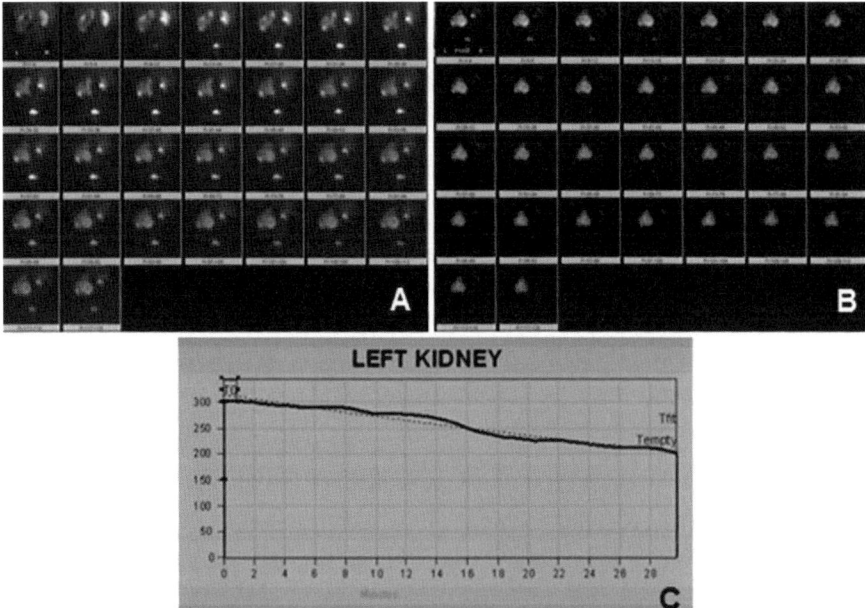

Fig. 12.8 MAG-3 scan demonstrating a ureteropelvic junction obstruction. (**a**) Pre-diuretic images reveal a central photopenic area in the left kidney due to the hydronephrosis in the first images. Prompt excretion of the radiotracer is seen by the right system with large volume retention of radiotracer in the left hydronephrotic system. (**b**) In the post-diuretic images, the dilated left kidney pelvis continues to retain the radiotracer. (**c**) This is further depicted by the very slow downward slope of the drainage curve compared to the steep downward slope in the non-obstructed system. The drainage T1/2 time is 51 min

tracer as indicated by a short T1/2 and a rapid downward slope of the drainage curve (Fig. 12.7). However, if the kidney is obstructed, the excretory phase will demonstrate a prolonged T1/2 associated with a slow and gradually declining or flattened curve, depending on the severity of the obstruction (Fig. 12.8). As obstruction becomes more severe, the relative renal function can become depressed and uptake of the radiotracer reduced. In cases of acute obstruction, prolonged cortical retention of radioisotope without filling of the collecting system may be visualized. Dehydration, poor renal function, and massive dilatation of the collecting system with urinary stasis may reduce the reliability of the diuretic renal scan.

The T1/2 has classically been used to determine drainage with <10 min considered normal drainage, 10–20 min considered indeterminate and >20 min considered obstructed. However, these values were determined in older children and adults. Recent studies have found that longer T1/2 in infants and young children may not indicate obstruction and may improve over time [16]. Since drainage half-times at one point in time have not been validated in infants, change in T1/2 over time is a more useful parameter to assess for progressive or persistent obstruction. The exception is when there is a flat or rising drainage curve and/or when delayed drainage is associated with ipsilateral reduced DRF below 35–40%, indicating high-grade obstruction.

Computed Tomography (CT)

CT scans have become an integral part of urologic practice for general conditions. However, its use for congenital genitourinary disorders is quite limited due to the relatively high amount of radiation exposure to an infant and possible nephrotoxicity of iodinated contrast. The basis of CT imaging is the attenuation of x-ray photons as they pass through different body tissues. A computer then reconstructs cross-sectional images of the body based on measurements of X-ray transmission through thin slices of the body tissue [17]. In general, three phases of a CT scan can be obtained in urologic practice. The initial, non-contrast CT phase is utilized to evaluate hydronephrosis, stones, renal parenchymal calcifications, or renal cysts. With the administration of intravenous contrast, an arterial and nephrogenic phase can be obtained to allow evaluation of vascular anatomy and abnormalities such as renal masses which notably enhance with the contrast. Finally delayed phase images, taken when the contrast enters and fills the renal collecting system, are used to detect filling defects, hydronephrosis, or extravasation of contrast from the collecting system. In spite of CT imaging advantages, it is rarely in infants used given the alternative imaging modalities of ultrasonography, nuclear medicine scans, and MRI scans which provide sufficient information with significantly less radiation to the developing child.

Magnetic Resonance Imaging

Improvements in technology and growing availability have led to an increase in the use of MRI in the evaluation of the genitourinary system. MRI acquires images based on proton density, T1 and T2 relaxation flow, magnetic susceptibility, and diffusion [4]. To obtain an MRI sequence, radiofrequency pulses are transmitted through the patient via a radiofrequency antenna or "coil." When the pulse stops, protons release their energy, and they are detected and processed to obtain the image. Weighting of the image is dependent on the energy imparted through the physics of the pulse sequence, and whether the energy is released slowly or quickly; images are described as being T1- or T2-weighted. On T1-weighted images, fluid has a low signal and appears dark, while on T2-weighted images signals are high and appear bright. Intravenous gadolinium contrast is administered to augment the relaxation of protons on T1-weighted images, making the kidney brighter and increasing the possibility of the detection and characterization of renal masses [1].

Currently MRI is reserved for evaluation of more complex pediatric urological anomalies. MRI can provide excellent details of the genitourinary system in the fetus or in neonates and children without radiation exposure [18]. It can delineate fine details to determine anatomic relationships making it a valuable imaging modality in the evaluation of congenital abdominal and pelvic masses, and duplicated collecting systems with ectopic ureters. Advances in MRI technology have allowed functional assessment of the renal system, including differential renal function and drainage of hydronephrotic kidneys. It has also been reported to be superior to renal scintigraphy for the diagnosis of pyelonephritis and renal scarring. However, direct comparison with histology in a refluxing infected piglet model showed similar accuracy between these imaging modalities [19, 20]. Limitations include its relative high expense and limited availability in comparison to other imaging modalities. Additionally, most children require heavy sedation or anesthesia.

Congenital Anomalies

Kidney/Adrenal

Congenital Hydronephrosis

Antenatal hydronephrosis is the most common urologic abnormality identified on prenatal ultrasonography [1]. Numerous grading systems have been developed in an attempt to adequately describe antenatal hydronephrosis. However, there is no consensus on the best method of reporting the degree of dilatation [1]. The most common method is the anterior–posterior diameter (APD) (Table 12.2). While this provides adequate information for pelvic dilatation, it does not adequately describe pelvic configuration or calyceal dilatation, and it offers little information on the appearance of the renal parenchyma. The 4-scale SFU grading system is the most commonly used system for postnatal ultrasound (Fig. 12.9) [21].

The differential diagnosis for antenatal hydronephrosis is expansive (Table 12.4). However the vast majority of cases (64 %) are due to non-obstructed, transient hydronephrosis which resolves spontaneously over time [7]. Patients diagnosed with hydronephrosis may require extensive prenatal imaging with serial ultrasounds or MRI. Postnatal studies are often required and include ultrasound, VCUG, and/or functional or diuretic renograms. The need for further testing is determined by the grade of hydronephrosis seen on postnatal ultrasound and any additional abnormalities such as hydroureter. Postnatal evaluation with diuretic renography or MRI is usually reserved for patients with persistent SFU grade 3 and grade 4 hydronephrosis. If a postnatal sonogram is performed within the first several days of life, a repeat exam is necessary to avoid underestimating the severity of hydronephrosis that can be caused by perinatal dehydration.

Ureteropelvic Junction (UPJ) Obstruction

The most common pathologic etiology of antenatal hydronephrosis is UPJ obstruction. Kidneys with UPJ obstruction may have varying degrees of renal pelvis dilation, variation in calyceal dilation and thinning of the renal parenchyma. In severe cases, cystic changes may also be seen indicating dysplasia. Congenital UPJ obstruction may present later in childhood or adolescence with flank or abdominal pain which is often cyclic and associated with nausea and vomiting. These symptoms are referred to as a Dietl's crisis and should prompt initial evaluation with renal ultrasonography. Other presentations in older children include urinary tract

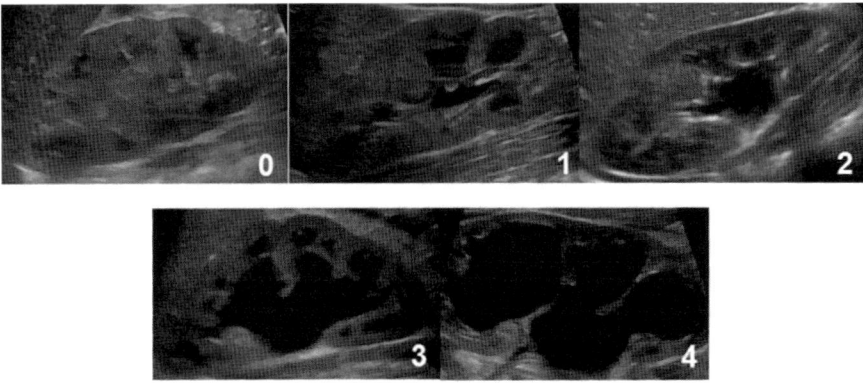

Grade of Hydronephrosis	Renal Pelvis	Renal Parenchymal Thickness
Grade 0	No dilatation	Normal
Grade 1	Mild dilatation; splitting of renal pelvis	Normal
Grade 2	Moderate dilatation but limited to renal pelvis	Normal
Grade 3	Marked dilatation, renal pelvis and calyces are dilated	Normal
Grade 4	Severe dilatation of renal pelvis and calyces	Thinned

Fig. 12.9 SFU grading system for hydronephrosis. With permission from Fernbach SK, Maizels M, Conway JJ. Ultrasound grading of hydronephrosis: introduction to the system used by the Society of Fetal Urology. Pediatr Radiol. 1993;23:478. (11)

Table 12.4 Differential diagnosis for antenatal hydronephrosis, categorized based on level of dilatation

Renal pelvis	Renal pelvis and ureter	Renal pelvis, ureter, bladder, and possibly urethra
UPJ obstruction	VUR	PUV
VUR	UVJ obstruction	Neuropathic bladder
MCDK	Nonobstructed megaureter	Urethral aplasia
ADPKD	Ectopic ureter	
	Ureterocele	
	Prune-belly syndrome	

infection or hematuria, especially following minor trauma, and less commonly, kidney stone formation.

If a UPJ obstruction is suspected on ultrasonography, a MAG-3 diuretic renal scan is the imaging modality of choice to confirm the diagnosis. This study provides a quantitative assessment of DRF as well as the drainage of the dilated collecting system. When MAG-3 imaging reveals a poorly draining system, two options are available: expectant surveillance or operative intervention. Surveillance is typically recommended for asymptomatic infants who have indeterminate drainage curves associated with preserved renal function of greater than 35–40 %. An indeterminate curve often slopes downward slowly, the T1/2 is greater than 20 min, and the collecting system may reveal incomplete emptying of the collecting system with retained radioisotope, even with gravity drainage. Spontaneous resolution or improvement of hydronephrosis has been reported in up to 78 % of kidneys with moderate or severe hydronephrosis and a differential function of greater than 35 %. However, careful follow-up is warranted because more than 30 % of UPJ obstruction cases may require pyeloplasty [22]. Follow-up includes serial sonograms with periodic MAG-3 diuretic renal scans at 6- to 12-month intervals, depending on the degree of obstruction and progression of hydronephrosis.

Indications for surgical intervention in the neonate with antenatal hydronephrosis include poor initial DRF (<35–40 %) or subsequent deterioration of DRF during follow-up, lack of significant drainage despite furosemide administration (flat or rising drainage curve), worsening drainage over time, and persistent obstruction with stable DRF but no evidence of improvement after 4–5 years of observation [10]. In contrast to asymptomatic infants, older children with UPJ obstruction who present with symptoms such as abdominal/flank pain, infection, or hematuria are usually managed by operative intervention.

Renal Cystic Disease

Multicystic dysplastic kidney (MCDK) is characterized sonographically by multiple noncommunicating cysts, minimal or absent parenchyma, and the absence of a central large cyst. By definition multicystic kidneys do not function. It is important to differentiate between a non-functioning MCDK and severe hydronephrosis with dysplasia where the renal pelvis and calyces communicate, and renal scintigraphy will reveal varying degrees of reduced renal function (Fig. 12.10) [1]. The natural history of MCDK is benign, and typically the kidney will spontaneously involute over time. Although the contralateral kidney usually demonstrates compensatory hypertrophy, in some cases the contralateral kidney may also be abnormal. Contralateral UPJ obstruction has been reported in 3–12 %, while VUR has been reported in as many as 18–43 % [1]. Radiographic evaluation of a MCDK can include a DMSA or MAG-3 scan to confirm the absence of function if the diagnosis of MCDK cannot be clearly established by sonography. A VCUG may also be considered to evaluate for contralateral reflux. However, some authors advocate that VCUG has little value in the absence of infection if sonography is consistent with a MCDK and the contralateral kidney appears normal [23]. Nonsurgical surveillance with a follow-up ultrasound in 6–12 months to monitor for involution is routinely recommended. Nephrectomy is rarely indicated due to the high rate of spontaneous involution and the absence of symptomatology associated with MCKD. Since hypertension has occasionally been noted in these children, yearly blood pressure monitoring is recommended.

Fig. 12.10 Ultrasound of multicystic dysplastic kidney. Classic findings of multiple non-communicating cysts and absent parenchyma are seen

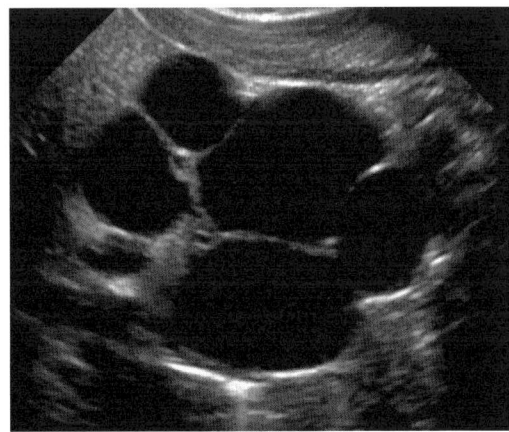

Fig. 12.11 Ultrasound of autosomal recessive polycystic kidney. Kidneys are typically massively enlarged and diffusely echogenic or bright. This kidney in a newborn measures 7 cm (normal size 4–6 cm)

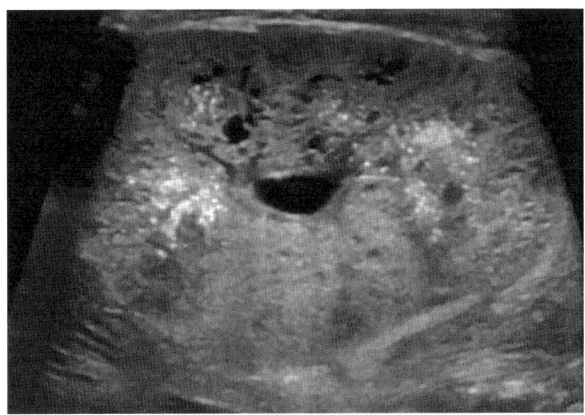

Autosomal recessive polycystic kidney disease (ARPKD) affects 1 in 10,000–50,000 live births. However as many as 50 % of affected newborns die in the first few days of life [1]. ARPKD may be detected prenatally with ultrasound imaging revealing symmetrically enlarged hyperechoic kidneys, enlarging fetal abdominal circumference, and oligohydramnios (Fig. 12.11). Postnatally imaging is required for evaluation of other organs such as the spleen and liver due to the presence of congenital hepatic fibrosis

Autosomal dominant polycystic kidney disease (ADPKD) is the most common inheritable form of renal cystic disease and affects 1 in 400–1000 live births [1]. While it is most commonly identified in adulthood, it has been reported in 2–5 % of newborns and infants [24]. When ADPKD is manifested in the fetus or neonate, 50 % of affected kidneys are large with identifiable macrocysts on ultrasound. Over time, cysts usually enlarge and increase in number [1]. Cysts are often noted in the liver, pancreas, spleen, and lungs; aneurysms of the circle of Willis, aortic aneurysms and mitral valve prolapse are common associated anomalies. Renal failure has been reported in 7–15 % of patients with ADPKD, most commonly in the adult population.

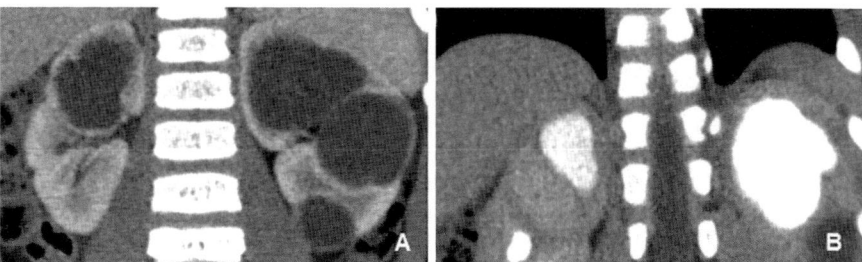

Fig. 12.12 CT scan of calyceal diverticulum with delayed images. (**a**) During the nephrogenic phase, the fluid filled structures within the kidneys appear as large simple cysts. (**b**) During the delayed phase, contrast is seen filtering into these fluid-filled structures, indicating calyceal diverticula

Simple cysts are rare but may occur in infants and present as round or ovoid, anechoic structures with sharply defined, smooth walls on ultrasound. Given the benign nature, long-term follow-up is not required. However, a repeat sonogram after 1 year of age is recommended to monitor for significant increases in size or changes in characteristics of the cyst. A calyceal diverticulum is often confused with a simple cyst. The calyceal diverticulum is an outpouching of the collecting system into the corticomedullary region of the kidney. It is connected to the renal pelvis via a narrow infundibulum. Calyceal diverticula are usually asymptomatic but may cause flank pain or result in stone formation due to stasis of urine. To differentiate between a simple cyst and a calyceal diverticulum, a MAG-3 renal scan or contrast CT with delayed images should be obtained. Delayed filling of the calyceal diverticulum or retention of radioisotope or contrast on imaging is diagnostic (Fig. 12.12).

Tumors

Solid masses in a newborn are rare but may be detected on prenatal ultrasound. Due to suboptimal visualization of masses on ultrasonography, contrast CT or MRI is often utilized to better characterize the mass and determine tumor consistency, extent of local disease, and distant organ involvement. Subtle differences may give some indication of the diagnosis. However, confirmatory histologic evaluation is necessary.

Although congenital mesoblastic nephroma is rare, it is the most common solid renal tumor in the neonatal period and the most common renal tumor diagnosed on prenatal imaging. Prenatal diagnosis via ultrasound has been made as early as 22 weeks of gestation and is suggested when a vascular ring sign or an anechoic ring surrounding the tumor is noted [25, 26]. Nephrectomy is considered curative in classic mesoblastic nephroma, although the cellular variant can recur locally or metastasize. Diagnosis in the newborn period is most often associated with the classic variant, while children diagnosed after 3 months of age may manifest the more aggressive cellular variant. Chaudry et al utilized CT, MRI and ultrasound imaging in 30 children (15 boys, 15 girls) with congenital mesoblastic nephroma to determine if imaging could characteristics could determine the classic versus cellular variant. They noted that findings suggestive of the classic variant included a peripheral hypoechoic ring or a large solid component, whereas cystic/necrotic changes and hemorrhage were more common in the cellular variant. They also noted that cystic components were readily identified on ultrasonography, central hemorrhage was easily identified on CT scanning, and MRI was highly sensitive for cystic components and central hemorrhage [27].

Congenital rhabdoid tumor of the kidney and Wilms tumor or renal nephroblastoma, are extremely rare congenital malignancies, but are quite aggressive when they occur. Rhabdoid tumor of the kidney is the most aggressive and lethal childhood renal tumor with a propensity to metastasize to the brain; therefore brain imaging with CT or MRI is vital. Case reports of Wilms tumor have been reported prenatally but typically present later in childhood. Initial screening is usually performed via ultrasound; however, if a suspicious lesion is present, contrast-enhanced CT or MRI should be performed.

The differential diagnosis of prenatally diagnosed adrenal masses includes neuroblastoma, adrenal hemorrhage, adrenal cysts, adrenal adenoma and carcinoma. Neuroblastoma is the most common extracranial solid tumor of childhood, and over half of children present with metastatic disease. Imaging studies play an important role in the evaluation of a child with neuroblastoma. Plain radiographs may demonstrate a calcified abdominal or posterior mediastinal mass. Contrast enhanced CT and MRI provide detailed information on the extent of disease. The finding of calcifications within the tumor and vascular encasement, or both, on CT is highly suggestive of neuroblastoma and helps differentiate it from Wilms tumor [28]. Currently the Children's Oncology Group protocols require both a radionuclide bone scan and meta-iodobenzylguanidine (MIBG) scan for staging [29]. While adrenal adenomas and carcinomas are extremely rare in the neonatal period, adrenal hemorrhage is relatively common and may occur in 1–2 % of healthy infants. Predisposing factors include prolonged labor, birth trauma, and large birth weight [1]. Ultrasonography reveals an echogenic suprarenal mass, with a late appearance of peripheral eggshell calcifications in contrast to stippled calcifications of neuroblastoma. Management of adrenal hemorrhage is always supportive and expectant.

Renal Anomalies

In utero, multiple anomalies can occur to the kidney ranging from complete absence to aberrant location, orientation, and shape of the kidney. These findings are often detected on prenatal ultrasound imaging or incidentally later in life. While bilateral renal agenesis is lethal, unilateral renal agenesis occurs in 1 in 1100 births, more frequently on the left side. The ipsilateral ureter is completely absent in about 60 % of cases [1]. It has been postulated that renal agenesis may be due to an involuted MCDK. The postnatal diagnosis is established by ultrasound which reveals a solitary kidney with compensatory hypertrophy. If renal agenesis is suspected, it is reasonable to confirm with a MAG-3 or DMSA renal scan to ensure a small ectopic kidney has not been missed.

Renal ectopia occurs when the kidney is outside of the normal anatomical location. Variants include anomalies of renal ascent where the kidney can be found in

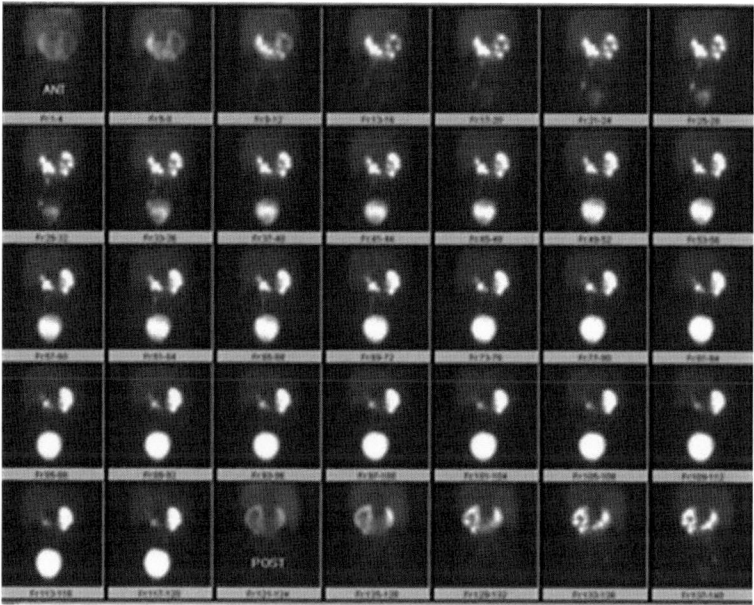

Fig. 12.13 MAG-3 scan demonstrating a horseshoe kidney. Due to the anterior location of horseshoe kidneys, a radiologist may invert the image anterior to posterior for better visualization of the kidneys as seen in the first four rows of this image. This pre-diuretic image demonstrates good drainage of the right system with retention of isotope within the dilated left system

the pelvis, lumbar region, or rarely the thoracic cage. In some cases, renal ectopia is associated with anomalies of renal fusion or form. The horseshoe kidney is the most common of all renal fusion anomalies and occurs in 1 in 400 births. It is possibly associated with an increased incidence of UPJ obstruction, and therefore a MAG-3 renal scan may be warranted to assess for urinary drainage if moderate or severe hydronephrosis is present (Fig. 12.13). In cases of crossed fused renal ectopia, the kidney crosses the midline to fuse with the contralateral kidney. These anomalies are often associated with aberrant vascular supply with an unpredictable pattern. This is important to note if surgical intervention is required. While ultrasonography detects these anomalies initially, DMSA or MAG-3 renal scan may provide further anatomical and functional confirmation.

Ureter

Vesicoureteral Reflux (VUR)

VUR is a common postnatal diagnosis for patients with antenatal hydronephrosis, although the severity of hydronephrosis itself may not be indicative of the presence of VUR and may not prompt the appropriate postnatal workup [7]. Authors have suggested that other parameters including hydroureter, renal duplication anomalies, and renal dysmorphia on initial sonography may be more useful for subsequent

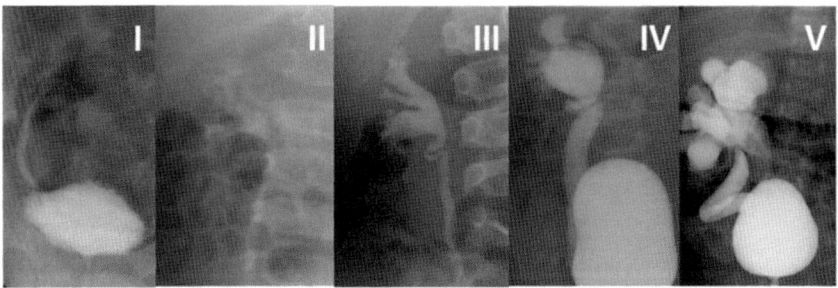

Grade of VUR	Description
Grade I	VUR does not reach the renal pelvis.
Grade II	VUR extends up to the renal pelvis without dilation.
Grade III	Mild or moderate dilation of the ureter and the renal pelvis. No or slight blunting of the fornices.
Grade IV	Moderate dilation of the ureter, renal pelvis, and calyces. Complete obliteration of the sharp angle of the fornices but maintenance of the papillary impression in most calyces.
Grade V	Gross dilation and tortuosity of the ureter. Gross dilation of the renal pelvis and calyces. The papillary impressions are not visible in most calyces.

Fig. 12.14 The international reflux grading system for VCUG. With permission from Fernbach SK, Feinstein KA, Schmidt MB. Pediatric voiding cystourethrography: a pictorial guide. Radiographics. 2000;20:155–71. (11)

detection of reflux [30]. Reflux is graded according to the International Reflux Study in Children (Fig. 12.14) [11]. While reflux alone does not harm the kidney, in the presence of infection and VUR significantly increases the risk of pyelonephritis and renal scarring. Since most VUR detected prenatally is high grade, newborns should remain on antibiotic prophylaxis to prevent infection until VUR is evaluated with VCUG. For higher grades of reflux, a DMSA scan is oftentimes obtained to assess for congenital reflux nephropathy and to determine differential renal function. Abnormalities on DMSA scan may be diffuse or segmental areas of decreased uptake of radioisotope resulting from congenital hypoplasia or dysplasia. These congenital defects may appear similar in some cases to those that are caused by post-pyelonephritic renal scarring. Differentiation between renal scarring and congenital reflux nephropathy is based on the presence or absence of a history of culture-documented urinary tract infection (UTI).

In contrast to infants diagnosed after UTI, prenatally diagnosed VUR occurs more frequently in males and is often high grade reflux [31]. Interestingly, prenatally detected VUR is associated with higher rates of spontaneous resolution or improvement compared with similar grades of VUR diagnosed following urinary infection, particularly in older infants and children. Spontaneous resolution of VUR over time has been reported in up to 43 % in patients with high grade reflux detected prenatally [32]. Follow-up recommendations include a VCUG or RNC at 18- to 24-month intervals and continuous antibiotic prophylaxis until resolution of the reflux or until sufficient improvement in a child who is toilet trained [33].

Megaureter

Megaureter is a generic term indicating the presence of an enlarged ureter measuring greater than 7 mm in diameter with or without concomitant dilatation of the renal collecting system. Megaureter is characterized as congenital primary megaureter or secondary megaureter when associated with anatomical or functional bladder outlet obstruction. Megaureter can be classified further as obstructed or non-obstructed, refluxing or non-refluxing, and, in rare cases, both refluxing and obstructed [34]. Initially the abnormal finding of a dilated ureter is found on ultrasonography. To further delineate the pathology, a VCUG is obtained to look for VUR and evaluate the bladder and urethra for other causes of ureteral dilation including ureterocele, ectopic ureter, PUV in boys, or neuropathic bladder. A MAG-3 renal scan is often necessary to evaluate the differential renal function and to determine drainage of the dilated ureter. The natural history of a non-refluxing, non-obstructed primary megaureter is spontaneous improvement or resolution in over 70 % [35, 36]. Serial ultrasonography is a safe and appropriate method for following these patients when there is preserved renal function of the involved kidney on MAG-3 renal scan and an established pattern of improving hydroureteronephrosis. Corrective surgery may become necessary if MAG-3 diuretic renal scintigraphy indicates high grade obstruction or if hydronephrosis worsens during follow-up. If the megaureter is associated with VUR and it does not improve or is associated with breakthrough UTIs, surgery may be indicated.

More extreme forms of megaureter are seen with anomalies such as megacystis-megaureter and prune-belly syndrome. Megacystis-megaureter occurs when massive bilateral reflux causes a gradual remodeling of the entire urinary tract as the urine yo-yo's between the bladder and ureters. This phenomenon can be identified initially via ultrasound as a massively dilated, thin-walled bladder and dilated upper tract. Diagnosis is confirmed with VCUG which reveals a large smooth-walled bladder associated with severe high grade VUR. Megacystis-megaureter can be confused with prune-belly syndrome where similar findings can be seen on VCUG. However, prune-belly syndrome presents with a constellation of other findings including lack of abdominal wall musculature, bilateral cryptorchidism, dilated posterior urethra due to prostatic hypoplasia, and other non-urologic abnormalities. In addition to severe bilateral hydroureteronephrosis which may be seen on ultrasound, patients with prune-belly syndrome may demonstrate increased renal parenchymal echogenicity, cystic changes, and poor corticomedullary differentiation indicative of renal dysplasia. Due to the risk of progressive renal insufficiency, these patients require long-term monitoring of the hydronephrosis as well as bladder and kidney function.

Ureteral Anomalies

Other ureteral anomalies can be identified with prenatal ultrasonography. Ureteral duplication is relatively common and may be characterized as simple or complex. A simple duplication is demonstrated by a larger-than-normal kidney associated with the sonographic finding of two central hyperechoic foci representing the renal perihilar fat separated by a band of normal echogenic renal parenchyma. There is no evidence of associated hydronephrosis or hydroureter, and the bladder is normal [34]. No additional imaging studies are indicated for these normal variants as they are not associated with an increased risk of infection.

Complex renal duplication occurs in approximately 4.7 % of patients with ureteral anomalies and is associated with dilatation of the fetal urinary tract [37]. More complex cases are associated with ureteroceles, ectopic ureters, UPJ obstruction, or VUR. Ultrasound may reveal variable degrees of hydronephrosis of the upper and/or lower pole moiety. Hydroureteronephrosis of the upper pole moiety is more often associated with an ectopic ureter or ureterocele. Ureterocele is a cystic dilation of the distal aspect of the terminal ureter and is seen on ultrasound as a thin-walled, balloon-like structure protruding into the bladder. Ureteroceles are most often associated with ureteral duplications (80 %) but can occur in single systems [1].

In the absence of a ureterocele, upper pole hydroureteronephrosis suggests an ectopic ureter [38]. Ectopic ureters may terminate in the bladder neck or proximal urethra in boys and girls, in the seminal vesicles or vas deferens in boys, or in the distal urethra or vagina in girls. Termination in girls below the external urethral sphincter will result in constant urinary incontinence most often noted after the child is toilet-trained. In boys, insertion of the ureter proximal to the external sphincter prevents continuous leakage. However, if the insertion site is in the vas deferens or seminal vesicles, UTI may be the presenting symptom. Dilation of the lower pole moiety is most often associated with high grade VUR and less commonly with lower pole UPJ obstruction [34]. VUR associated with a duplex system usually is only seen into the lower moiety unless the duplication is incomplete and both ureters empty into a short common stem near the bladder or in a submucosal segment of the ureter. The risk of urinary infection is significantly increased in these anomalies.

Following initial ultrasound, a VCUG should be obtained to evaluate the presence of reflux and to evaluate the bladder for abnormalities such as ureteroceles. VUR into the lower moiety of a duplex system typically is associated with a "drooping lily" appearance of the lower pole collecting system caused by lateral and downward dis-

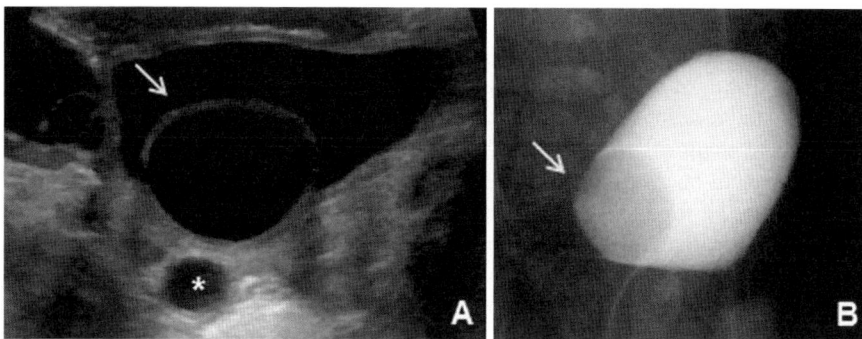

Fig. 12.15 Ultrasound and VCUG demonstrating a ureterocele. (**a**) The ultrasound demonstrates a thin-wall cystic structure within the bladder (*arrow*) with an associated dilated ureter (*asterisk*). (**b**) VCUG demonstrates a filling defect near the trigone, early in filling (*arrow*)

placement by the non-visualized upper moiety. The collecting system opacified by contrast usually demonstrates only two major infundibula and an incomplete set of calyces which are more laterally positioned and associated with a more vertical axis. Ureteroceles are typically detected during the early filling phase of the bladder as a smooth, round filling defect (Fig. 12.15). It is prudent to evaluate the voiding phase of the VCUG as reflux into an upper pole ectopic ureter may only occur while the bladder neck is open during voiding. In complex duplicated collecting systems, a MAG-3 renal scan can provide both functional and drainage information for each system. Typically the upper pole moiety associated with an ectopic ureter or uretero-cele will reveal severely diminished function and delayed drainage. However, some upper pole moieties with non-obstructing ureteroceles or ectopic ureters in the blad-der will have better preservation of function and non-obstructed drainage on a furo-semide MAG-3 renal scan. A DMSA scan may be useful to assess renal function in cases where reflux is present in the duplex system. Magnetic resonance urography is less commonly used but may be helpful in defining complex anatomic relationships.

Bladder

Diverticula

Bladder diverticula are found in approximately 1.7 % of children [39]. A paraure-teral diverticulum can develop dorsal or lateral to the ureteral orifice and is often associated with VUR. Stasis within a large, poorly draining diverticulum with a narrow neck is often associated with an increased risk of UTI. While ultrasonogra-phy may detect these lesions, they are best viewed on a VCUG with oblique views. This provides anatomical detail and can assess emptying of the diverticulum after voiding. While bladder masses occur rarely in children, they are almost never con-genital and therefore are not discussed.

Urachal Anomalies

Anomalies of the urachus, the embryonic remnant of the communication between the bladder and umbilicus, include urachal sinus, urachal cyst, patent urachus, and urachal diverticulum. Patients most often present after birth with periumbilical discharge. In these cases the differential diagnosis includes an umbilical granuloma or patent omphalomesenteric duct. Older patients are more likely to present with a periumbilical mass or cyst and abdominal or periumbilical pain. Ultrasonography is the initial diagnostic imaging modality of choice and may reveal a cystic appearing mass at the most superior aspect of the bladder. VCUG is often necessary to determine if there is communication between the bladder and the urachal remnant or if there is a blind-ending sinus. Alternatively, a sinogram can be performed by instilling contrast into the umbilical opening. CT or MRI may also be used if the ultrasound or VCUG is non-diagnostic.

Exstrophy

The exstrophic complex of anomalies of the bladder ranges from the mildest form of epispadias to cloacal exstrophy. The most common anomaly is classic bladder exstrophy. Prenatal ultrasound may suggest bladder exstrophy in a fetus by absence of bladder filling or non-visualization of the bladder, a low-set umbilicus, widening of the pubic rami, and diminutive genitalia [1]. Cloacal exstrophy is the most severe manifestation of the exstrophy–epispadias complex, carrying all the findings associated with bladder exstrophy and renal, spinal, and bowel involvement in the form of a lateral enterovesical fistula. Complex cysts in the pelvis noted on prenatal ultrasound raise suspicion for cloacal exstrophy. However, like the classic variant, cloacal exstrophy is possible when the bladder is not visualized. Because of prolapsed ileum, cloacal exstrophy may be confused on prenatal sonography with omphalocele. Although sonography is an excellent modality to evaluate the fetus, factors such as maternal body habitus and/or oligohydramnios can prevent an adequate assessment of fetal anatomy, and ultrasound may not be adequate. Prenatal MRI has become an important imaging study in these cases. Children born with any exstrophic complex abnormality will require complex treatment and full evaluation of the skeletal, genitourinary, and reproductive systems.

Neuropathic Bladder

The most common cause of a neuropathic bladder in infants is due to spina bifida. This may initially be detected on prenatal screening with α-fetoprotein and ultrasonography where a small posterior fossa, small cerebellum, effaced cisterna magna, or ventriculomegaly may be visualized. Diagnosis may be made postnatally based on physical examination of the lower back as well as on plain film as an abnormality of the spine or sacrum or on spinal ultrasound or MRI. Along with the other neurologic implications of the entity, a neuropathic bladder and bowel commonly develop which manifest as significant bladder and bowel dysfunction. Infants with spina bifida should be evaluated by renal/bladder ultrasound to evaluate the upper tracts for hydronephrosis or hydroureteronephrosis that may be secondary to a high pressure bladder associated with functional bladder outlet obstruction from an overactive or dyssynergic external sphincter. In these cases, the bladder may be thick-walled or trabeculated. The ultrasound should be repeated yearly to monitor the urinary tract for progressive changes. A VCUG is also warranted to diagnose secondary VUR which occurs due to elevated bladder pressures. It may confirm bladder wall trabeculations with diverticula that may not be appreciated on ultrasound [33].

Urethra

Posterior Urethral Valve

Posterior urethral valve (PUV) can result in prenatally detected hydronephrosis in male fetuses. Prenatal ultrasound findings may include a distended bladder with a thickened bladder wall and unilateral or bilateral hydronephrosis or hydroureter. Prenatal sonography of the bladder may show a "keyhole" sign, representing the dilated prostatic urethra immediately below the distended bladder. In severe cases, kidneys may be severely hydronephrotic with increased echogenicity or cystic changes in renal parenchyma suggestive of dysplasia. Oligohydramnios may be noted. Postnatal outcomes are worse when these findings are detected before 24 weeks of gestation.

Postnatally, a 5–6 French feeding tube or urethral catheter without a balloon should be placed, and urine output and renal function should be monitored closely. A definitive diagnosis is made with a VCUG which demonstrates a dilated posterior urethra and an abrupt transition point with a narrow caliber distal urethra at the location of the valve (Fig. 12.16). The bladder neck is often prominent due to hypertrophy and may appear as an annular band. The valve bladder can be irregular with trabeculations, diverticula, and bladder wall thickening. VUR is present in 50 % of cases and is often severe [40].

The function of each renal unit can vary and may be equal or asymmetrical. In some cases unilateral high-grade reflux is present and secondary to the high bladder pressure. The "pop-off" mechanism to relieve the high intravesical pressure allows the contralateral kidney to develop normally but often sacrifices the function of the refluxing kidney. This phenomenon is called VURD syndrome (posterior urethral valve, unilateral vesicoureteral reflux, and renal dysplasia). Bladder diverticula, a patent urachus, and urinoma may also act as "pop-off" mechanisms, preserving renal function by lowering bladder pressures. While MAG-3 renal scintigraphy may be useful in assessing drainage and differential renal function, children are often followed by serial serum creatinine and ultrasound. A nadir serum creatinine higher than 1.0 mg/dL after a period of bladder decompression indicates a higher risk of progressive deterioration in renal function as the patient ages [41].

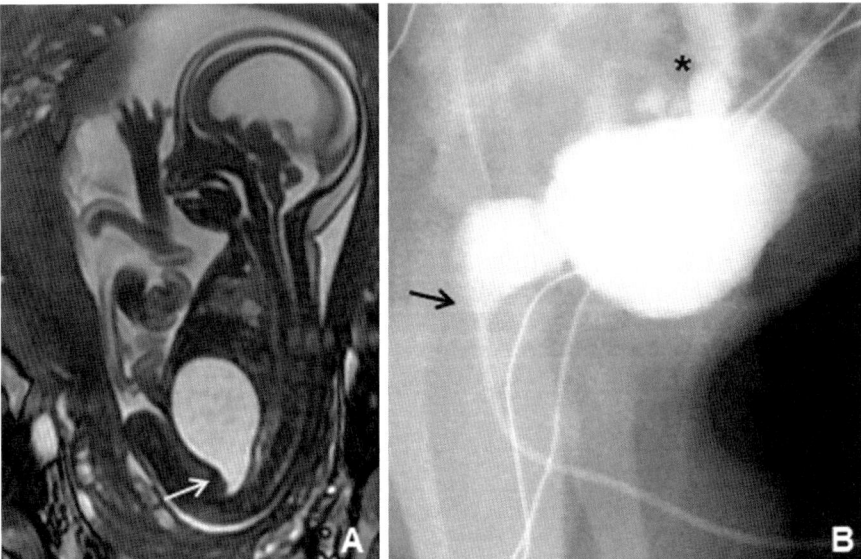

Fig. 12.16 MRI and VCUG showing PUV. (**a**) This prenatal MRI demonstrates a markedly distended bladder which is bright on T2-weighted imaging and a classic "keyhole" sign, as demonstrated by the *arrow*. (**b**) On postnatal VCUG, the posterior urethra is dilated with a distinct transition point at the area of the valve, indicated by the *arrow*. High grade reflux is also demonstrated (*asterisk*)

Prune-belly syndrome can also present with similar prenatal findings of severe bilateral hydroureteronephrosis and a distended, thick-walled bladder. The kidneys may appear hyperechoic or even cystic in severe cases. Postnatally, the posterior urethral may also be dilated in a patient with prune-belly syndrome; however the transition to the posterior urethra in prune-belly syndrome is more tapered than the abrupt transition seen with PUV. The bladder neck is often gaping and patulous due to aplasia of the prostate in prune-belly syndrome. Clinical diagnosis of prune-belly syndrome is established postnatally by the triad of deficiency of the abdominal wall musculature, bilateral non-palpable undescended testes, and an anomalous urinary tract including varying degrees of hydronephrosis, vesicoureteral reflux, renal dysplasia, dilated tortuous ureters, and an enlarged bladder.

Anterior Urethral Valve

An anterior urethral valve is a rare cause of obstruction in male infants. Much like PUV, bilateral hydronephrosis, bladder thickening, and oligohydramnios may be detected. Postnatally, patients may void with a weak stream and a midline scrotal bulge with voiding may be appreciated. In older children urinary frequency or UTI may be the presenting symptoms. VCUG will demonstrate an obstructing valve at the penoscrotal, bulbar, or penile urethra [34]. As with all cases of bladder outlet obstruction, VUR is often present. Other rare urethral anomalies such as a dilated prostatic utricle which is commonly associated with severe hypospadias, megalourethra usually seen in prune-belly syndrome, and congenital urethral diverticulum are diagnosed with VCUG.

Summary

Imaging in the pediatric patient is critical to the diagnosis and management plan for many congenital urologic anomalies. One must be familiar with the possible conditions and various imaging modalities, including their risks and benefits as well as their limitations. Combined with a thorough history and physical exam, imaging is an invaluable adjunct to the workup of congenital genitourinary conditions.

References

1. Campbell MF, Walsh PC, Retik AB. Campbell's urology. 10th ed. Philadelphia: Saunders; 2012.
2. Hsieh MH, Lai J, Saigal CS. Trends in prenatal sonography use and subsequent urologic diagnoses and abortions in the United States. J Pediatr Urol. 2009;5:490–4.
3. Grandjean H, Larroque D, Levi S. Sensitivity of routine ultrasound screening of pregnancies in the Eurofetus database. The Eurofetus Team. Ann N Y Acad Sci. 1998;847:118–24.
4. Sty JR, Pan CG. Genitourinary imaging techniques. Pediatr Clin North Am. 2006;53:339–61.
5. Gloor JM. Management of prenatally detected fetal hydronephrosis. Mayo Clin Proc. 1995;70:145–52.
6. Cohen HL, Cooper J, Eisenberg P, et al. Normal length of fetal kidneys: sonographic study in 397 obstetric patients. Am J Roentgenol. 1991;157:545–8.
7. Lee RS, Cendron M, Kinnamon DD, et al. Antenatal hydronephrosis as a predictor of postnatal outcome: a meta-analysis. Pediatrics. 2006;118:586–93.
8. Corteville JE, Gray DL, Crane JP. Congenital hydronephrosis: correlation of fetal ultrasonographic findings with infant outcome. Am J Obstet Gynecol. 1991;165:384–8.
9. Nguyen HT, Herndon CD, Cooper C, et al. The Society for Fetal Urology consensus statement on the evaluation and management of antenatal hydronephrosis. J Pediatr Urol. 2010;6:212–31.
10. Belman AB, King LR, Kramer SA. Clinical pediatric urology. 4th ed. London: Martin Dunitz; 2002.
11. Fernbach SK, Feinstein KA, Schmidt MB. Pediatric voiding cystourethrography: a pictorial guide. Radiographics. 2000;20:155–71.
12. Goldfarb CR, Srivastava NC, Grotas AB, et al. Radionuclide imaging in urology. Urol Clin North Am. 2006;33:319–28.
13. Willi U, Treves S. Radionuclide voiding cystography. Urol Radiol. 1983;5:161–73.
14. Rushton HG, Majd M, Chandra R, Yim K. Evaluation of 99mTechnetium-dimercapto-succinic acid renal scans in experimental acute pyelonephritis in piglets. J Urol. 1988;140:1169–74.
15. Majd M, Rushton HG, Chandra R, et al. Technetium-99m-DMSA renal cortical scintigraphy to detect experimental acute pyelonephritis in piglets: comparison of planar (pinhole) and SPECT imaging. J Nucl Med. 1996;37:1731–4.
16. Ross SS, Kardos S, Krill A, et al. Observation of infants with SFU grades 3-4 hydronephrosis: worsening drainage with serial diuresis renography indicates surgical intervention and helps prevent loss of renal function. J Ped Uro. 2011;7:266–71.

17. Brant WE, Helms CA. Fundamentals of diagnostic radiology. 4th ed. Baltimore: Williams & Wilkins; 2012.
18. Caire JT, Ramus RM, Magee KP, et al. MRI of fetal genitourinary anomalies. Am J Roentgenol. 2003;181:1381–5.
19. Cerwinka WH, Grattan-Smith JD, Kirsch AJ. Magnetic resonance urography in pediatric urology. J Pediatr Urol. 2008;4:74–82.
20. Madj M, Nussbaum Blask AR, Markle BM, et al. Acute pyelonephritis: comparison of diagnosis with 99mTc-DMCA, SPECT, spiral CT, MR imaging, and power Doppler US in an experimental pig model. Radiology. 2001;218:101–8.
21. Fernbach SK, Maizels M, Conway JJ. Ultrasound grading of hydronephrosis: introduction to the system used by the Society of Fetal Urology. Pediatr Radiol. 1993;23:478.
22. Bajpai M, Chadrasekharam VV. Nonoperative management of neonatal moderate to severe bilateral hydronephrosis. J Urol. 2002;167:662–5.
23. Calaway AC, Whittam B, Szymanski KM, et al. Multicystic dysplastic kidney: is an initial voiding cystourethrogram necessary? Can J Urol. 2014;21:7510–4.
24. Avner ED, Sweeney Jr WE. Renal cystic disease: new insights for the clinician. Pediatr Clin North Am. 2006;53:889–909.
25. Chen WY, Lin CN, Chao CS, et al. Prenatal diagnosis of congenital mesoblastic nephroma in mid-trimester by sonography and magnetic resonance imaging. Prenat Diagn. 2003;23:927–31.
26. Kelner M, Droulle P, Didier F, et al. The vascular "ring" sign in mesoblastic nephroma: report of two cases. Pediatr Radiol. 2003;33:123–8.
27. Chaudry G, Perez-Atayde AR, Ngan BY, Gundogan M, Daneman A. Imaging of congenital mesoblastic nephroma with pathological correlation. Pediatr Radiol. 2009;39:1080–6.
28. Dickson PV, Sims TL, Streck CJ, et al. Avoiding misdiagnosing neuroblastoma as Wilms tumor. J Pediatr Surg. 2008;43:1159–63.
29. Naranjo A, Parisi MT, Shulkin BL, et al. Comparison of ^{123}I-metaiodobenzylguanidine (MIBG) and ^{131}I-MIBG semi-quantitative scores in predicting survival in patients with stage 4 neuroblastoma: a report from the Children's Oncology Group. Pediatr Blood Cancer. 2011;56:1041–5.
30. Lee NG, Rushton HG, Peters CA, et al. Evaluation of prenatal hydronephrosis: novel criteria for predicting vesicoureteral reflux on ultrasonography. J Urol. 2014;192:914–8.
31. Yeung CK, Godley ML, Dhillon HK, et al. The characteristics of primary vesico-ureteric reflux in male and female infants with pre-natal hydronephrosis. Br J Urol. 1997;80:319–27.
32. Martin AD, Iqbal MW, Sprague BM, et al. Most infants with dilating vesicoureteral reflux can be treated nonoperatively. J Urol. 2013;191:1620–7.
33. Skoog SJ, Peters CA, Arant BS, et al. Pediatric vesicoureteral reflux guidelines panel summary report: clinical practice guidelines for screening siblings of children with vesicoureteral reflux and neonates/infants with prenatal hydronephrosis. J Urol. 2010;184:1145–51.
34. Palmer LS. Pediatric urologic imaging. Urol Clin North Am. 2006;33:409–23.
35. Shukla AR, Cooper J, Patel RP, et al. Prenatally detected primary megaureter: a role for extended followup. J Urol. 2005;173:1353–6.
36. McLellan DL, Retik AB, Bauer SB, et al. Rate and predictors of spontaneous resolution of prenatally diagnosed primary nonrefluxing megaureter. J Urol. 2002;168:2177–80.
37. Ismaili K, Hall M, Donne C, et al. Results of systematic screening for minor degrees of fetal renal pelvis dilatation in an unselected population. Am J Obstet Gynecol. 2003;188:242–6.
38. Abuhamad AZ, Horton CE, Horton SH, et al. Renal duplication anomalies in the fetus: clues for prenatal diagnosis. Ultrasound Obstet Gynecol. 1996;7:174–7.
39. Blane CE, Zerin JM, Bloom DA. Bladder diverticula in children. Radiology. 1994;190:695–7.
40. Berrocal T, Lopez-pereira P, Arjonilla A, et al. Anomalies of the distal ureter, bladder, and urethra in children: embryologic, radiologic, and pathologic features. Radiographics. 2002;22:1139–64.
41. DeFoor W, Clark C, Jackson E, et al. Risk factors for end stage renal disease in children with posterior urethral valves. J Urol. 2008;180:1705–8.

Chapter 13
Prenatal Diagnosis of Congenital Anomalies of the Kidney and Urinary Tract

Rebecca S. Zee and C.D. Anthony Herndon

Abbreviations

APD	Anteroposterior diameter
DMSA	Tc-dimercaptosuccinic acid
fUTI	Febrile urinary tract infection
GA	Gestational age
MAG3	Tc-mercaptoacetyltriglycine
MCDK	Multicystic dysplastic kidney
MRU	Magnetic resonance urography
PA	Prophylactic antibiotics
SFU	Society for Fetal Urology
UPJ	Ureteropelvic junction obstruction
UTD	Urinary tract dilation
UTI	Urinary tract infection
VCUG	Voiding cystourethrogram
VUR	Vesicoureteral reflux

R.S. Zee, M.D., Ph.D.
Department of Urology, University of Virginia School of Medicine,
P.O. Box 800422, Charlottesville, VA 22908-0422, USA

C.D.A. Herndon, M.D., F.A.C.S., F.A.A.P. (✉)
Departments of Urology and Pediatrics, University of Virginia School of Medicine,
Charlottesville, VA, USA
e-mail: cdaherndon23@gmail.com

© Springer International Publishing Switzerland 2016
A.J. Barakat, H. Gil Rushton (eds.), *Congenital Anomalies of the Kidney
and Urinary Tract*, DOI 10.1007/978-3-319-29219-9_13

Table 13.1 Etiology and incidence of obstructive etiologies that affect the kidney, ureter, and/or bladder [1]

Etiology	Incidence (%)
Transient UTD	41–88
UPJ obstruction	10–30
VUR	10–20
UVJ/megaureter	5–10
MCDK	4–6
Duplex/ureterocele/ ectopic	5–7
PUV/urethral atresia	1–2

Introduction

The fetal kidney first begins development around the 8th week of gestation. Quantifiable urine production can be visualized as early as the 14th week of gestation. Major obstructive urologic anomalies may present this early but most diseases encountered postnatally will not be detected until the first screening US that is performed in the USA around 20 weeks [1]. This chapter focuses on diseases that present early in the second trimester as well as those encountered in the later stages of pregnancy.

A meta-analysis by Lee et al. documented that the severity of urological disease had a linear relationship with the degree of prenatal UTD. As the kidney became more dilated so did the likelihood of diagnosing significant urological disease. This held true for most urological conditions and was most consistent with ureteropelvic junction (UPJ) obstruction and least consistent with vesicoureteral reflux (VUR). The differential diagnosis represents a spectrum of disease that ranges from transient UTD to obstructive etiologies that affect the kidney, ureter and/or bladder (Table 13.1) [2].

Meaningful research for prenatal UTD has been hampered by the discrepancy in grading systems for UTD amongst physicians that treat the patient before and after delivery [3]. Most obstetricians will rely on anteroposterior pelvic diameter (APD) first pioneered by Corteville. Several other centers have substantiated appropriate thresholds during the second and third trimester that are representative of urological disease. Classically, >4 mm during the second trimester and >7 mm during the third trimester were thresholds used to represent potentially significant dilation [4–6]. Postnatally, practitioners are more inclined to use a combination of the APD and Society for Fetal Urology systems to grade UTD [3].

Anteroposterior Diameter (APD) Measurement

APD measurement should be reliable, objective and reproducible. Although for minor dilation it can be useful, it is unfortunately operator-dependent for more significant disease. Measurement of APD must occur within the confines of the renal parenchyma; otherwise, a compliant extrarenal pelvis may overestimate disease state. Several papers have demonstrated the effectiveness of APD cutoffs to be predictive of for both urological disease and the need for surgical intervention. In the classic study from Great Ormond Street, patients were randomized to observation or surgery for UPJ obstruction. When the APD threshold was >40 mm, all patients observed required surgical intervention as compared to none of the observed patients with less than 20 mm [4]. Other centers have demonstrated similar results but used a lower threshold to be predictive of disease. The St. Louis group of Coplen et al. found that a 15 mm APD measurement in the third trimester translated to a specificity of 82% and sensitivity of 73% for predicting UPJ obstruction [5]. Utilizing prospective data collected in the Society for Fetal Urology Hydronephrosis Registry, Shamshirsaz identified a second trimester cutoff of 9.5 mm and a similar third trimester cutoff of 15 mm to represent significant disease [6]. Postnatally, Burgu et al. found that APD <20 mm is predictive of preserved renal function at a mean of 1.6 weeks [7]. An interesting recent publication by Sharma and Sharma demonstrated the positional differences observed with UTD when imaging in both the supine and prone position. Surgery was required in all patients with an APD of 40 mm, which was similar to the Great Ormond street data. However, when looking at kidneys that demonstrated a decrease in renal APD in the prone compared to supine position, 7/16 with 30–40 mm and 11/15 15–30 mm improved without surgery [8]. It is interesting to postulate that positional change of the UPJ facilitates drainage and this may be why we observe spontaneous improvement with longitudinal follow-up of UPJ obstruction and transient UTD once infants become ambulatory.

Society for Fetal Urology

In 1993, the Society for Fetal Urology (SFU) introduced a 5-point system to grade UTD based on urinary dilation as well as the integrity of the renal parenchyma (Table 13.1) [9]. The system is based on a subjective assessment of the degree of UTD dilation ranging from primarily the renal pelvis to the entire calyceal collecting system. Differentiating factors for grade 3 and 4 are based on the presence of renal thinning which is an objective assessment. This system is simple and yet has been found to be predictive of both the need for surgical intervention as well as preservation of renal function [10, 11]. The Chicago group demonstrated in a moderate series that all (33/33) patients with SFU grade 3 demonstrated retained renal function (>40% differential function). The SFU grading system has been proven to demonstrate good intrarater and interrater variability. Additionally, the use of Computer Enhanced Visual Learning (CEVL) has been proven as an effective means to disseminate a learning module for grading hydronephrosis [12]. Recently, the Children's National group used the SFU grading system as a predictor of early versus late surgical intervention for UPJ obstruction. They retrospectively reviewed a total of 125 patients with SFU grade 3 or 4 hydronephrosis. For the early surgery group ($n=27$), most patients (89%) demonstrated grade 4 hydronephrosis. The delayed surgical intervention group was also predominated by SFU grade 4 but to a lesser degree (62%). The continually observed group was more represented by grade 3 hydronephrosis (78%) [13].

Urinary Tract Dilation (UTD)

Summary of Consensus Conference for Prenatal UTD

In March 2014, a consortium of health care providers including maternal fetal medicine physicians, pediatric radiologists, pediatric nephrologists, and pediatric urologists met with the fundamental goal of formulating a unified position on prenatal UTD. The underlying goals were to achieve a consensus on terminology, prenatal follow-up as well as postnatal recommendations for imaging and institution of prophylactic antibiotics.

For terminology, the group felt the use of the term Urinary Tract Dilation (UTD) was the most consistent with the disease process. The use of terms such as hydronephrosis, caliectasis, pelviectasis, and pelvicaliectasis was discouraged. When imaging the kidney, they recommended a combination of both objective and subjective variables that included six measurements that should be reported with each US: APD measurement, integrity of renal parenchyma, degree of calyceal dilation, and presence of ureteral or bladder abnormalities [14]. In addition, a statement was developed to standardize the technique both prenatally and postnatally. The spine should be oriented either in the 6 or 12 o'clock position and most importantly postnatally, notation of prone or supine position should be made. The same position should be used for serial imaging in the postnatal time period.

Normative Values for UTD (Prenatal and Postnatal)

A number of normative values for UTD were given based on the prenatal gestational trimester as well as postnatal assessment (Table 13.2). In summary, APD <4 mm at <27 weeks, <7 mm at ≥28 weeks, and <10 mm in the postnatal period all were considered to represent acceptable physiologic dilation of the renal pelvis [14]. Although normative values have been recognized and influence prenatal assessment

Table 13.2 Normal values for urinary tract dilation classification system [14]

Normal values for urinary tract dilation classification system	16–27 GA	≥27 GA	>48 h
Anterior–posterior renal pelvis diameter (APRPD)	<4 mm	<7 mm	<10 mm
Calyceal dilation			
Central	No	No	No
Peripheral	No	No	No
Parenchymal thickness	Normal	Normal	Normal
Parenchymal appearance	Normal	Normal	Normal
Ureter(s)	Normal	Normal	Normal
Bladder	Normal	Normal	Normal
Unexplained oligohydramnios	No	No	NA

and follow-up, postnatal normative values simply do not exist. Equally, it is recognized that UTD represents a spectrum of disease in the postnatal period and significant disease processes such as vesicoureteral reflux may exist in the absence of postnatal UTD [15].

Urinary Tract Infection

Although UTD has been associated with postnatal UTI, the exact correlation is yet to be determined. A number of studies have looked at this but they are confounded by the lack of uniform patient populations with respect to the administration of PA. Additionally, UTD is not a diagnosis and certainly patients with obstruction or VUR may have higher risk of UTI when compared to those without. These populations cannot be identified by US alone and this clouds the interpretation of its impact on UTI. Despite these cofounding variables, there appears to be a linear relationship between the degree of UTD and risk of developing UTI. In the meta-analysis of prenatal UTD by Lee, a 4, 14, 33, and 40 % incidence of UTI was found with SFU grades of 1–4, respectively [2]. In looking at single institutional studies, Szymanski looked at 206 patients and reported a significantly higher rate of UTI for high grade (SFU 3 or 4) UTD as compared to low grade (SFU 1 or 2) UTD, 13.8 % vs. 4.1 % ($p=0.03$), respectively [16]. Coelho demonstrated a similar linear correlation with UTD and UTI in his review of 192 patients. UTI rates were 11, 18, and 39 %, respectively, for mild, moderate, and severe degrees of UTD [17]. None of these studies are prospective or are controlled for use of uroprophylaxis. Finally, Zareba et al. identified risk factors for febrile UTI by reviewing their database of prenatal UTD. On multivariate analysis, high grade UTD, female gender and uncircumcised status were all significant risk factors [18]. Looking at these studies it appears fairly clear that the presence of moderate to severe UTD does place the neonate at risk of UTI and this should be discussed with the family prenatally or postnatally. Of course, this conversation must take place within the context of the use of prophylaxis in preventing UTI and other anatomical considerations.

Prophylactic Antibiotics (PA)

The recommendation for prophylactic antibiotics for prenatal UTD should consider the degree of UTD, risk of UTI and proposed anatomical studies. A recent survey of pediatric urologists demonstrated a clear lack of consensus for the use of prophylactic antibiotics for prenatal UTD. A number of factors influenced the decision to prescribe prophylactic antibiotics including APD measurement, SFU grade, and demographics of the respondents. A minority of respondents, 3 and 4 %, respectively, would recommend PA for APD less than 4 mm or SFU grade 1. This compares to 70 and 66 % for APD greater than 10 mm and SFU grade IV, respectively. American pediatric urologists were more likely to prescribe PA when compared to their European counterparts for two scenarios that included indiscriminant use of PA regardless of degree of UTD (77% vs. 40% $p < 0.001$) and with the complete absence of hydronephrosis on initial postnatal imaging (29% vs. 5% $p < 0.001$) [19]. A similar lack of consensus was seen in Canada with a survey of pediatric nephrologists and pediatric urologists that demonstrated significant differences for recommendations for PA in the scenario of bilateral low grade UTD (29.6% vs. 11.4% $p = 0.02$) and isolated high grade UTD (73% vs. 38.2% $p = 0.02$), respectively [20].

Several studies have addressed the utility of prophylactic antibiotics. Braga performed a systematic review of the literature, which included 3876 infants. PA did not influence UTI rates for low grade UTD, 2.2% vs. 2.8%. However, when looking at high grade UTD a significant decrease in the rate of UTI was seen with the administration of PA; PA 14.6% versus no PA 28.9% $p < 0.01$. With high grade UTD, the estimated number to treat was 7 in order to prevent one UTI [20]. Herz et al. reported a 10-year retrospective experience in patients with prenatally detected UTD. The incidence of febrile UTI on PA was 7.9% vs. 18.7% without PA ($p = 0.02$). In looking at independent risk factors on multi-regression analysis, ureteral dilation, high grade VUR, and UVJ obstruction all were significant predictors of UTI. Finally, ureteral dilation of over 11 mm in patients not maintained on PA afforded a fivefold higher risk of developing a febrile UTI [21].

Postnatal Imaging

Renal Ultrasound

Renal sonography affords an opportunity to monitor UTD in a safe and readily available manner that allows a smooth transition to the postnatal period. A number of factors such as technician experience, hydration status, positioning of the patient (supine versus prone), and degree of bladder distension impact the reliability of imaging [8]. Despite the ability to accurately detect urological anomalies prenatally, there is little evidence to suggest that this modality positively impacts patient outcome as represented by recent documentation of its increased utilization. You et al. reported a threefold increase over a 10-year interval in the proportion of patients receiving at least four prenatal ultrasounds within the second or third trimester. This increase was not correlated to maternal risk [22].

One of the important facets of renal ultrasound is that it allows for longitudinal follow-up with serial imaging in the absence of radiation or invasive testing. This allows for both specific measurement of APD of the renal pelvis and an assessment of the degree of dilation within the collecting system compared to previous imaging. The absence of discomfort from catheter insertion and ionizing radiation make it an excellent modality for close interval follow-up. It is important for the practitioner to not only assess the degree of UTD in comparison to the last image recorded but also relative to the initial ultrasound. This will allow proper classification of the degree of UTD as improving, stable or worsening. Kidneys that are improving, such as an infant that has improved to SFU grade 2, can be safely monitored at extended intervals of follow-up from 6 to 12 months [23].

The practitioner should be aware that the presence of a normal renal US in a patient with prenatal hydronephrosis does not always equate to the absence of urological pathology. Besides VUR, which can be present in up to 25 % of patients with a normal postnatal US, patients may have subsequent UTD in the presence of a normal initial postnatal US 28 % of the time, or occasionally even present as a late UPJ obstruction [15, 24, 25]. Therefore, it is recommended for patients that demonstrate a normal renal US to have a subsequent follow-up US within 3–6 months to confirm resolution.

Voiding Cystourethrogram (VCUG)

The decision to obtain a VCUG should be based on a cost–benefit analysis that factors in the utility of the study, morbidity of the procedure as well as a balance of the impact on disease with asymptomatic detection in the early postnatal period. For neonates, the study does not require sedation although there is a slight risk of UTI as well as exposure to ionizing radiation. It should be considered a safe and effective procedure to evaluate the lower urinary tract. In addition to the identification of VUR, other anatomical considerations such as the presence of a ureterocele or bladder wall thickening should be the basis for imaging. Recently, there has been a paradigm shift away from indiscriminate screening for any grade of UTD detected in the pre or postnatal period [26].

The degree of prenatal UTD correlates poorly with the presence of VUR [2, 27]. However, some centers recommend VCUG only for SFU grade 3 and 4 hydronephrosis. Recently, Lee et al. reported that a similar degree of sensitivity could be achieved with half the number of patients requiring screening with a VCUG by using the criteria of associated ureteral dilatation, evidence of duplication, or renal dysmorphia on ultrasound [28]. Furthermore, the absence of UTD on the initial postnatal US does not exclude VUR which can be present in up to 25 % of children with a normal postnatal US [15, 29]. The main issue yet to be resolved is the benefit of identifying asymptomatic VUR in the neonatal period.

Renal Scintigraphy

A number of agents are used for renal scintigraphy including Tc-mercaptoacetyltriglycine (Tc-Mag3), Tc-dimercaptosuccinic acid (DMSA), and less commonly Tc-diethylenetriamine pentaacetic acid (DTPA). These agents are selected based on their characteristics. Classically, DMSA is used to assess cortical defects for dysplasia, scarring or for the confirmation of a solitary functioning kidney or Multicystic Dysplastic Kidney (MCDK). The agent binds to the proximal convoluted tubule. MAG3 is cleared by renal tubular secretion and is the ideal choice to evaluate drainage of the kidney. Differential function can also be assessed but is not as reliable as DMSA. Imaging for MAG3 uses only a posterior camera view which does not offer as a complete evaluation of the parenchyma for the assessment of differential renal function. DTPA is used in a similar manner to MAG3 and is cleared by glomerular filtration [1].

Renal scintigraphy for the evaluation of prenatal UTD is mainly used to identify surgical obstruction as well as differential renal function. The two most common scenarios involve evaluating drainage/differential function of a UPJ obstruction or confirmation of the lack of function in the case of a MCDK.

In terms of the evaluation of UTD detected prenatally, recent recommendations have called for a more selective approach with the use of longitudinal renal US instead [23]. Most would agree that renal scintigraphy is indicated for SFU grade 3 and 4 hydronephrosis. When indicated, a "well tempered" diuretic renogram should follow a strict protocol which allows for bladder decompression with a catheter, hydration, as well as the administration of a diuretic [30]. Despite this protocol, the ability to identify obstruction and accurately document function is less than ideal. The main pitfall for this test occurs with a large capacious renal pelvis that may require a longer interval to collect radiotracer prior to the administration of diuretic. In this situation, the drainage curve is still on an upslope because the kidney is filling, which can lead to the curve being misinterpreted as obstructed. This can be avoided if the diuretic is not administered until the dilated collecting system is visualized to have filled with radiotracer. Additionally, poorly functioning kidneys may not respond well to the diuretic or demonstrate a phenomenon known as "hyperfiltration" which may lead to falsely increased differential function. Also, the region of interest for background subtraction of radiotracer may be incorrectly drawn leading to overestimation of function. In some situations, bilateral UPJ obstruction may coexist and the differential renal function may not be representative of overall renal function. Lastly, it important to recognize that UPJ obstruction is a dynamic condition that can worsen or improve over time. Therefore, serial monitoring with imaging studies is often necessary to determine if and when surgical intervention is required. Surgical indications for UPJ obstruction include a differential function of less than 40 % or the presence of a worsening and/or highly obstructive drainage curve. In situations of bilateral UPJ, the kidney with least function should be addressed first [1].

Magnetic Resonance Urography (MRU)

Magnetic resonance urography (MRU) provides excellent anatomic detail as well as functional assessment and drainage for the evaluation of UTD. Most pediatric urologic data stems from the group in Emory that has demonstrated the utility of MRU for a variety of urological conditions. Renal transit time and Patlak score have been used to determine single nephron GFR [31, 32]. Additionally, superior correlations have been reported with MRU when compared to standard evaluation of UTD with RUS, VCUG, and renal scintigraphy [33]. Although MRU is a proven modality to follow outcomes after pediatric pyeloplasty, the cost, need for sedation, and software requirements likely make its widespread use unlikely for the standard evaluation of prenatally detected UTD [34].

Commentary on Febrile UTI, Prophylactic Antibiotics (PA), and VCUG

The decision to administer prophylactic antibiotics and obtain a VCUG for prenatal UTD lacks consensus amongst pediatric urologists [19]. Currently, the decision to place patients with prenatally detected UTD on PA is not evidence-based and this decision should be made with this in mind. An informed discussion with the parents should encompass the incidence of fUTI, impact of fUTI on the developing kidney, the risk–benefit of the administration of PA as well as the natural history of prenatally detected VUR and contrast this with VUR that presents symptomatically with UTI. The latter group has a defined risk of UTI and the former has a correlation of fUTI based on the degree of prenatal UTD [15, 35]. One important and difficult facet to this conversation is that it must take place in temporal relationship to delivery. Frequently, the pediatric urologist is not present or even within the same institution and therefore the primary care team must partake in these conversations.

Future endeavors should focus on providing recommendations for each risk profile that are evidence-based that will allow for protocol-based management for patients with prenatal UTD. The Society for Fetal Urology prenatal hydronephrosis registry should provide a means to acquire such data to formulate evidence based recommendations [6].

Differential Diagnosis, Evaluation and Management Strategy

The differential diagnosis and treatment strategy for UTD should take into account a number of factors such as the presence of normal amniotic fluid, family history of urological conditions and anatomic considerations such as solitary kidney or bladder abnormalities such as ureteroceles. Fortunately, oligohydramnios in the presence of UTD is not a common condition but should be used as the primary consideration for establishing a differential diagnosis. The following diagnoses including transient UTD, UPJ obstruction, VUR, megaureter, and duplication anomalies are discussed with the understanding of normal amniotic fluid. Conditions associated with oligohydramnios such as posterior urethral valves, prune belly syndrome, and urethral atresia are not discussed in this chapter. Lee et al. demonstrated through their meta-analysis that the degree of UTD severity had a direct correlation with the presence of pathologic urologic conditions [36].

Transient UTD

Transient dilation of the urinary tract is the most common condition seen prenatally. The degree to which this occurs likely is under appreciated due to the benign nature of the condition. Several institutions documented this phenomenon in the early 1990s for prenatal UTD that often resolved within the third trimester and shortly after birth [37–39]. Most of these studies used a threshold of >4 mm APD under 33 weeks and >7 mm after 33 weeks. The Mandell study used >5 mm under 20 weeks and >8 mm after 20 weeks. These three studies likely are representative of the same population of patients. Collectively, about 1/3rd (21–31%) of cases of UTD resolved within the 3rd trimester, which increased in the early postnatal period to over one half (55%) of patients in the study reported by Mandell [38].

Postnatally, several recent studies have demonstrated similar findings to the earlier prenatal studies [40–43]. In the Maayan-Metzger review of 178 patients with prenatal UTD, 97.5% of mild prenatal UTD resolved or remained mild with follow-up while 80% of moderate UTD improved and 20% of severe [40]. A similar finding was demonstrated with the Barbosa group with 25% resolving prenatally, and 90 and 75% of mild and moderate UTD, respectively, demonstrating resolution postnatally. This is in contrast to severe UTD, which demonstrated only 28% resolution postnatally [42]. Tombesi et al. reviewed a total of 193 newborns with prenatally detected UTD, which demonstrated complete resolution within the first year of life [43]. In the Madden-Fuentes review of 416 patients, SFU I hydronephrosis ($n=398$ renal units) demonstrated resolution in 67%, stability in 30%, and progression in only 3% at a mean of 9.3 months. For SFU II hydronephrosis ($n=225$ renal units), resolution occurred in 48%, improved in 31%, remained stable in 20%, and progressed in 1% at a mean of 8.4 months. This review was important because it was one of the first to document expected timing for the above conditions which is a common question asked by parents and pediatricians [40].

UPJ Obstruction

UPJ represents the most common pathologic urological condition that presents with prenatal UTD (Fig. 13.1). Lee et al. demonstrated a linear correlation between the degree of UTD and presence of UPJ obstruction with severe UTD having the best correlation at 54% [2]. Several studies have tried to identify certain thresholds of APD or SFU classification that are predictive of the need for surgical correction of UPJ obstruction (see Fig. 5.3). The presence of severe UTD does not always equate to surgery as demonstrated by Koff. In his series comprised of 104 neonates with severe UTD, a resolution rate of 69% was observed at a mean of 2.5 years. A minority (22%) of these patients required surgical intervention [44].

In the late 1990s Dhillon and colleagues from Great Ormond Street conducted a randomized trial of UTD based on APD measurement as well as differential renal function. A total of 75 patients were randomized to upfront surgery ($n=39$) versus observation ($n=36$) with the inclusion criteria of >15 mm APD and ≥40% differential

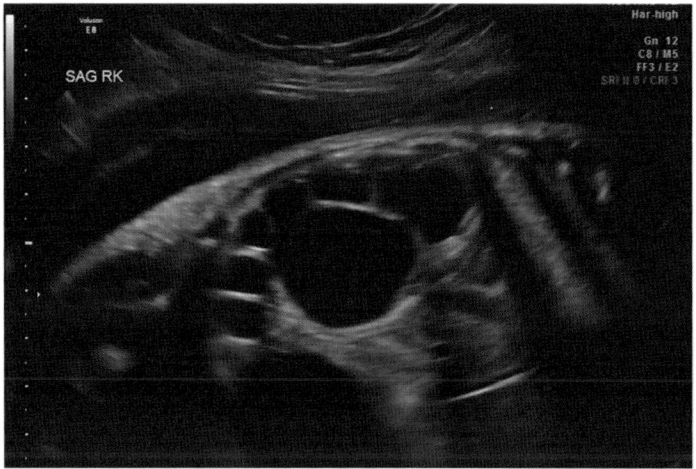

Fig. 13.1 UPJ obstruction

renal function. Renal preservation was maintained in all but one patient in the surgical arm. For the observation group, 7/36 demonstrated a significant decrease in function requiring surgery and the APD was >20 mm in all patients. Equally, spontaneous resolution was seen in 17/36, 9 of which initially had an APD >20 mm [4]. Other centers have demonstrated similar results using APD cutoff as a predictor of surgery. Coplen reviewed 257 neonates with prenatal UTD. Of this group, a mean prenatal APD of 11.8 mm was seen for the nonoperative group which was significantly less than the operative cohort that demonstrated a mean prenatal APD of 22.8 mm. His analysis revealed that a prenatal threshold APD of 15 mm carried a 73 % sensitivity and 82 % specificity for obstruction requiring surgical intervention [5]. Using the Society for Fetal Urology Hydronephrosis Registry, Shamshirsaz identified a similar APD threshold of 15 mm in the third trimester as well as a unique APD threshold in the second trimester of 9.5 mm [6]. Finally, the SFU classification system was used by Ross et al. to predict the need and timing of surgical intervention as well as preservation of renal function. This retrospective study reviewed outcomes for 125 patients with either SFU III or SFU IV UTD. Early surgical intervention was required in a minority (20 %) of patients. Most (89 %) in this early surgery group demonstrated SFU IV UTD. For the remaining 80 %, delayed surgery occurred in a minority and was less represented with SFU IV (62 %). For the group that did not have surgery and was continually observed, 78 % demonstrated SFU III UTD [13].

Recommendations for Ureteropelvic Junction (UPJ) Obstruction

A majority of patients with UPJ obstruction can be followed clinically without surgical intervention. Thus, most patients can safely be followed with US alone. This allows for comparison of longitudinal imaging which gives the clinician a basis for determination of progression of disease. An assessment of dilation in the calyceal system may be a useful adjunct but may not be reproducible given its subjective nature. In addition, it does not assess function or drainage. The clinician should be selective with the use of renal scintigraphy [23]. Due to the invasiveness of the study, radiation exposure and inherent flaws with interpretation of both drainage of the kidney and differential function assessment it should be used with some caution. Candidates for renal scintigraphy include SFU IV UTD or P3 classification. Other considerations may include SFU III or P2 or increasing dilation within the collecting system compared to previous imaging or symptomatic UTD [14].

Ideally the selection interval of follow-up, use of prophylactic antibiotics and invasive testing of the upper and lower urinary tract should be based on a risk assessment. Patients with severe UTD (SFU IV or P3) are considered high risk and should be considered increased potential for the development of fUTI and managed with PA. Renal ultrasound should be performed at 1–2 month intervals and a well-tempered renogram performed as well. The lower urinary tract should be assessed with a VCUG. Patients with moderate UTD (SFU III or P2) are considered intermediate risk and can be followed with renal ultrasound at 3-month intervals. Because of moderate risk, PA and lower urinary tract imaging are recommended. A "well tempered" renogram should be used selectively in patients with P2 risk [14].

Vesicoureteral Reflux (VUR)

Prenatal VUR represents the third most common urological condition that presents with prenatal UTD. Prenatal VUR is more common in boys and typically is represented by bilateral high grade disease. The natural history of prenatal VUR is much different than the VUR that presents in girls with UTI and bowel and bladder dysfunction [15, 35]. UTD severity is equally a poor predictor of VUR in contrast to other urological conditions such as UPJ obstruction. Lee et al. meta-analysis reported that the incidence of VUR was 4 % for mild, 14 % for moderate, and 8.5 % for severe UTD [2]. In fact, up to 25 % of patients with prenatal UTD and VUR may have a normal postnatal US [15]. Boys with prenatal VUR have known higher voiding pressures which may be related to a delay in bladder neck development over the first year of life. This maturation correlates with an increased rate of resolution for high grades of VUR [45].

Herndon et al. used the SFU Prenatal Hydronephrosis Registry data sheets to perform a multicenter review of prenatal VUR. A total of 71 patients (56 male) representing 116 renal units with prenatal UTD were confirmed postnatally to have VUR. Of these, the initial postnatal US was normal in 25 %, with most patients demonstrating SFU I/II UTD. Febrile UTI occurred more significantly in uncircumcised boys (10/19) despite the use of PA. High grade VUR (III-V) was found in 74/116 units of which 15 demonstrated resolution at a mean age of 0.9 years for boys and 2.1 years for girls [15]. Other centers have demonstrated similar findings [46].

Recommendations for Prenatal VUR

The clinician should use a selective approach towards the use of lower urinary tract imaging to identify prenatal VUR. The practice of routine VCUG imaging for prenatal UTD is not evidence-based. As we move forward, the focus of risk should move away from the probability of identifying disease, which may be as high as 21 % and shift towards identifying those at risk of UTI. Some centers have reported the selective use of VCUG imaging without increasing patient harm [47].

A practical approach would limit VCUG imaging to those patients with intermediate (P2) or high (P3) UTD or those with the ureteral dilation detected prenatally. As previously mentioned, an informed discussion pertaining to the inherent benefits and risks of both the omission of and inclusion of the diagnosis of VUR should take place with the parents.

Multicystic Dysplastic Kidney (MCDK)

MCDK is a congenital form of cystic kidney disease that is not progressive and is expected to involute in the early postnatal period. It may be confused with a severe UPJ obstruction and likely represents a severe form of this process, which occurs very early in kidney development. The diagnosis is suspected because of the absence of a reniform shape of the kidney that is replaced with varying sized cysts (Fig. 13.2). Associated conditions in the contralateral kidney are common and include both VUR and UPJ obstruction [48–50].

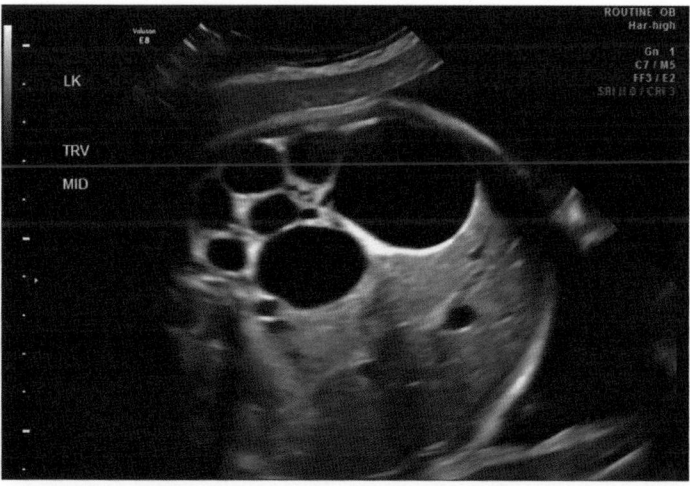

Fig. 13.2 Multicystic dysplastic kidney

The postnatal evaluation should include a renal ultrasound to confirm the presence and quality of cyst seen prenatally. Because of the prevalence of VUR which can be as high as 20 %, consideration should be given to a VCUG although recently some centers have challenged this practice [51]. Furthermore, the utility of routine use of a DMSA renal scan to confirm the absence of function has been called into question [52]. Certainly, in today's health care costs crisis, every effort should be made to minimize cost without negatively impacting care and the selective use of imaging for the diagnosis of MCDK is in line with this approach.

Historically, simple nephrectomy was customary for the persistence MCKD. However, a systematic review of the literature failed to demonstrate any increased risk for Wilms' tumor development and this practice has fallen out of favor [53]. Yearly renal US should be used to longitudinally follow both the involution of cyst as well as maintaining surveillance of the contralateral kidney. Interestingly, Perez et al. recommended early nephrectomy based on a cost analysis that demonstrated this to be most efficient option if one elects to pursue serial imaging of the contralateral kidney [54]. Annual blood pressure monitoring has also been suggested although the level of increased risk for hypertension is relatively low.

Recommendations for MCDK

Postnatal evaluation of MCDK should include an initial renal ultrasound and strong consideration given to a DMSA as well as a VCUG. The use of PA is not recommended as the MCDK is not considered to be at increased risk of fUTI.

Duplication Anomalies (Ureterocele/Ectopic Ureter)

The prenatal presentation of duplication anomalies usually involves the identification of the dilated upper pole ureter. At the level of the kidney, cystic changes may be seen and is more common with high-grade obstruction. The differentiation of an ectopic ureter from an ureterocele is based on the visualization of a cystic mass within the bladder that correlates to a ureterocele (Fig. 13.3). This may be difficult to assess prenatally given its dependence on fetal position during imaging. On rare occasion, ureterocele disproportion may be seen, which represents the presence of a large ureterocele in the presence of minimal upper urinary tract dilation [55]. Most ureteroceles will be unilateral and associated with duplex collecting systems in females.

Although the cystic nature of the ureterocele makes it an attractive target for prenatal intervention it should not be considered the standard of care [56, 57]. Early postnatal puncture of the ureterocele traditionally has been reserved for bladder outlet obstruction or patients experiencing sepsis. However, primary elective

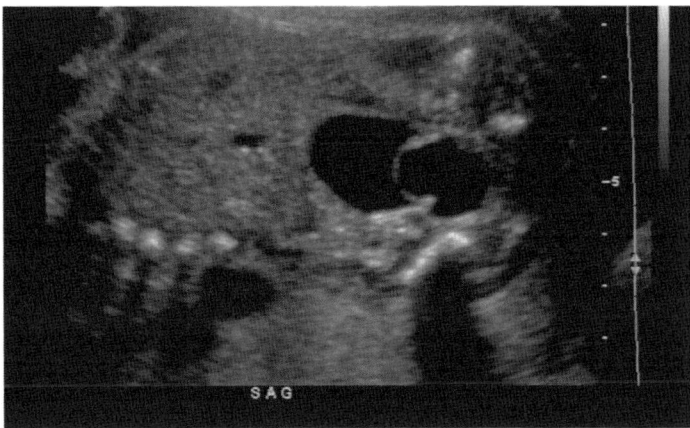

Fig. 13.3 Ureterocele within bladder

puncture has gained recent popularity as a first line treatment option [58–60]. Additionally, some centers have reported success with elective puncture and expectant management of resultant reflux [61]. Furthermore, success has been reported with a watchful waiting protocol in select patients that obviates the need for puncture of the ureteroceles [62, 63].

The preservation of the lower pole of a duplex system associated with an ectopic ureterocele or ectopic ureter should be the primary objective of any treatment strategy. For the ureterocele population, this may involve extensive bladder reconstruction with excision of ureterocele and ureteral reimplantation. There is some controversy pertaining to the surgical approach to the obstructed nonfunctioning duplicated system. The approach to the upper urinary tract has shifted towards a minimally invasive approach with both nephron ablative and sparing techniques demonstrating success [64–66]. An informed discussion should take place with parents when presenting options for the management of the obstructed nonfunctioning upper pole moiety. The advantage of a nephron-sparing approach is the mitigation of inadvertent injury to the lower pole. The advantages of a nephron ablative approach include minimization of risk of UTI development secondary to urinary stasis in a dilated upper pole ureter.

The decision to proceed with surgery at the level of the bladder is based on the risk of fUTI which correlates with the presence and severity of VUR. For the Mayo group, the absence of VUR allowed all patients to be treated with a single kidney level procedure with removal of the upper pole. For patients with low grade VUR, excision of the ureterocele with ureteral reimplantation was performed in 40 % because of fUTI. For patients with high grade VUR, 96 % underwent a procedure to excise the ureterocele with reimplantation of the ureter [67]. For the management of ectopic ureters, most patients will require only a kidney level procedure with a minority requiring subsequent surgery for removal of the distal ureteral stump [68].

Recommendations for Duplex Anomalies

The postnatal evaluation of duplication anomalies should include an early postnatal renal ultrasound and examination of the introitus to ensure the absence of a prolapsed ureterocele. PA should be instituted due to the increased risk for UTI and a VCUG obtained to assess the size of the bladder defect, its impact on voiding and the presence of vesicoureteral reflux. An informed discussion with the family should include all available treatment options including ureterocele puncture and procedures at the level of the kidney and/or bladder.

Megaureter

Primary megaureter is an uncommon condition that represents a minority of patients with prenatal UTD [1]. It must be differentiated from a single system ectopic ureter which usually can be accomplished based on an assessment of the integrity of renal parenchyma as well as its insertion into the bladder (Fig. 13.4). The classification system includes obstructed, non-obstructed, refluxing, and non-refluxing.

Most patients with prenatally detected megaureter will not require surgical intervention and can be managed with observation alone. Shukla et al. reviewed 40 patients and demonstrated resolution of hydronephrosis in 50 % of patients with an average follow-up of 7 years. In a sub-cohort of 10 patients with 13.4-year follow-up, resolution occurred in 4 patients but renal deterioration occurred in 1 that resulted in nephrectomy [69]. McLellan et al. presented similar findings on 54 patients with a 2-year follow-up. She reported a resolution rate of 72 % and identified ureteral dilation of 1.32 cm as predictive of the need for surgery [70]. Finally, Chertin reported a 31 % surgical intervention rate at an average age of 14.3 months and identified differential function of less than 30 % and ureteral diameter of 1.33 cm as risk factors for surgery [60].

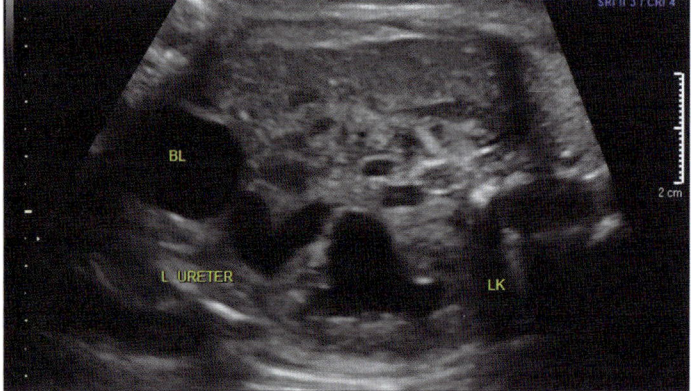

Fig. 13.4 Primary megaureter. *BL* bladder, *LK* left kidney

Recommendations for Megaureter

The British Association of Pediatric Urologists published a consensus statement on the evaluation and management of primary obstructive megaureter [71]. A summary of their recommendations include:

1. Evaluation-ureteral diameter of ≥ 7 mm after 30 weeks as threshold for postnatal renal ultrasound, initiation of PA, VCUG in all patients with special consideration for timing in those suspected to potentially have posterior urethral valves, and consideration of renal scintigraphy to assess function and obstruction at the level of the UVJ.
2. Surgical intervention will be required in a minority and reserved for decreased renal function (<40 %), fUTI, or pain. Temporizing procedures such a cutaneous ureterostomy, cutaneous pyelostomy, or refluxing ureteral reimplantation should be performed for patients under 1 year of age. Ideally, the procedure should be deferred until a year of age and allow for a definitive ureteral reimplantation.
3. Follow-up BAPU recommends long-term follow-up into adulthood because of the risk of late asymptomatic deterioration.

Summary

Prenatal UTD is a relatively common condition and thus the evaluation and management should be a defined process that is practical and strives to minimize invasiveness while maintaining the ability to identify significant urologic disease. Most of the early postnatal evaluation is not evidence-based and simply represents practice patterns, which are aimed to identify disease. Recently, there has been a shift towards a more selective approach to both the initiation of prophylactic antibiotics and evaluation of the lower urinary tract for reflux. The degree of UTD dilation not only correlates with the presence of significant urological disease but also appears to be predictive of the risk for UTI and thus should drive the decision for PA and lower urinary tract imaging. The recent multidisciplinary consensus conference developed and presented a risk stratification system, which serves as a foundation for recommendations. Future studies utilizing resources such as the Society for Fetal Urology (SFU) prenatal hydronephrosis registry appear to be a means to further develop and enhance these recommendations.

Appendix

Risk Stratification (Prenatal UTD)

Prenatally, APD measurement thresholds exist for two periods before and after 28 weeks of gestation. Based on the multidisciplinary consensus conference, Low risk (A1) was defined as 4–7 mm APD between 16 and 27 weeks and as 7–10 mm

APD at >28 weeks with normal central calyceal dilation values for the 5 remaining data points. Increased risk (A2/3) was defined as ≥7 mm APD for 16–27 weeks and as ≥10 mm APD for ≥28 weeks with central calyceal dilation associated with the presence of other positive values for the 5 remaining data points [14] (see Fig. 5.9).

Risk Stratification (Postnatal UTD)

Postnatally, APD measurements are integral to stratifying risk into low (P1), intermediate (P2), and high (P3). Based on the multidisciplinary consensus conference, a value greater than 15 mm was considered to be a benchmark for risk of urological disease. The assessment of UTD should be made at 48 h after birth to account for underestimation of UTD caused by physiological dehydration in the early postnatal period. If possible, the practitioner should personally review the image or the report should be formatted to include all 6 data points which will allow for risk assessment. P1 risk is similar to A1 risk and includes APD (10 to <15 mm) with central calyceal dilation. P2 risk includes APD ≥ 15 mm, peripheral calyceal dilation as well as ureteral dilation with P3 risk including other data points that were positive such as parenchymal abnormalities, the presence of cysts or an abnormality in the bladder [14] (see Fig. 5.10).

Management Strategy

Prenatal UTD

The level of risk was used to provide a standardized recommendation for prenatal follow-up of urologic conditions. For A1 risk, the recommendation was to perform an additional US after 32 weeks followed by one postnatally between age 48 h and 1 month. For A2/3 risk, the recommendation was to perform a repeat fetal US in 4–6 weeks and one postnatally between 48 h and 1 month (see Fig. 5.9).

Postnatal UTD

The postnatal recommendations were made with the assumption that the first US was performed after 48 h of age, and these results were used to classify into risk groups (P1-P3). For low risk (P1), a second US is recommended prior to 6 months of age. For intermediate risk (P2), a second US is recommended between 1 and 3 months of age. For both P1 and P2 risk, prophylactic antibiotics and a VCUG are left up to the discretion of the physician. For P3 risk, a second US is recommended at 1 month, prophylactic antibiotics should be instituted and a VCUG should be performed. A MAG3 scan is left to the discretion of the treating physician [14] (see Fig. 5.10).

References

1. Nguyen HT, Herndon CD, Cooper C, Gatti J, Kirsch A, Kokorowski P, et al. The Society for Fetal Urology consensus statement on the evaluation and management of antenatal hydronephrosis. J Pediatr Urol. 2010;6:212–31. doi:10.1016/j.jpurol.2010.02.205.
2. Lee RS, Cendron M, Kinnamon DD, Nguyen HT. Antenatal hydronephrosis as a predictor of postnatal outcome: a meta-analysis. Pediatrics. 2006;118:586–93. doi:10.1542/peds.2006-0120.
3. Zanetta VC, Rosman BM, Bromley B, Shipp TD, Chow JS, Campbell JB, et al. Variations in management of mild prenatal hydronephrosis among maternal-fetal medicine obstetricians, and pediatric urologists and radiologists. J Urol. 2012;188:1935–9. doi:10.1016/j.juro.2012.07.011.
4. Dhillon HK. Prenatally diagnosed hydronephrosis: the Great Ormond Street experience. Br J Urol. 1998;81 Suppl 2:39–44.
5. Coplen DE, Austin PF, Yan Y, Blanco VM, Dicke JM. The magnitude of fetal renal pelvic dilatation can identify obstructive postnatal hydronephrosis, and direct postnatal evaluation and management. J Urol. 2006;176:724–7. doi:10.1016/j.juro.2006.03.079. discussion 727.
6. Shamshirsaz AA, Ravangard SF, Egan JF, Prabulos AM, Ferrer FA, Makari JH, et al. Fetal hydronephrosis as a predictor of neonatal urologic outcomes. J Ultrasound Med. 2012;31:947–54.
7. Burgu B, Aydogdu O, Soygur T, Baker L, Snodgrass W, Wilcox D. When is it necessary to perform nuclear renogram in patients with a unilateral neonatal hydronephrosis? World J Urol. 2012;30:347–52. doi:10.1007/s00345-011-0744-6.
8. Sharma G, Sharma A, Maheshwari P. Predictive value of decreased renal pelvis anteroposterior diameter in prone position for prenatally detected hydronephrosis. J Urol. 2012;187:1839–43. doi:10.1016/j.juro.2011.12.093.
9. Fernbach SK, Maizels M, Conway JJ. Ultrasound grading of hydronephrosis: introduction to the system used by the Society for Fetal Urology. Ped Rad. 1993;23(6):478–80.
10. Palmer LS, Maizels M, Cartwright PC, Fernbach SK, Conway JJ. Surgery versus observation for managing obstructive grade 3 to 4 unilateral hydronephrosis: a report from the Society for Fetal Urology. J Urol. 1998;159:222–8.
11. Erickson BA, Maizels M, Shore RM, Pazona JF, Hagerty JA, Yerkes EB, et al. Newborn society of fetal urology grade 3 hydronephrosis is equivalent to preserved percentage differential function. J Pediatr Urol. 2007;3:382–6. doi:10.1016/j.jpurol.2007.01.196.
12. Marks A, Maizels M, Mickelson J, Yerkes E, Anthony Herndon CD, Lane J, et al. Effectiveness of the computer enhanced visual learning method in teaching the society for fetal urology hydronephrosis grading system for urology trainees. J Pediatr Urol. 2011;7:113–7. doi:10.1016/j.jpurol.2010.09.009.
13. Ross SS, Kardos S, Krill A, Bourland J, Sprague B, Majd M, et al. Observation of infants with SFU grades 3-4 hydronephrosis: worsening drainage with serial diuresis renography indicates surgical intervention and helps prevent loss of renal function. J Pediatr Urol. 2011;7:266–71. doi:10.1016/j.jpurol.2011.03.001.
14. Nguyen HT, Benson CB, Bromley B, Campbell JB, Chow J, Coleman B, et al. Multidisciplinary consensus on the classification of prenatal and postnatal urinary tract dilation (UTD classification system). J Pediatr Urol. 2014;10:982–98. doi:10.1016/j.jpurol.2014.10.002.
15. Herndon CD, McKenna PH, Kolon TF, Gonzales ET, Baker LA, Docimo SG. A multicenter outcomes analysis of patients with neonatal reflux presenting with prenatal hydronephrosis. J Urol. 1999;162:1203–8.
16. Szymanski KM, Al-Said AN, Pippi Salle JL, Capolicchio JP. Do infants with mild prenatal hydronephrosis benefit from screening for vesicoureteral reflux? J Urol. 2012;188:576–81. doi:10.1016/j.juro.2012.04.017.
17. Coelho GM, Bouzada MCF, Pereira AK, Figueiredo BF, Leite MRS, Oliveira DS, et al. Outcome of isolated antenatal hydronephrosis: a prospective cohort study. Pediatr Nephrol. 2007;22:1727–34. doi:10.1007/s00467-007-0539-6.

18. Zareba P, Lorenzo AJ, Braga LH. Risk factors for febrile urinary tract infection in infants with prenatal hydronephrosis: comprehensive single center analysis. J Urol. 2014;191:1614–8. doi:10.1016/j.juro.2013.10.035.

19. Merguerian PA, Herz D, McQuiston L, Van Bibber M. Variation among pediatric urologists and across 2 continents in antibiotic prophylaxis and evaluation for prenatally detected hydronephrosis: a survey of American and European pediatric urologists. J Urol. 2010;184:1710–5. doi:10.1016/j.juro.2010.03.115.

20. Braga LHP, Ruzhynsky V, Pemberton J, Farrokhyar F, Demaria J, Lorenzo AJ. Evaluating practice patterns in postnatal management of antenatal hydronephrosis: a national survey of Canadian pediatric urologists and nephrologists. Urology. 2014;83:909–14. doi:10.1016/j.urology.2013.10.054.

21. Herz D, Merguerian P, McQuiston L. Continuous antibiotic prophylaxis reduces the risk of febrile UTI in children with asymptomatic antenatal hydronephrosis with either ureteral dilation, high-grade vesicoureteral reflux, or ureterovesical junction obstruction. J Pediatr Urol. 2014;10:650–4. doi:10.1016/j.jpurol.2014.06.009.

22. You JJ, Alter DA, Stukel TA, McDonald SD, Laupacis A, Liu Y, et al. Proliferation of prenatal ultrasonography. CMAJ. 2010;182:143–51. doi:10.1503/cmaj.090979.

23. Herndon CD. The role of ultrasound in predicting surgical intervention for prenatal hydronephrosis. J Urol. 2012;187:1535–6. doi:10.1016/j.juro.2012.02.011.

24. Aksu N, Yavascan O, Kangin M, Kara OD, Aydin Y, Erdogan H, et al. Postnatal management of infants with antenatally detected hydronephrosis. Pediatr Nephrol. 2005;20:1253–9.

25. Gatti JM, Broecker BH, Scherz HC, Perez-Brayfield MR, Kirsch AJ. Antenatal hydronephrosis with postnatal resolution: how long are postnatal studies warranted? Urology. 2001;57:1178.

26. St Aubin M, Willihnganz-Lawson K, Varda BK, Fine M, Adejoro O, Prosen T, et al. Society for fetal urology recommendations for postnatal evaluation of prenatal hydronephrosis: will fewer voiding cystourethrograms lead to more urinary tract infections? J Urol. 2013;190 Suppl 4:1456–61. doi:10.1016/j.juro.2013.03.038.

27. Phan V, Traubici J, Hershenfield B, Stephens D, Rosenblum ND, Geary DF. Vesicoureteral reflux in infants with isolated antenatal hydronephrosis. Pediatr Nephrol. 2003;18:1224–8. doi:10.1007/s00467-003-1287-x.

28. Lee NG, Rushton HG, Peters CA, Groves DS, Pohl HG. Evaluation of prenatal hydronephrosis: novel criteria for predicting vesicoureteral reflux on ultrasonography. J Urol. 2014;192:914–8. doi:10.1016/j.juro.2014.03.100.

29. Zerin JM, Ritchey ML, Chang AC. Incidental vesicoureteral reflux in neonates with antenatally detected hydronephrosis and other renal abnormalities. Radiology. 1993;187:157–60.

30. Conway JJ, Mazeils M. The "well tempered" diuretic renogram: a standard method to examine the asymptomatic neonate with hydronephrosis or hydroureteronephrosis. A report from combined meetings of The Society for Fetal Urology and members of The Pediatric Nuclear Medicine Council. J Nucl Med. 1992;33(11):2047–51.

31. Jones RA, Perez-Brayfield MR, Kirsch AJ, Grattan-Smith JD. Renal transit time with MR urography in children. Radiology. 2004;233(1):41–50.

32. McMann LP, Kirsch AJ, Scherz HC, Smith EA, Jones RA, Shehata BM, et al. Magnetic resonance urography in the evaluation of prenatally diagnosed hydronephrosis and renal dysgenesis. J Urol. 2006;176:1786–92. doi:10.1016/j.juro.2006.05.025.

33. Perez-Brayfield MR, Kirsch AJ, Jones RA, Grattan-Smith JD. A prospective study comparing ultrasound, nuclear scintigraphy and dynamic contrast enhanced magnetic resonance imaging in the evaluation of hydronephrosis. J Urol. 2003;179(4 pt 1):1330–4.

34. Kirsch AJ, McMann LP, Jones RA, Smith EA, Scherz HC, Grattan-Smith JD. Magnetic resonance urography for evaluating outcomes after pediatric pyeloplasty. J Urol. 2006;176:1755–61. doi:10.1016/j.juro.2006.03.115.

35. Herndon CD, DeCambre M, McKenna PH. Changing concepts concerning the management of vesicoureteral reflux. J Urol. 2001;166:1439–43. doi:10.1097/00005392-200110000-00065.

36. Lee JH, Choi HS, Kim JK, Won HS, Kim KS, Moon DH, et al. Nonrefluxing neonatal hydronephrosis and the risk of urinary tract infection. J Urol. 2008;179:1524–8. doi:10.1016/j.juro.2007.11.090.
37. Corteville JE, Gray DL, Crane JP. Congenital hydronephrosis: corrleation of fetal ultrasonographic findings with infant outcome. Am J Obs Gynecol. 1992;165(2):384–8.
38. Mandell J, Kinard HW, Mittelstaedt CA, Seeds JW. Prenatal diagnosis of unilateral hydronephrosis with early postnatal reconstruction. J Urol. 1984;132:303–7.
39. Adra AM, Mejides AA, Dennaoui MS, Beydoun SN. Fetal pyelectasis: is it always "physiologic"? Am J Obstet Gynecol. 1995;173:1263–6.
40. Maayan-Metzger A, Lotan D, Jacobson JM, Raviv-Zilka L, Ben-Shlush A, Kuint J, et al. The yield of early postnatal ultrasound scan in neonates with documented antenatal hydronephrosis. Am J Perinatol. 2011;28:613–8. doi:10.1055/s-0031-1276735.
41. Madden-Fuentes RJ, McNamara ER, Nseyo U, Wiener JS, Routh JC, Ross SS. Resolution rate of isolated low-grade hydronephrosis diagnosed within the first year of life. J Pediatr Urol. 2014;10:639–44. doi:10.1016/j.jpurol.2014.07.004.
42. Barbosa JABA, Chow JS, Benson CB, Yorioka MA, Bull AS, Retik AB, et al. Postnatal longitudinal evaluation of children diagnosed with prenatal hydronephrosis: insights in natural history and referral pattern. Prenat Diagn. 2012;32:1242–9. doi:10.1002/pd.3989.
43. Tombesi MM, Alconcher LF. Short-term outcome of mild isolated antenatal hydronephrosis conservatively managed. J Pediatr Urol. 2012;8:129–33. doi:10.1016/j.jpurol.2011.06.009.
44. Ulman I, Jayanthi VR, Koff SA. The long-term follow-up of newborns with severe unilateral hydronephrosis managed non-operatively. J Urol. 2000;164(3 Pt 2):1101–5.
45. Yeung CK, Godley ML, Dhillon HK, Duffy PG, Ransley PG. Urodynamic patterns in infants with normal lower urinary tracts or primary vesico-ureteric reflux. Br J Urol. 1998;81:461–7.
46. Upadhyay J, McLorie GA, Bolduc S, Bagli DJ, Khoury AE, Farhat W. Natural history of neonatal reflux associated with prenatal hydronephrosis: long-term results of a prospective study. J Urol. 2003;169:1837–41. doi:10.1097/01.ju.0000062440.92454.cf. discussion 1841; author reply 1841.
47. Yerkes EB, Adams MC, Pope IV JC, Brock III JW. Does every patient with prenatal hydronephrosis need voiding cystourethrography? J Urol. 1999;162(3 pt 2):1218–20.
48. al-Khaldi N, Watson AR, Zuccollo J, Twining P, Rose DH. Outcome of antenatally detected cystic dysplastic kidney disease. Arch Dis Child. 1994;70:520–2.
49. Atiyeh B, Hussman D, Baum M. Contralateral renal abnormalities in multicystic-dysplastic kidney disease. J Ped. 1992;121:65–7.
50. Heikkinen ES, Herva R, Lanning P. Multicystic kidney. A clinical and histological study of 13 patients. Ann Chir Gynaecol. 1980;69:15–22.
51. Calaway AC, Whittam B, Szymanski KM, Misseri R, Kaefer M, Rink RC, et al. Multicystic dysplastic kidney: is an initial voiding cystourethrogram necessary? Can J Urol. 2014;21:7510–4.
52. Whittam BM, Calaway A, Szymanski KM, Carroll AE, Misseri R, Kaefer M, et al. Ultrasound diagnosis of multicystic dysplastic kidney: Is a confirmatory nuclear medicine scan necessary? J Pediatr Urol. 2014;10:1059–62. doi:10.1016/j.jpurol.2014.03.011.
53. Narchi H. Risk of Wilms' tumor with multicystic kidney disease: a systemic review. Arch Dis Child. 2005;90:147–9.
54. Pérez LM, Naidu SI, Joseph DB. Outcome and cost analysis of operative versus nonoperative management of neonatal multicystic dysplastic kidneys. J Urol. 1998;160:1207–11. discussion 1216.
55. Share JC, Lebowitz RL. Ectopic ureterocele without ureteral and calyceal dilatation (ureterocele disproportion): findings on urography and sonography. Am J Roentgenol. 1989;152:567–71. doi:10.2214/ajr.152.3.567.
56. Godinho AB, Nunes C, Janeiro M, Carvalho R, Melo MA, da Graça LM. Ureterocele: antenatal diagnosis and management. Fetal Diagn Ther. 2013;34:188–91. doi:10.1159/000353388.

57. Quintero RA, Homsy Y, Bornick PW, Allen M, Johnson PK. In-utero treatment of fetal bladder-outlet obstruction by a ureterocele. Lancet. 2001;357:1947–8. doi:10.1016/S0140-6736(00)05084-4.
58. Chertin B, de Caluwe D, Puri P. Is primary endoscopic puncture of ureterocele a long-term effective procedure? J Pediatr Surg. 2003;38:116–9.
59. Chertin B, Rolle U, Farkas A, Puri P. Does delaying pyeloplasty affect renal function in children with a prenatal diagnosis of pelvi-ureteric junction obstruction? BJU Int. 2002;90:72–5.
60. Chertin B, Pollack A, Koulikov D, Rabinowitz R, Shen O, Hain D, et al. Long-term follow up of antenatally diagnosed megaureters. J Pediatr Urol. 2008;4:188–91. doi:10.1016/j.jpurol.2007.11.013.
61. Jesus LE, Farhat WA, Amarante ACM, Dini RB, Leslie B, Bägli DJ, et al. Clinical evolution of vesicoureteral reflux following endoscopic puncture in children with duplex system ureteroceles. J Urol. 2011;186:1455–8. doi:10.1016/j.juro.2011.05.057.
62. Direnna T, Leonard MP. Watchful waiting for prenatally detected ureteroceles. J Urol. 2006;175:1493–5. doi:10.1016/S0022-5347(05)00676-2. discussion 1495.
63. Han MY, Gibbons MD, Belman AB, Pohl HG, Majd M, Rushton HG. Indications for nonoperative management of ureteroceles. J Urol. 2005;174:1652–6.
64. Storm DW, Modi A, Jayanthi VR. Laparoscopic ipsilateral ureteroureterostomy in the management of ureteral ectopia in infants and children. J Pediatr Urol. 2011;7:529–33. doi:10.1016/j.jpurol.2010.08.004.
65. Mason MD, Anthony Herndon CD, Smith-Harrison LI, Peters CA, Corbett ST. Robotic-assisted partial nephrectomy in duplicated collecting systems in the pediatric population: techniques and outcomes. J Pediatr Urol. 2014;10:374–9. doi:10.1016/j.jpurol.2013.10.014.
66. McLeod DJ, Alpert SA, Ural Z, Jayanthi VR. Ureteroureterostomy irrespective of ureteral size or upper pole function: a single center experience. J Pediatr Urol. 2014;10:616–9. doi:10.1016/j.jpurol.2014.05.003.
67. Husmann DA, Ewalt DH, Glenski WJ, Bernier PA. Ureterocele associated with ureteral duplication and a nonfunctioning upper pole segment: management by partial nephro-ureterectomy alone. J Urol. 1995;154:723–6. doi:10.1016/S0022-5347(01)67144-1.
68. De Caluwe D, Chertin B, Puri P. Fate of the retained ureteral stump after upper pole heminephrectomy in duplex kidneys. J Urol. 2002;168:679–80.
69. Shukla AR, Cooper J, Patel RP, Carr MC, Canning DA, Zderic SA, et al. Prenatally detected primary megaureter: a role for extended followup. J Urol. 2005;173:1353–6. doi:10.1097/01.ju.0000152319.72909.52.
70. McLellan DL, Retik AB, Bauer SB, Diamond DA, Atala A, Mandell J, et al. Rate and predictors of spontaneous resolution of prenatally diagnosed primary nonrefluxing megaureter. J Urol. 2002;168:2177–80. doi:10.1097/01.ju.0000034943.31317.2f. discussion 2180.
71. Farrugia M-K, Hitchcock R, Radford A, Burki T, Robb A, Murphy F. British Association of Paediatric Urologists consensus statement on the management of the primary obstructive megaureter. J Pediatr Urol. 2014;10:26–33. doi:10.1016/j.jpurol.2013.09.018.

Chapter 14
Clinical Consequences of Congenital Anomalies of the Kidney and Urinary Tract

Donna J. Claes and Prasad Devarajan

Abbreviations

ABPM	Ambulatory blood pressure monitoring
ARBs	Angiotensin II receptor blockers
BP	Blood pressure
CKD	Chronic kidney disease
CKiD	Chronic kidney disease in children
ESA	Erythropoietin stimulating agent
ESRD	End stage renal disease
GFR	Glomerular filtration rate
KDIGO	Kidney disease improving global outcomes
KDOQI	Kidney disease outcomes quality initiative
LVH	Left ventricular hypertrophy
MAP	Mean arterial blood pressure
NAPRTCS	North American Pediatric Renal Trials and Collaborative Studies
UPEC	Uropathogenic *E. coli*
USRDS	United States Renal Data System
UTI	Urinary tract infection
VUR	Vesicoureteral reflux

D.J. Claes, M.D., M.S., B.S.Pharm.
Division of Pediatric Nephrology and Hypertension, Cincinnati Children's Hospital
Medical Center, 3333 Burnet Avenue, Cincinnati, OH 45229, USA

P. Devarajan, M.D., F.A.A.P. (✉)
Division of Nephrology and Hypertension, Cincinnati Children's Hospital Medical Center,
University of Cincinnati College of Medicine, Cincinnati, OH, USA
e-mail: prasad.devarajan@cchmc.org

© Springer International Publishing Switzerland 2016
A.J. Barakat, H. Gil Rushton (eds.), *Congenital Anomalies of the Kidney and Urinary Tract*, DOI 10.1007/978-3-319-29219-9_14

287

Introduction

The management of CAKUT is evolving. Prenatal diagnosis and supportive or corrective surgical inventions have improved survival of affected newborns, allowing them to live well beyond previous historical projections. However, as a consequence, these children will often have significant medical comorbidities. The most common comorbidities in this patient population include chronic kidney disease (CKD) and its complications (especially hypertension and proteinuria), as well as recurrent urinary tract infections (UTIs).

CKD is a state of irreversible kidney damage that can lead to end stage renal disease (ESRD). ESRD patients require renal replacement therapy in the form of either dialysis or transplantation to maintain survival. Currently, there is no cure for CKD, and treatment is supportive in nature. As approximately 70 % of pediatric patients with CKD progress to ESRD before reaching adulthood, the care of patients with CKD focuses on interventions to preserve native renal function. Current evidence suggests that optimizing the care for the common complications of pediatric CKD—such as high blood pressure, proteinuria, metabolic acidosis, and/or anemia—may slow native kidney deterioration and thus delay the progression to ESRD. In addition, adequately identifying, treating, and preventing urinary tract infections is another important cornerstone to preserving renal health in patients with underlying CAKUT. This chapter discusses the diagnosis, morbidity and mortality, and overall medical support needed in the pediatric CKD patient, emphasizing the importance of a multidisciplinary approach among pediatric urologists, nephrologists, and pediatricians for children with congenital anomalies of the kidney and urinary tract. This chapter also highlights emerging evidence regarding the treatment of UTIs in children with underlying CAKUT, specifically focusing on issues related to recurrent UTIs.

Chronic Kidney Disease

Epidemiology

Much of what we know about the epidemiology of pediatric CKD is obtained from various registries and reporting systems. The pediatric populations represented within these registries may be limited to just ESRD patients (such as the United States Renal Data System (USRDS), European Dialysis and Transplant Registry, or Australia and New Zealand Dialysis and Transplant Registry). They may include pre-dialysis CKD patients in addition to the ESRD population (i.e., North American Pediatric Renal Trials and Collaborative Studies (NAPRTCS) or the ItalKid registry). These databases have inherent limitations in the ability to provide accurate epidemiological information pertaining to the entire spectrum of pediatric CKD (both pre-ESRD and ESRD) populations, including selection bias from registries that require voluntary permission for enrollment and reporting clinical information. Furthermore, many patients with CKD are asymptomatic and may go undiagnosed for many years until kidney disease becomes advanced. The true incidence of pediatric CKD is therefore difficult to ascertain and is likely underestimated by registry data.

Understanding the inherent limitations of database registries, the ItalKids registry estimated the overall prevalence of pediatric CKD in Italian children <20 years of age at 74.7 cases per million of the age-related population, with about 12.1 new cases diagnosed per million of the population per year [1]. Based on the data from the 2014 USRDS report, about 7500 US children under the age of 20 years are living with ESRD (including approximately 1200 incident cases diagnosed in the year 2012), with almost three-fourths of this total population represented by those with a functioning renal transplant. Worldwide, CAKUT are the most common cause of pediatric CKD, responsible for 50–60 % of all cases [1, 2].

Definition and Staging of Pediatric CKD

The National Kidney Foundation's (NKF) Kidney Disease Outcomes Quality Initiative (KDOQI) Clinical Practice Guidelines define CKD in the pediatric population as [3]:

- Kidney damage for ≥3 months, as defined by structural or functional abnormalities of the kidney, with or without decreased glomerular filtration rate (GFR), manifest by 1 or more of the following features:

  - Abnormalities in the composition of the blood or urine (i.e., proteinuria, hematuria).
  - Abnormalities in imaging tests (i.e., ultrasound, CT, MRI).
  - Abnormalities on kidney biopsy.

- GFR ≤60 ml/min/1.73 m² for ≥3 months, with or without the other signs of kidney damage as described above.

Patients with normal kidney function but with findings of persistent renal damage—most notably those with persistent proteinuria—are included in the CKD definition as these patients are at increased risk of developing the adverse outcomes associated with CKD. CKD is further staged based on severity of renal dysfunction in those patients 2 years of age or greater, irrespective of underlying diagnosis (Table 14.1). Children younger than 2 years of age cannot be accurately

Table 14.1 Classification of the stages of CKD in children ≥2 years of age [3]

Stage	GFR (ml/min/1.73 m²)
1	≥90
2	60–89
3	30–59
4	15–29
5	≤15

Table 14.2 KDIGO classification of CKD in adults according to GFR category

GFR category	GFR (ml/min/1.73 m²)	Terms
G1	≥90	Normal or high
G2	60–89	Mildly decreased
G3a	45–59	Mildly to moderately decreased
G3b	30–44	Moderately to severely decreased
G4	15–29	Severely decreased
G5	<15	Kidney failure

Table 14.3 KDIGO classification of albuminuria in adults with CKD

Category	Albumin excretion rate (mg/24 h)	Albumin–creatinine ratio (ACR), MG/G	Terms
A1	<30	<30	Normal to mildly increased
A2	30–300	30–300	Moderately increased
A3	>300	>300	Severely increased

staged for CKD because renal development and maturation is still occurring. However, these young patients can be classified as moderate or severe CKD if the serum creatinine is above 2 or 3 standard deviations above the general population, respectively. Because accurate assessment of kidney function is necessary to correctly classify CKD, it is important to discuss the methods of GFR measurement used in clinical practice.

Classification of CKD in adult patients per the Kidney Disease Improving Global Outcomes (KDIGO) guidelines is derived using the "CGA" classification system—*c*ause of kidney disease, *G*FR category, and *a*lbuminuria category (Tables 14.2 and 14.3, respectively) [4, 5]. Combining these three elements predicts overall prognosis in adult CKD patients in regard to disease progression, morbidity (such as hospitalization rates), and mortality (including cardiovascular events and mortality)—and thus plays an integral role in guiding treatment and other medical intervention decisions in the adult CKD patient.

Measuring Versus Estimating GFR

Kidney function is most commonly assessed by GFR, which is defined as the transudation of plasma across the glomerular filtration barrier. GFR is estimated by measuring the renal clearance of a substance from the plasma that has the following properties: (1) it is completely filtered by the renal glomerulus, and (2) it is not secreted, metabolized, or transported by the kidney. As renal clearance is affected by renal size (which correlates with body surface area), renal clearance of any substance is further scaled to the body surface area of a "standard" adult, resulting in the measurement of renal clearance in milliliters per minute per 1.73 m^2 (ml/min/1.73 m^2). The renal clearance of a substance is measured by the formula [6]:

$$\text{Clearance of } X = (Ux \times V)/Px$$

in which X substance being measured, Ux urine concentration of the substance, V urine volume over time (ml/min), Px plasma concentration of the substance being measured.

Inulin, the gold standard in measuring GFR, is a non-protein bound substance that has all the properties of an ideal marker of GFR. It is freely filtered by the glomerulus, and it is not secreted, metabolized or transported by the kidney. Unfortunately, inulin is not readily available at present and requires urinary collection in addition to plasma collections to measure renal function (which is less than ideal in pediatric patients who may not be fully toilet trained, or have associated abnormalities of the bladder and other voiding issues). Thus, newer agents such as iohexol (a low osmolar, low-toxicity intravenous contrast agent) or nuclear-medicine based radioisotopes (^{99m}Tc-DTPA, ^{51}Cr-EDTA, or [125]Iothalamate) are considered the new standards to measure GFR.

Measuring creatinine clearance using 24 h urine collections has historically been a common and relatively economical method to calculate renal function [3]. Creatinine is produced at a relatively constant rate by muscle cells and is freely filtered at the glomerulus. Most importantly, serum creatinine is routinely measured by the general medical community, which improves its practicality for use. Unfortunately, creatinine is an imperfect marker to estimate renal function because its production is reflective of muscle mass as well as diet (and thus can be falsely low in those with poor muscle mass, amputations, or those with strict vegetarian diets). Furthermore, creatinine is known to be secreted and absorbed by renal tubules, especially in those with severely decreased GFR. In addition, timed urinary collections are fraught with error, especially in the pediatric population, where many children may not be toilet trained or have abnormal bladders and urinary voiding.

Many GFR estimating equations that provide a simpler and more convenient method to quantify kidney function have been developed. These formulas are easier to use in the day-to-day clinical setting given the complex logistics and time (sometimes up to 5–9 h in length) required for formal GFR testing. One of the first GFR estimating formulas was derived by Schwartz et al in the 1970s. At the time the original Schwartz formula was derived, serum creatinine was measured using the Jaffe method, a method known to over-estimate serum creatinine at the low values commonly seen in the pediatric population. Today, most clinical laboratories use enzymatic-based assays which measure serum creatinine more accurately. To account for this, the original Schwartz formula has been recently updated based on data from the Chronic Kidney Disease in Children (CKiD) study [7].

$$\text{Schwartz formula: eGFR}\left(\text{ml/min/1.73m}^2\right)$$
$$= \left[0.413 \times \text{height}\left(\text{cm}\right)\right]/\text{plasma creatinine}\left(\text{mg/dL}\right)$$

This formula demonstrates improved estimation of GFR in a patient population with a measured GFR between 15 and 75 ml/min/1.73 m². However, it lacks precision and continues to over-estimate GFR in the CKD population and under-estimate GFR in children with normal renal function [8, 9].

As serum creatinine has many undesirable qualities for its use in assessing renal function, cystatin C is gaining more popularity as its surrogate for estimating renal function in both the pediatric and adult populations. Cystatin C, a low-molecular weight protein (13 kDa) discovered in the mid-1980s, belongs to a family of endogenous cystine protease inhibitors that are thought to be involved with regulation of proteases released by the lysosomes of injured or dying cells [10]. Cystatin C has many properties that appear to make it an more suitable surrogate maker as compared to serum creatinine to estimate renal function. Cystatin C is produced by all cells of the body at a relatively constant rate, it is freely filtered by the glomerulus, it is absorbed and then degraded by the proximal tubular cells of the nephron without tubular absorption or secretion, and it has minimal extra-renal elimination. Cystatin C measurement is also independent of muscle mass, and displays less inter-patient and intra-patient variability as compared to serum creatinine measurements. However, many conditions can alter endogenous cystatin C production and may therefore affect GFR estimations based on cystatin C. For example, increased inflammation (such as in the setting of administration of glucocorticoids or immunosuppression in solid organ transplant patients), increased "cellular load" (i.e., malignancy), or increased metabolic activity (i.e., hyperthyroidism) have all been associated with increased cystatin C levels [11]. Other possible conditions that may explain cystatin C variability in the general population include obesity and cigarette smoking. A recent analysis of healthy 12–19-year-old adolescents enrolled in the NHANES research study showed that demographic characteristics also affect cystatin C levels. Higher cystatin C values were found in males and non-Hispanic white participants' cystatin C concentration also decreased with age [12]. Finally, variations in cystatin C values can also be related to differences in methods of its laboratory measurement [10].

There are multiple GFR estimating formulas that use only serum creatinine, only cystatin C, a combination of cystatin C plus serum creatinine, or a large number of laboratory values and various clinical variables. The most important factor in choosing the "best" estimating formula—whether a creatinine based or cystatin C based formulas—is understanding if the patient population from which the formula was derived "fits" the patient population to which the estimating formula is being applied. Most of these pediatric estimating equations have been derived from primarily CKD populations, and may lose accuracy and precision when applied to non-CKD patient populations [8, 9, 13].

Morbidity and Mortality Associated with Pediatric CKD

Although pediatric CKD is relatively rare and pediatric ESRD patients represent <5 % of the total ESRD population in the US, children with CKD share one factor in common with their adult CKD counterparts—an increased mortality risk.

Pediatric patients with CKD have a 30- to 150-fold higher death rate as compared to age-matched healthy peers [14]. World-wide patient cohorts from countries including the United States, Germany, Netherlands, Australia and New Zealand have all demonstrated that cardiovascular disease is the leading cause of death in the pediatric ESRD population. Cardiovascular disease is responsible for 32, 28 and 22 % of deaths seen in US pediatric hemodialysis, peritoneal dialysis, and transplant patients, respectively [15]. Overall, pediatric patients with ESRD carry a 100–1000-fold increased risk of cardiovascular death as compared to the general pediatric population. Cardiovascular death from arrhythmias, asystole/cardiac arrest, valvular disease, or cardiomyopathy occurs amongst all pediatric age groups, including infants under age 1 year [16]. Factors associated with increased risk of cardiovascular death in pediatric ESRD patients include black race and increased age; in contrast, a functioning renal transplant is associated with a 78 % lower risk of cardiovascular death as compared to patients receiving any form of dialysis [14]. Cardiovascular disease, which can be appreciated even in the early stages of CKD, is evidenced in the form of left ventricular hypertrophy (LVH) and dysfunction, large arterial stiffness, and/or coronary vessel calcification [15]. Thus, a strong focus on reducing both "traditional" (hypertension, obesity, dyslipidemia, and insulin resistance) and "uremic" cardiovascular risk factors (abnormal mineral metabolism which can include hyperphosphatemia, hypercalcemia, and secondary hyperparathyroidism; anemia; inflammation; and hypoalbuminemia) in this patient population is necessary to reduce future mortality and morbidity in the pediatric CKD population.

Growth failure commonly occurs in children with CKD and is also associated with significant morbidity and mortality. According to the NAPRTCS 2005 annual report, nearly one-third of pediatric CKD patients had evidence of severe growth failure (a height SDS <−1.88, or height <3 % for age and gender) at the time of entry into NAPRTCS, and less than 20 % of children had a height greater than a SDS >0 [17, 18]. Unfortunately, many CKD patients continue to have sub-optimal growth velocity throughout childhood, which leads to a stunted final adult height. For example, in a retrospective study of 52 German children who underwent renal transplantation before age 15 years, approximately 75 % failed to reach a final adult height above the 3rd percentile. This severe short stature appears to carry a significant burden of global health-related quality of life, as the final adult height in pediatric CKD patients has been found to be positively associated with the ability to marry and level of education, and negatively associated with level of employment. Unfortunately, poor growth is not just "a cosmetic issue," but it is associated with increased mortality, increased hospitalization, and less full-time school attendance in the pediatric ESRD population [19].

Factors associated with poor growth include young age, degree/severity of renal impairment, uncontrolled metabolic acidosis, having structural renal abnormalities or other underlying renal tubular disorders (non-glomerular disorder), and renal bone disease (such as secondary hyperparathyroidism) [18]. All of these result in reduced caloric intake and abnormal protein metabolism. Advanced CKD is also associated with growth hormone resistance and delayed puberty, both of which can further impair linear growth. The initial treatment of growth failure focuses on opti-mizing caloric and protein intake (which often involves the use of gastrostomy tubes in infants and toddlers with CKD), correction of metabolic acidosis and sec-ondary hyperparathyroidism, and use of additional sodium supplementation in those patients with excessive renal salt wasting. However, for CKD patients with continued short stature refractory to initial medical management therapies, recom-binant growth hormone is a safe and effective treatment option. Recombinant growth hormone use has been extensively studied and is FDA approved for use in the pediatric CKD population. Growth hormone use has been shown to improve growth in all stages of CKD (pre-ESRD, dialysis, and post-transplantation), and many children with CKD are able to achieve normal adult height with long-term growth hormone use. The NAPRTCS database demonstrates that CKD patients using growth hormone did not have an accelerated rate of renal loss as compared to non-growth hormone users; likewise, growth hormone use in kidney transplant recipients is not associated with an increased frequency of allograft rejection. Further evaluation of the NAPRTCS database did not reveal an increased frequency of growth-hormone related adverse events—such as avascular necrosis (AVN), slipped capital femoral epiphysis (SCFE), glucose intolerance, pancreatitis, malig-nancy, and intracranial hypertension, as compared to untreated patients. Growth hormone use appears to be most effective in terms of overall height gain in pre-ESRD CKD patients as compared to use during dialysis or following renal trans-plantation, but its use in this population remains under-utilized, as reports from the CKiD study has demonstrated that less than one-fourth of pediatric CKD patients with a height SDS score of <-1.88 are currently prescribed growth hormone [20].

Progression of CKD and Its Medical Management

Whether renal impairment is secondary to congenital anomalies of the kidney and urinary tract or an acquired glomerular disease, the timing of progression of CKD from minimal renal injury to onset of ESRD can be variable. This variable time course presents challenges in medical practice, especially when having discussion with patients and families in regard to the timing to initiate renal replacement therapy, including preemptive kidney transplantation. The CKiD study has reported the median GFR change over time to be -4.3 ml/min/1.73 m^2 per year and -1.5 ml/min/1.73 m^2 per year in children with glomerular and non-glomerular etiologies, respectively [21].

Nonmodifiable risk factors associated with faster CKD progression include older age, glomerular etiology of renal disease, and more advanced CKD [22, 23]. Onset of puberty is also an important risk factor associated with CKD risk progression. In an analysis of Italian children with CKD with predominantly congenital renal and/or urological abnormalities, the risk of developing ESRD prior to 10 years of age was less than 10%, but this risk increased to 50% by age 18 years. Furthermore, there was a tenfold increased loss of renal function when comparing change in renal function prior to and then following onset of the pubertal growth spurt [24].

Modifiable risk factors associated with CKD progression include hypertension, proteinuria, anemia, and acidosis. Both hypertension and proteinuria have been independently associated with more rapid CKD progression in various pediatric CKD observational studies [23]. The prevalence of hypertension in children with CKD is high, even when the GFR is only mildly reduced, and increases progressively with further declines in GFR. In children with CKD from any etiology, strict blood pressure control has been shown to slow the progression of kidney disease and reduce the risk of cardiovascular disease. In particular, both angiotensin converting enzyme (ACE) inhibitors and angiotensin receptor blockers (ARBs) have been proven effective in controlling blood pressure, reducing proteinuria, and slowing progression of CKD in these patients. However, despite this knowledge, many pediatric CKD patients continue to have under-recognized as well as under-treated blood pressure. Thirty-seven percent of pediatric CKiD participants had documented blood pressures >90th percentile for age, gender and height, and one-third of those with elevated blood pressure were not prescribed any antihypertensive medication. Of those receiving antihypertensive medications, 36 % continued to have elevated systolic or diastolic blood pressures >90 % [25]. In addition, up to 30 % of pediatric CKD patients have masked hypertension, defined as a normal office blood pressure (<90th percentile) but abnormally elevated blood pressures as recorded by 24 h ambulatory blood pressure monitoring (ABPM) [26]. Thus, close nephrology follow up with interventions focusing on methods to improve the recognition and continued treatment of blood pressure elevation are needed.

In 2009, the ESCAPE study was the first randomized control trial in the pediatric CKD population to demonstrate that intensive blood pressure control (i.e., a 24 h mean arterial blood pressure (MAP), below the 50th percentile for age, gender, and height) is associated with slower CKD progression as compared to those with more conventional blood pressure control (24 h MAP between the 50th and 90th percentile) at 5 year follow up [27]. Patients in both the intensive as well as conventional blood pressure treatment arm of the study were prescribed a maximum dose of the ACE inhibitor ramipril; additional antihypertensive medications were prescribed to participants of the intensive treatment arm as indicated to achieve a 24 h MAP <50 % as per 24 h ABPM. Patients in the intensive blood pressure control arm were 35 % less likely to reach the clinical endpoint (defined as a 50 % decrease in eGFR, an eGFR <10 ml/min/1.73 m^2, or initiation of renal replacement therapy) by the end of the 5 year study; patients with a baseline GFR of <45 ml/min/1.73 m^2, a pre-study eGFR loss of >3 ml/year, a 24 h MAP >90 %, and proteinuria >0.5 mg/mg creatinine appeared to benefit the most from intensive blood pressure management. There was no difference in adverse events between the two groups (intensive versus conventional therapy).

Since the ESCAPE study results have been published, goals of blood pressure control in pediatric CKD patients in regard to when to initiate antihypertensive therapy, target blood pressure goals, as well as method of blood pressure measurement upon which to base treatment management decisions (auscultatory office blood pressure reading versus 24 h ABPM) has been controversial. In children with CKD, the National Kidney KDOQI guidelines have traditionally recommended target systolic and diastolic blood pressures of less than 90th percentile for age, gender, and height, or less than 120/80 mmHg, whichever is lower, based on office measurements. A post hoc analysis of the ESCAPE study revealed similar improvements in renal outcomes with any 24-h MAP <75 %. Based on this information plus the improved benefit of slower CKD progression with intensive blood pressure control to <50 % in CKD patients with proteinuria, European guidelines for pediatric CKD patients recommend a target blood pressure of <75 % for age, gender, and height in patients without proteinuria, and a target blood pressure of <50 % in those patients with proteinuria [28]. Although slightly different, 2012 KDIGO guidelines recommend initiating antihypertensive therapy in pediatric CKD patients whose office blood pressure is consistently >90 % for age, gender, and height; with a suggested blood pressure treatment target of <50 % (especially in those patients with proteinuria) [29]. With regard to the method of blood pressure measurement, both guidelines recognize the benefits of 24 h ABPM use in the pediatric CKD patient population, especially given its unique ability to diagnose white coat hypertension and masked hypertension. However, both guidelines lack specific recommendations in regard to the frequency of ABPM use in this population. In addition to absence of data in regard to answering this specific question, other barriers to recommending routine ABPM use include anticipated costs—both directly to the patient (especially regarding insurance reimbursement) as well as the indirect department costs of supporting an ABPM program.

It seems reasonable for pediatric nephrologists to integrate the use of ABPM, office blood pressure readings, and home blood pressure readings as a way to facilitate blood pressure management in pediatric CKD patients. In our practice, we recommend performing ABPMs in children with CKD at baseline and at relatively reasonable intervals based on office and/or home blood pressure readings (up to every 2–3 years if the BP is defined as well controlled, and at minimum every year if office BPs are not a reliable method of blood pressure assessment or are suggestive of poor BP control). We have also recommend that the target blood pressure goal for all pediatric CKD patients is at minimum <75 %, with the goal of maximizing antihypertensive therapy to <50 % for any patient currently prescribed antihypertensive therapy management unless limited by signs and symptoms of hypotension.

Treatment of hypertension is directed at both pharmacologic as well as non-pharmacologic therapies. Non-pharmacologic therapies include weight reduction, exercise, stress control, and dietary salt reduction. When pharmacologic therapy is indicated, ACE inhibitors or angiotensin II receptor blockers (ARBs) are the preferred agents given their combined antihypertensive effect, antiproteinuric effect, and documented reduction in progression of CKD as compared with other antihypertensive drugs. We recommend initiating therapy with an ACE inhibitor as there are more data on the safety and efficacy of this class of drugs compared with ARBs in children. We use ARBs in patients who have side effects to ACE inhibitors. We avoid combination therapy of ACE inhibitors and ARBs, as data from adults suggest an increased likelihood of adverse events. We use ACE inhibitors and ARBs cautiously in those patients with advanced CKD. Since any decline in GFR induced by these agents typically occurs within the first few days after the onset of therapy, we measure serum creatinine and potassium concentrations within a week of institution of therapy. The potential of these agents to cause birth defects also should be discussed in detail with any adolescent female prior to administration of ACE inhibitor or ARB therapy. Finally, addressing nonadherence issues is extremely important in any patient with CKD, especially in regard to blood pressure management.

Proteinuria is an important risk factor associated with CKD progression in both glomerular and non-glomerular CAKUT etiologies of pediatric CKD. With CKD progression, proteinuria is the result of both glomerular damage from hyperfiltration as well as tubular damage leading to impaired tubular reabsorption. Accumulating experimental and clinical evidence indicates that chronic proteinuria by itself is detrimental to the kidney, irrespective of the etiology. In clinical studies, proteinuria is independently associated with worsening severity of renal impairment, glomerular cause of CKD, and African American race [30]. In assessing CKD progression in those with non-glomerular etiology such as CAKUT, even normotensive CKiD participants with proteinuria (urine protein-to-creatinine ratio >0.5) had an almost two-fold increase rate of CKD progression as compared to those without proteinuria (GFR decline of 1.8 ml/min/1.73 m^2 per year versus 0.8 ml/min/1.73 m^2 per year respectively) [31]. In the ESCAPE study, one of the most important predictors of a slower CKD progression rate was a 50 % reduction in proteinuria within the first 2 months of ACE inhibitor therapy [27]. For children with CKD, we recommend the use of ACE inhibitors (or ARBs if ACE inhibitors are not tolerated well) with a goal of maintaining the urine protein–creatinine ratio at <0.5. In contrast with adults, in children with CKD, there is no evidence that a low protein diet slows the progression of kidney disease. There is also concern that such a diet may impair growth. We recommend that children with CKD be given a daily diet containing 100 % of the dietary protein requirement based upon age and gender, irrespective of the degree of proteinuria. Indeed, additional protein supplementation should be considered if the protein intake is inadequate to maximize growth and neurodevelopment.

Anemia in pediatric CKD and ESRD patients is associated with significant mortality and morbidity, including a decreased quality of life, LVH, and increased hospitalization. Studies focusing on the relationship between anemia and morbidity and mortality in the pediatric dialysis population have shown that patients whose serum hemoglobin was ≥11 g/dL were 62 % less likely to die over a 2–3 year follow-up period; [32] likewise, pediatric patients with a hematocrit <33 % within 30 days of starting dialysis had an increase likelihood of prolonged hospitalization and death as compared to those whose hematocrit was ≥33 % [33]. The prevalence of anemia in the pre-ESRD population (defined as a hematocrit <33 %) from the NAPRTCS database ranges from approximately 20 % (CKD stage II) to 60 % (CKD stage V) [34]. Anemia in the pre-dialysis CKD population has been associated with faster CKD progression: patients with a hematocrit <33 % at the time of NAPRTCS registry enrollment had a 52 % higher risk of progression to ESRD as compared to those with a hematocrit ≥33 % [22].

There have been no studies focusing on correction of anemia and long-term outcomes (LVH, hospitalization rates, CKD progression, and/or death) in the pediatric

CKD population. Thus, current guidelines defining the hemoglobin level at which to initiate erythropoietin stimulating agent (ESA) therapy recommend an "individualized" approach that balances individual patient symptoms with the risks and benefits of therapy [35]. Recommended hemoglobin targets for pediatric patients on ESA therapy are generally in the range of 11–12 g/dL, with a hemoglobin value no greater than 13 g/dL.

Metabolic acidosis is a relatively common complication seen in the pediatric and adult CKD populations, and it increases in prevalence with increased renal impairment. Patients in the CKiD study with a measured GFR <30 ml/min/1.73 m^2 have a threefold higher rate of metabolic acidosis as compared to those with a GFR >50 ml/min/1.73 m^2 [21]. In a randomized control trial in 134 adult CKD patients with moderately to severely depressed renal function (eGFR of 15–30 ml/min/1.73 m^2), improvement of metabolic acidosis utilizing oral sodium bicarbonate supplementation resulted in a significantly slowed CKD progression as compared to those patients whose metabolic acidosis was not treated with oral supplementation, without an increase in adverse events such as worsening blood pressure [36]. In addition, patients who received oral sodium bicarbonate supplementation had improved nutritional parameters. Therefore, improving bicarbonate supplementation appears to be a relatively easy intervention that could delay onset of ESRD. However, similar to that seen with uncontrolled blood pressure, many pediatric CKD patients have unrecognized and undertreated metabolic acidosis despite the positive effects its reversal can achieve.

Indications to Initiate Maintenance Renal Replacement Therapy

Indications for initiating maintenance dialysis typically include uremic symptoms (such as fatigue, weakness, nausea, vomiting, anorexia, and poor sleep patterns), electrolyte abnormalities (hyperkalemia, hyperphosphatemia), and malnutrition (including poor linear growth in infants and young toddlers with CKD) [37]. There is no consensus among various national guidelines regarding the exact timing to initiate dialysis. Generally, renal replacement therapy is considered as the GFR approaches 15 ml/min/1.73 m^2. However, imprecision with GFR estimation and variability in CKD comorbid conditions among patients with similar kidney function (such as decreased muscle mass secondary to malnutrition and anorexia) preclude using an exact GFR cutoff to determine the need for dialysis.

Despite the survival benefits associated with preemptive renal transplantation, many pediatric patients require dialysis prior to renal transplantation. The choice of dialysis modality can be complex. Contraindications to hemodialysis may include small size and the associated challenges in obtaining hemodialysis access, as well as limitations imposed by the geographic distance from a hemodialysis facility that can appropriately manage a pediatric hemodialysis patient. Peritoneal dialysis contraindications include anatomic complications (such as significant surgical adhesions, omphalocele or gastroschisis, or bladder exstrophy), peritoneal membrane failure associated with previous severe peritoneal infections (especially fungal peritonitis), or lack of an appropriate caregiver who can reliably perform peritoneal dialysis in the home.

Urinary Tract Infection

In 2011, the American Academy of Pediatrics (AAP) revised their clinical practice guideline for the diagnosis and management of the initial urinary tract infection (UTI) in febrile infants and children between the ages of 2–24 months. The AAP guideline recommendations include: (a) obtaining a urinalysis and urine culture prior to antibiotic administration, (b) using only urine specimens from either a clean catheterization or suprapubic aspiration in non-toilet trained infants for urine culture results, and (c) diagnosis of UTI should be made only in patients who have both pyuria and at least 50,000 colony-forming units per ml of a uropathogen obtained by either urinary catheterization or suprapubic catheterization [38]. However, the biggest change was a reversal in the prior recommendation to obtain routine voiding cystourethrogram (VCUG) after the first UTI. Presently, the AAP recommends that febrile infants (2–24 months of age) with a febrile UTI undergo renal and bladder ultrasonography as a routine screen; VCUG is reserved for patients with either evidence of anatomic abnormality on ultrasound (such as hydronephrosis) or for those infants with recurrent UTIs.

Much of the change in regard to obtaining VCUG testing was based on previous studies which questioned the utility of prophylactic antibiotics to prevent recurrent UTIs and renal scarring in patients with underlying VUR. Many of these studies had limitations—such as accepting bag urine specimens for culture results as well as including patients without pyuria at UTI presentation or underlying VUR. Almost 3 years following this AAP statement, the results of the Randomized Intervention for Children with Vesicoureteral Reflux (RIVUR) study were published. In this study, 607 children under the age of 7 years with underlying VUR (Grade II–IV) were randomized to either daily low-dose trimethoprim–sulfamethoxazole prophylaxis or placebo following their first or second UTI [39]. Evidence of pyuria in addition to a positive uropathogen from a urine catheterization culture sample was required. After 2 years of follow-up, patients receiving antibiotic prophylaxis had 50% fewer UTIs as compared to the patients receiving placebo, although with a threefold increased rate of trimethoprim-sulfamethoxazole resistance in those receiving UTI prophylaxis. UTI reduction in the prophylaxis group was even more pronounced in those patients who had underlying bladder dysfunction or whose index UTI was febrile. Although there was no obvious difference in the evidence of renal scarring after 2 years of follow-up, the overall rate of renal scarring was low in both groups (10%), limiting the ability to draw significant conclusions regarding the utility of prophylaxis and prevention of long-term renal damage. Thus, antibiotic prophylaxis does indeed prevent UTI recurrence in young children with VUR, but at the cost of increased antibiotic resistance and with unclear benefits in preventing underlying renal damage. Antibiotic prophylaxis most likely has its greatest benefit in prevention of new renal damage in higher risk patients such as those with high grade VUR, voiding and bowel dysfunction, and a history of recurrent UTIs.

The utility of long-term antibiotic prophylaxis may be related to the ability of certain uropathogenic *E. coli* (UPEC) strains to invade bladder epithelial cells [40]. Although originally thought of as a host defense mechanism, bladder epithelial uptake of UPEC is associated with a survival advantage for UPEC organisms. Once within the bladder epithelium, UPEC can either replicate (often up to quite high levels) or can "hibernate," entering a quiescent state within the cytoplasm. Intracellular UPEC can also move in and out of bladder epithelial cells, disseminating a low-level of UPEC colonization that can serve as the nidus for recurrent UTIs over time.

When to Consult a Pediatric Nephrologist

Given the complex medical issues associated with CKD, it is important that pediatric nephrologists and urologists work together with the general pediatrician to optimize medical care of these patients. Medical management of issues such as malnutrition and/or anemia prior to planned surgical interventions of the urologic tract can dramatically improve postoperative outcomes. Nutritional issues are closely related to fluid and electrolyte replacement issues that are part of the day-to-day practice of a pediatric nephrologist. In addition, many children with congenital anomalies of the kidney and urinary system have urinary concentration defects, resulting in increased free water excretion and polyuria. These patients are at increased risk to develop hypernatremic dehydration if prescribed intravenous fluids at a rate insufficient to replace their ongoing free water losses while NPO during the perioperative and postoperative periods. Finally, there are many other nuances of CKD care, such as hypertension, proteinuria, anemia, and electrolyte management, which are best managed by a pediatric nephrology team. As there is a limited time to intervene on specific medical issues, it is important to consult a pediatric nephrologist early upon diagnosis of underlying renal disorders. Patients with mild CKD benefit from at minimum yearly screening for CKD-related medical complications, with an increased frequency of medical visits needed for those with more severe renal impairment.

References

1. Ardissino G, Dacco V, Testa S, Bonaudo R, Claris-Appiani A, Taioli E, et al. Epidemiology of chronic renal failure in children: data from the ItalKid project. Pediatrics. 2003;111:e382–7.
2. Seikaly MG, Ho PL, Emmett L, Fine RN, Tejani A. Chronic renal insufficiency in children: the 2001 Annual Report of the NAPRTCS. Pediatr Nephrol. 2003;18:796–804.
3. Hogg RJ, Furth S, Lemley KV, Portman R, Schwartz GJ, Coresh J, et al. National Kidney Foundation's Kidney Disease Outcomes Quality Initiative clinical practice guidelines for chronic kidney disease in children and adolescents: evaluation, classification, and stratification. Pediatrics. 2003;111:1416–21.

4. [No authors listed]. Chapter 1: definition and classification of CKD. Kidney Int Suppl. 2013;3:19–62.
5. [No authors listed]. Chapter 2: definition, identification, and prediction of CKD progression. Kidney Int Suppl. 2013;3:63–72.
6. Schwartz GJ, Work DF. Measurement and estimation of GFR in children and adolescents. Clin J Am Soc Nephrol. 2009;4:1832–43.
7. Schwartz GJ, Munoz A, Schneider MF, Mak RH, Kaskel F, Warady BA, et al. New equations to estimate GFR in children with CKD. J Am Soc Nephrol. 2009;20:629–37.
8. Staples A, LeBlond R, Watkins S, Wong C, Brandt J. Validation of the revised Schwartz estimating equation in a predominantly non-CKD population. Pediatr Nephrol. 2010;25:2321–6.
9. Fadrowski JJ, Neu AM, Schwartz GJ, Furth SL. Pediatric GFR estimating equations applied to adolescents in the general population. Clin J Am Soc Nephrol. 2011;6:1427–35.
10. Newman DJ, Cystatin C. Ann Clin Biochem. 2002;39:89–104.
11. Rule AD, Bergstralh EJ, Slezak JM, Bergert J, Larson TS. Glomerular filtration rate estimated by cystatin C among different clinical presentations. Kidney Int. 2006;69:399–405.
12. Groesbeck D, Kottgen A, Parekh R, Selvin E, Schwartz GJ, Coresh J, et al. Age, gender, and race effects on cystatin C levels in US adolescents. Clin J Am Soc Nephrol. 2008;3:1777–85.
13. Sharma AP, Yasin A, Garg AX, Filler G. Diagnostic accuracy of cystatin C-based eGFR equations at different GFR levels in children. Clin J Am Soc Nephrol. 2011;6:1599–608.
14. Parekh RS, Carroll CE, Wolfe RA, Port FK. Cardiovascular mortality in children and young adults with end-stage kidney disease. J Pediatr. 2002;141:191–7.
15. Mitsnefes MM. Cardiovascular disease in children with chronic kidney disease. J Am Soc Nephrol. 2012;23:578–85.
16. Chavers BM, Li S, Collins AJ, Herzog CA. Cardiovascular disease in pediatric chronic dialysis patients. Kidney Int. 2002;62:648–53.
17. Seikaly MG, Salhab N, Warady BA, Stablein D. Use of rhGH in children with chronic kidney disease: lessons from NAPRTCS. Pediatr Nephrol. 2007;22:1195–204.
18. Mahan JD, Warady BA, Consensus C. Assessment and treatment of short stature in pediatric patients with chronic kidney disease: a consensus statement. Pediatr Nephrol. 2006;21:917–30.
19. Furth SL, Stablein D, Fine RN, Powe NR, Fivush BA. Adverse clinical outcomes associated with short stature at dialysis initiation: a report of the North American Pediatric Renal Transplant Cooperative Study. Pediatrics. 2002;109:909–13.
20. Rodig NM, McDermott KC, Schneider MF, Hotchkiss HM, Yadin O, Seikaly MG, et al. Growth in children with chronic kidney disease: a report from the Chronic Kidney Disease in Children Study. Pediatr Nephrol. 2014;29:1987–95.
21. Furth SL, Abraham AG, Jerry-Fluker J, Schwartz GJ, Benfield M, Kaskel F, et al. Metabolic abnormalities, cardiovascular disease risk factors, and GFR decline in children with chronic kidney disease. Clin J Am Soc Nephrol. 2011;6:2132–40.
22. Staples AO, Greenbaum LA, Smith JM, Gipson DS, Filler G, Warady BA, et al. Association between clinical risk factors and progression of chronic kidney disease in children. Clin J Am Soc Nephrol. 2010;5:2172–9.
23. Staples A, Wong C. Risk factors for progression of chronic kidney disease. Curr Opin Pediatr. 2010;22:161–9.
24. Ardissino G, Testa S, Dacco V, Paglialonga F, Vigano S, Felice-Civitillo C, et al. Puberty is associated with increased deterioration of renal function in patients with CKD: data from the ItalKid Project. Arch Dis Child. 2012;97:885–8.
25. Flynn JT, Mitsnefes M, Pierce C, Cole SR, Parekh RS, Furth SL, et al. Blood pressure in children with chronic kidney disease: a report from the Chronic Kidney Disease in Children study. Hypertension. 2008;52:631–7.
26. Mitsnefes M, Flynn J, Cohn S, Samuels J, Blydt-Hansen T, Saland J, et al. Masked hypertension associates with left ventricular hypertrophy in children with CKD. J Am Soc Nephrol. 2010;21:137–44.

27. Group ET, Wuhl E, Trivelli A, Picca S, Litwin M, Peco-Antic A, et al. Strict blood-pressure control and progression of renal failure in children. N Engl J Med. 2009;361:1639–50.
28. Lurbe E, Cifkova R, Cruickshank JK, Dillon MJ, Ferreira I, Invitti C, et al. Management of high blood pressure in children and adolescents: recommendations of the European Society of Hypertension. J Hypertens. 2009;27:1719–42.
29. [No authors listed]. Chapter 6: blood pressure management in children with CKD ND. Kidney Int Suppl. 2012;2:372–6.
30. Wong CS, Pierce CB, Cole SR, Warady BA, Mak RH, Benador NM, et al. Association of proteinuria with race, cause of chronic kidney disease, and glomerular filtration rate in the chronic kidney disease in children study. Clin J Am Soc Nephrol. 2009;4:812–9.
31. Fathallah-Shaykh SA, Flynn JT, Pierce CB, Abraham AG, Blydt-Hansen TD, Massengill SF, et al. Progression of pediatric CKD of nonglomerular origin in the CKiD cohort. Clin J Am Soc Nephrol. 2015;10(4):571–7.
32. Amaral S, Hwang W, Fivush B, Neu A, Frankenfield D, Furth S. Association of mortality and hospitalization with achievement of adult hemoglobin targets in adolescents maintained on hemodialysis. J Am Soc Nephrol. 2006;17:2878–85.
33. Warady BA, Ho M. Morbidity and mortality in children with anemia at initiation of dialysis. Pediatr Nephrol. 2003;18:1055–62.
34. Staples AO, Wong CS, Smith JM, Gipson DS, Filler G, Warady BA, et al. Anemia and risk of hospitalization in pediatric chronic kidney disease. Clin J Am Soc Nephrol. 2009;4:48–56.
35. [No authors listed]. IV. NKF-K/DOQI clinical practice guidelines for anemia of chronic kidney disease: update 2000. Am J Kidney Dis. 2001;37:S182–238.
36. de Brito-Ashurst I, Varagunam M, Raftery MJ, Yaqoob MM. Bicarbonate supplementation slows progression of CKD and improves nutritional status. J Am Soc Nephrol. 2009;20:2075–84.
37. Warady BA, Schaefer F, Alexander S. Pediatric dialysis. 2nd ed. New York: Springer Science and Business Media; 2011.
38. Subcommittee on Urinary Tract Infection SCoQI, Management, Roberts KB. Urinary tract infection: clinical practice guideline for the diagnosis and management of the initial UTI in febrile infants and children 2 to 24 months. Pediatrics. 2011;128:595–610.
39. Investigators RT, Hoberman A, Greenfield SP, Mattoo TK, Keren R, Mathews R, et al. Antimicrobial prophylaxis for children with vesicoureteral reflux. N Engl J Med. 2014;370:2367–76.
40. Mulvey MA, Schilling JD, Martinez JJ, Hultgren SJ. Bad bugs and beleaguered bladders: interplay between uropathogenic Escherichia coli and innate host defenses. Proc Natl Acad Sci U S A. 2000;97:8829–35.

Chapter 15
Genetics of Congenital Anomalies of the Kidneys and Urinary Tract

Asaf Vivante and Friedhelm Hildebrandt

Abbreviations

CAKUT   Congenital anomalies of the kidney and urinary tract
CKD   Chronic kidney disease
VUR   Vesicoureteral reflux

Definition and Phenotypic Appearance of CAKUT

Congenital anomalies of the kidneys and urinary tract (CAKUT) cover a wide range of structural malformations that result from a defect in the morphogenesis of the kidney and/or urinary tract [1]. About 50 % of chronic kidney disease (CKD) in individuals before the age of 18 years is caused by CAKUT [2]. The most common phenotypic forms of CAKUT include renal agenesis, renal hypodysplasia, multicystic dysplastic kidney, hydronephrosis, ureteropelvic junction obstruction, megaureter, ureter duplex, vesicoureteral reflux (VUR), and posterior urethral valves. In the same individual multiple different malformations may coexist. CAKUT may

A. Vivante, M.D., Ph.D.
Division of Nephrology, Boston Children's Hospital,
300 Longwood Ave., Boston, MA 02115, USA
e-mail: Asaf.Vivante@childrens.harvard.edu

F. Hildebrandt, M.D. (✉)
Division of Nephrology, Boston Children's Hospital, Boston, MA, USA

Division of Nephrology, Harvard Medical School, Boston, MA, USA

Division of Nephrology, Howard Hughes Medical Institute,
Enders 561, 300 Longwood Avenue, Boston, MA, USA
e-mail: Friedhelm.Hildebrandt@childrens.harvard.edu

© Springer International Publishing Switzerland 2016
A.J. Barakat, H. Gil Rushton (eds.), *Congenital Anomalies of the Kidney and Urinary Tract*, DOI 10.1007/978-3-319-29219-9_15

appear as an isolated feature without extrarenal involvement ("isolated CAKUT") or as part of a more generalized malformation syndrome in association with extra-renal manifestations ("syndromic CAKUT"). Many observations strongly suggested that CAKUT may frequently be caused by single-gene (monogenic) mutations ("monogenic CAKUT"). This notion is supported by a large number of monogenic mouse models that exhibit CAKUT phenotypes, by human multiorgan monogenic syndromes that may include CAKUT, and by the fact that developmental nephro-genesis of the kidney and urinary tract is strongly governed by hundreds of develop-mental genes. CAKUT may appear with familial aggregation in up to 15 % of cases [3–6]. Table 15.1 provides definitions of some common genetic terms to help address the genetic terminology discussed herein.

Genetic and Molecular Control of Kidney Morphogenesis

The molecular control of the morphogenesis of the kidney and urinary tract is gov-erned by a large number of genes and related signaling pathways that coordinate this complex process [7–9]. The pathogenesis of CAKUT is based on the disturbance of normal nephrogenesis, and can be due to genetic abnormalities in renal develop-mental genes that direct this process. CAKUT phenotypes cover a wide spectrum of malformations that ranges from mild to severe phenotypes. Different structural mal-formations can appear in different individuals of the same family, or in both kidneys of the same individual, even if the causative single-gene mutation is identical. The latter is genetically known as "variable expressivity" of a phenotype (Table 15.1). Understanding the related molecular control mechanisms of kidney development has led to a paradigm shift away from classic anatomic theories to the current cell biological and genetic approaches to the etiology of CAKUT (Fig. 15.1) [1].

Genetic Causality in CAKUT

Single-gene (monogenic) diseases, also known as Mendelian disorders, are caused by mutations in a single causative gene. Even though gene and mutation may differ between different individuals, in each individual mutation(s) in a single (mono-genic) gene will be sufficient to cause disease. Monogenic disorders include three main modes of inheritance: autosomal dominant, autosomal recessive, and X-linked.

In dominant diseases mutation of one copy of an autosomal gene (for each of which we carry two copies, one inherited from the mother and one from the father) is sufficient to cause disease. Therefore, as a rule, one parent and the parent ances-tors will express the disease as they carry the same-single copy (heterozygous) mutation. In contrast, in recessive genes, both parental copies of a gene need to be mutated to cause disease. Therefore, both parents will be healthy heterozygous car-riers and no one in the ancestry will have had the disease.

Table 15.1 Glossary of genetic terms

Term	Definition
Allele	Specific DNA sequence variant in a given gene. Alleles can be designated according to their frequency as common or rare alleles
Exon	The protein coding part of a gene. Exons are spliced together following gene transcription to form messenger RNA, which is translated into protein
Exome	The protein coding sequences of the entire genome (about 1 % of the human genome)
Expressivity	Variation of the expression of the phenotype among affected individuals with the same genotype. Variable expressivity refers to different degrees of severity and/or organ involvement in different affected individuals that carry identical mutation
Genotype	The set of alleles (variants of genes) that structure an individual's genetic makeup
Homozygosity	The presence of identical alleles in the two copies of a gene or locus. The presence of different alleles is referred to as heterozygosity
Homozygosity mapping	A technique in which the homozygous region across the genome are identified. This is an effective strategy for the discovery of autosomal recessive monogenic diseases genes in consanguineous families
Next-generation sequencing	This is a DNA sequencing method, also known as massively parallel sequencing, which allows to simultaneously sequence multiple DNA segments in a high-throughput manner
Phenotype	The observable characteristics of an individual as a morphological, clinical or biochemical trait. A phenotype can also be the presence or absence of a disease
Penetrance	The proportion of individuals that express a certain phenotype in relation to the number of individuals that carry the pathogenic variant(s). It can be age dependent. Incomplete penetrance refers to the observation that some individuals with the mutation do not develop the diseases phenotype at all
Sanger sequencing (first generation sequencing)	DNA sequencing method (invented by Frederick Sanger) that involves termination of polymerized DNA strands at the position of specific labeled nucleotides
Variant filtering	Variant filtering refers to the process of excluding variants between the individual examined and a "normal reference individual" from further consideration as disease causing. For instance, very common variants and variants which do not alter the protein sequence are excluded
Variant	A difference in a DNA sequence as compared to normal reference sequence. A variant may be benign, i.e., single nucleotide polymorphism (SNP) or disease causing (i.e., mutation)
Whole exome sequencing	Targeted capture and sequencing of the exome (exons of all genes) using next-generation sequencing. This method offers a powerful approach towards identification monogenic disease causing genes

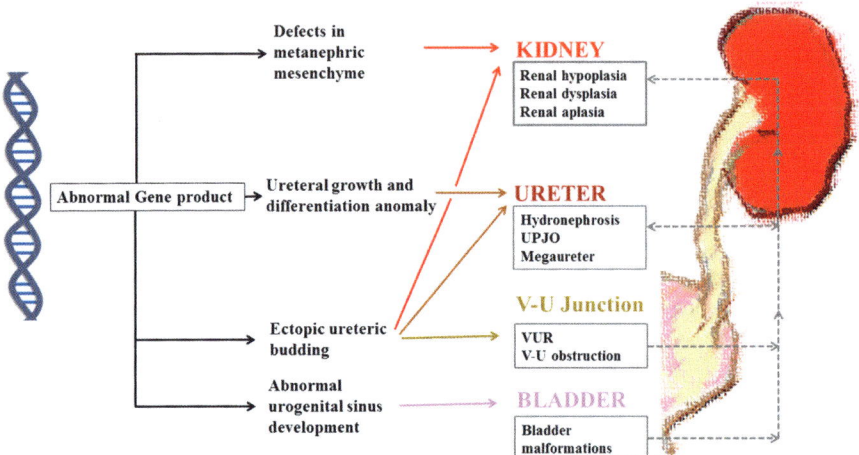

Fig. 15.1 Overview of the phenotypic variability of CAKUT. Single-gene mutations cause a wide spectrum of CAKUT. The phenotypic variability of CAKUT in the presence of an identical mutation may be due to stochastic gene dosage effects of the gene products involved or secondary to their multiple biological actions during different stages of morphogenesis. Alternatively, phenotypic variability may be caused by a so-called genetic "sequence," in which the primary genetic defect causes urinary tract obstruction, which then mechanically leads to developmental defects such as renal hypodysplasia. (Image redrawn from Ichikawa: Paradigm shift from classic anatomic theories to contemporary cell biological views of CAKUT: Kidney Int 2002; 61:889–98). UPJO: ureteropelvic junction obstruction; VUR:vesicoureteral reflux; V-U: vesicoureteral

The degree to which causality is ascribed to a certain genetic variant can be classified according to the penetrance of a given disease-causing mutation (Table 15.2)."Full penetrance" means that 100 % of individuals that carry a genetic variant also express the disease phenotype. At one end of the range of genetic causality are autosomal recessive single-gene disorders. They feature a tight genotype–phenotype correlation, so that the disease phenotype is almost entirely determined by disease-causing mutations in a monogenic disease gene (full penetrance) (Table 15.2). In autosomal dominant single-gene disorders there is a weaker genotype–phenotype correlation due to the features of incomplete penetrance and variable expressivity (see Table 15.1 for glossary). At the other end of the spectrum of genetic causality are more common conditions that are due to genetic variants of low-penetrance, so-called "risk alleles" [10]. Those conditions, which often are referred to as "complex" or "polygenic diseases" have a weak genotype–phenotype correlation (Table 15.2). Thus, usually only a small fraction of the statistical variance for a disease phenotype can be assigned to a risk allele. The role of risk alleles in the pathogenesis of non-monogenic CAKUT is mostly unknown.

Table 15.2 Degrees of genetic causality

	Monogenic recessive diseases	Monogenic dominant diseases	Risk alleles (polygenic/complex) diseases
Penetrance	Full	Full or incomplete	Low
Predictive power of a mutation	Almost 100%	High	Low
Onset	Predominantly during childhood	Childhood and adulthood	Predominantly during adulthood
Disease frequency	Low	Low	High
Number of affected subjects needed for gene discovery	Few	Few	100–10,000
Gene mapping approaches include	Homozygosity mapping or linkage analysis	Linkage analysis	Genome-wide association studies (GWAS)
Whole exome sequencing (WES)	In consanguinity, single affected individuals are sufficient	WES in distant relatives to minimize shared variants	N/A
Functional analysis in animal models (mice, zebrafish)	Easily feasible (knockdown, knockout)	Feasible	Difficult
Examples of genes mutated in patients with CAKUT	*FRAS1, ITGA8*	*PAX2, HNF1B*	?

Strategies for Gene Identification

Discovery of disease-causing mutations in recessive or dominant monogenic CAKUT genes reveals the primary cause (etiology) of the disease. Strategies chosen for identification of monogenic genes depend on the mode of inheritance (Table 15.2). The most frequently chosen strategies are high-throughput exon sequencing of candidate genes and whole exome sequencing combined with homozygosity mapping or linkage analysis.

High-Throughput Candidate Gene Sequencing

In a candidate gene approach exon sequencing is performed in genes that are hypothesized to cause disease, if mutated. For instance, candidate genes for isolated CAKUT can be selected for mutation analysis based on previous knowledge about genes that if mutated cause syndromic form of CAKUT in humans (e.g., *HNF1B* and *PAX2*) [11–13]. This approach is exemplified in a European multicenter study, in which five genes known to cause syndromic CAKUT if mutated were screened in 100 children with renal hypodysplasia [14]. In this study, novel variants were detected in 17 % of patients mostly in the genes *HNF1B* and *PAX2*.

Next-generation sequencing technologies have recently made the candidate gene approach more efficient, as screening of a large number of genes (gene panels) across a large number of individuals is now feasible in a relatively short period of time [15]. We established a cost-effective mutation analysis screen of large patient cohorts [16, 17]. We have developed a microfluidic technique (Fluidigm™) for multiplex PCR-based amplification of ~600 exons of 30 target genes, with barcoding of individual DNAs followed by next-generation sequencing [16]. We applied this technology to examine a large international cohort of 650 unrelated families with CAKUT for the presence of mutations in 17 autosomal dominant and 6 autosomal recessive known CAKUT-causing genes [15, 18]. Our results showed that over 10 % of cases with CAKUT are caused by single-gene mutations in one of the 17 genes. In the meantime, over 34 monogenic CAKUT genes have been recognized (Table 15.3).

Whole Exome Sequencing

The human exome is the entirety of all protein-coding sequences of the human genome. Whole exome sequencing (WES) (Table 15.1) is a very powerful tool that can be applied to molecular genetic diagnostics in known disease genes as well as for the discovery of novel disease genes. A detailed description of the WES technique can be found elsewhere [19, 20]. The application of whole-exome sequencing to diagnostics or gene discovery is challenged by the large number of genetic variants that result when comparing the exome sequences of the studied individual to the normal genome reference sequence. This problem can be overcome by restricting variant filtering (Table 15.1) to smaller regions of interest that are generated for instance by homozygosity mapping or linkage analysis [21], or by analyzing only shared variants across several affected individuals within the same family. In addition, comparison of WES data from an affected individual and the parents ("trio analysis") has been also shown to strongly improve the variant filtering process [22, 23].

Genes that cause monogenic kidney disease if mutated are found mutated usually only in one family within hundreds [24, 25]. The rarity of single-gene causes of recessive kidney diseases relates also to CAKUT [15, 18]. Therefore it is necessary that disease-causing mutations can be identified in single families. Consequently, combining whole exome sequencing (WES) with genetic mapping strategies [21] enables identification of disease genes in those rare monogenic causes of CAKUT. For instance, application of homozygosity mapping has permitted us to identify recessive CAKUT causing genes [26].

The rarity of individuals with mutations in the same CAKUT gene suggests that CAKUT may be caused by a multitude of different disease-causing genes, each gene representing a rare monogenic recessive or dominant cause of CAKUT [3].

Table 15.3 Single gene causes of human CAKUT phenotype

Gene symbol	Renal phenotype*	Extrarenal phenotype (facultative)	Human disease [OMIM#]	Mode of inheritance
BMP4	Renal hypodysplasia	Cleft lip, microphthalmia	Microphthalmia, syndromic 6 [*607932], Orofacial cleft 11 [*600625]	AD
CHD1L	Renal hypodysplasia, VUR, UPJO	None	–	AD
DSTYK	Renal hypodysplasia, UPJO	Epilepsy in 2 out of 7 affected	CAKUT [#610805]	AD
EYA1	Multicystic dysplastic kidney, renal aplasia	Deafness, ear malformations, branchial cysts	Anterior segment anomalies with or without cataract [113650], Branchiootic syndrome 1 [*602588], Branchiootorenal syndrome 1, with or without cataracts [*113650], Otofaciocervical syndrome [*166780]	AD
GATA3	Renal dysplasia	Hypoparathyroidism, heart defects, immune deficiency, deafness	Hypoparathyroidism, sensorineural deafness, and renal dysplasia [*146255]	AD
HNF1B	Renal hypodysplasia, single kidney, horseshoe kidney	Diabetes mellitus (MODY5) hyperuricemia, hypomagnesaemia, elevated LFT	Diabetes mellitus, noninsulin-dependent [*125853] Renal cysts and diabetes syndrome [*137920]	AD
MUC1	Medullary cystic kidney disease type 1	None	Medullary cystic kidney disease 1 [#1740]	AD
PAX2	Vesicoureteral reflux, renal hypoplasia	Optic nerve colobomas, hearing loss	Papillorenal syndrome [*120330] Renal hypoplasia, isolated [*191830]	AD
RET	Renal agenesis	See OMIM# in the next column	Central hypoventilation syndrome, congenital [*209880] Medullary thyroid carcinoma [*155240], Multiple endocrine neoplasia IIA [*171400], Multiple endocrine neoplasia IIB, [*162300] Pheochromocytoma [*171300], Renal agenesis [*191830]	AD

(continued)

Table 15.3 (continued)

Gene symbol	Renal phenotype*	Extrarenal phenotype (facultative)	Human disease [OMIM#]	Mode of inheritance
ROBO2	VUR, ureterovesical junction defects	None	Vesicoureteral reflux 2 [*610878]	AD
SALL1	Renal hypodysplasia, renal agenesis	Limb, ear, anal abnormalities	Townes–Brocks syndrome [*107480]	AD
SIX1	Renal hypodysplasia, VUR	Deafness, ear defects, branchial cysts	Branchiootic syndrome 3 [*608389], Deafness, autosomal dominant 23 [*605192]	AD
SIX2	Renal hypodysplasia	None	–	AD
SIX5	Renal hypodysplasia, VUR	Deafness, ear defects, branchial cysts	Branchiootorenal syndrome 2 [*610896]	AD
SOX17	VUR, UPJO	None	Vesicoureteral reflux 3 [*613674]	AD
SRGAP1	CAKUT	None	–	AD
TBX18	Obstructive uropathy (e.g., UPJO) and other forms of CAKUT	None	[*604613]	AD
TNXB	VUR	Joint hypermobility	Ehlers–Danlos syndrome, autosomal dominant, hypermobility type [*130020] Ehlers–Danlos syndrome, autosomal recessive, due to tenascin X deficiency [*606408]	AD
UMOD	Medullary cystic kidney disease type 2	Hyperuricemia	MCKD2—Medullary cystic kidney disease type 2 [#603860], HNFJ2—Hyperuricemic nephropathy, familial juvenile 2 [#6130925], [#613092]	AD
UPK3A	Renal adysplasia	Subtle facial and limb defects	Renal adysplasia [*191830]	AD
WNT4	Renal hypodysplasia	Female-to-male sex reversal, adrenal dysplasia, lung dysplasia (SERKAL)	Mullerian aplasia and hyperandrogenism [*158330] SERKAL syndrome [*611812]	AD

(continued)

Table 15.3 (continued)

Gene symbol	Renal phenotype*	Extrarenal phenotype (facultative)	Human disease [OMIM#]	Mode of inheritance
Autosomal Recessive				
ACE	Absence or incomplete differentiation of proximal tubules	Pulmonary hypoplasia (Potter sequence), skull abnormalities	Renal tubular dysgenesis (RTD) [*267430]	AR
AGT	Similar to *HPSE2*	Similar to *HPSE2*	Renal tubular dysgenesis (RTD) [*267430]	AR
AGTR1	Similar to *ACE*	Similar to *ACE*	Renal tubular dysgenesis (RTD) [*267430]	AR
CHRM3	Prune Belly syndrome	–	Abdominal Muscle, absence of, with urinary tract abnormality and cryptorchidism [#100100]	AR
FGF20	Bilateral renal agenesis	None	–	AR
FRAS1	Renal agenesis	Cryptophthalmos, nose ear and larynx malformations. Mental retardation and syndactyly.	Fraser Syndrome [*219000]	AR
FREM2	Renal agenesis	Cryptophthalmos, nose ear and larynx malformations. Mental retardation and syndactyly.	Fraser Syndrome [*219000]	AR
FREM1	Renal anomalies	Bifid nose and anorectal malformations	Manitoba oculotrichoanal syndrome (MOTA) [#248450], bifid nose with or without anorectal and renal anomalies BNAR syndrome [608980]	AR
GRIP1	Similar to *FRAS1*	Similar to *FRAS1*	Fraser Syndrome [*219000]	
HSPE2	Urofacial Syndrome (Ochara syndrome). Bladder abnormalities	Distorted facial expression with smiling	Urofacial Syndrome 1 [*613469]	AR
ITGA8	Bilateral renal agenesis	Potter sequence	Renal hypodysplasia/ aplasia 1 [#191830]	AR
LRIG2	Similar to *HPSE2*	Similar to *HPSE2*	Urofacial Syndrome 2 [#615112]	AR
REN	Similar to *ACE*	Similar to *ACE*	Renal tubular dysgenesis [*267430]	AR

(continued)

Table 15.3 (continued)

Gene symbol	Renal phenotype*	Extrarenal phenotype (facultative)	Human disease [OMIM#]	Mode of inheritance
TRAP1	VUR, renal agenesis	VACTERL association	–	AR
X-Linked				
KAL1	Renal agenesis	Micropenis, bilateral cryptorchidism, anosmia	Hypogonadotropic hypogonadism 1 with or without anosmia (Kallmann syndrome 1) [*308700]	XL

ACE angiotensin converting enzyme; *AD* autosomal dominant; *AR* autosomal recessive; *LFT* liver function tests; *MODY 5* maturity onset diabetes of the young type 5; *OMIM* Online Mendelian Inheritance in Man; *SERKAL* sex reversal, kidneys, adrenals, and lungs dysgenesis; *UPJO* uretero-pelvic junction obstruction; *VACTERL* vertebra, anal, cardiac, trachea-esophageal, renal, and limb anomalies; *VUR* vesicoureteral reflux. *XL* X-linked

CAKUT is Caused by Single Gene Mutations

Several lines of evidence have supported the notion that CAKUT may be caused by single-gene mutations ("monogenic CAKUT"). These lines of evidence include the existence of transgenic mouse models of CAKUT, the congenital nature of CAKUT, the involvement of CAKUT in monogenic genetic syndromes, as well as familial occurrence of CAKUT [6]. In familial cases of CAKUT, the documented mode of inheritance in most published pedigrees is compatible with autosomal dominant with variable expressivity and incomplete penetrance. Nonetheless, several CAKUT-causing genes with autosomal recessive mode of inheritance, have been recently identified [18, 26, 27]. To date more than 34 different single-gene causes for isolated CAKUT in humans have been described which account for ~12% of cases (Table 15.3). In addition, more than 100 genes that if mutated cause syndromic variants of CAKUT have been described (Online Mendelian Inheritance in Man (OMIM), http://www.omim.org.). Most of the known genes that cause CAKUT if mutated are transcription factors and genes encoding proteins that are involved in early developmental stages of nephrogenesis [3, 7, 28]. Table 15.3 summarizes single-gene causes of CAKUT, and provides phenotypic details about extrarenal manifestations, which can direct molecular genetic diagnostics towards specific disease-causing gene. Mutations in the genes in the table may cause human isolated CAKUT or syndromes with a predominant CAKUT phenotype. In the following sections we review some of the main CAKUT-causing genes as well as important genetic concepts relevant to patients with CAKUT.

HNF1B—Renal Cysts and Diabetes Syndrome

Hepatocyte nuclear factor 1B (HNF1B) is a homeodomain-containing transcription factor, which is involved in the development of the kidneys, liver, pancreas and the urogenital tract [29]. Heterozygous mutations in *HNF1B* may cause "isolated CAKUT" or "syndromic CAKUT" that is associated with one or more of the following extrarenal manifestations: maturity onset diabetes of the young (MODY type 5), pancreatic hypoplasia, genital malformations, elevated liver function tests, hyperuricemia, and hypomagnesaemia (Table 15.3) [30]. Dominant mutations in *HNF1B* have initially been described as the genetic cause of "renal cysts and diabetes syndrome (RCDS)" [12]. Later, heterozygous *HNF1B*-mutations and deletions were reported among individuals with isolated CAKUT that encompassed various forms of renal malformations such as prenatal bilateral hyperechogenic kidneys, renal hypodysplasia, multicystic dysplastic kidney, cystic kidney disease, single kidney, horseshoe kidney, collecting system abnormalities, and oligomeganephronia [14, 31–33]. Furthermore, it is increasingly recognized now that heterozygous contiguous gene deletions in the 17q12 region (which includes the gene *HNF1B*) can result in CAKUT with a neurologic phenotype of the autism spectrum disorder, or of cognitive impairment or schizophrenia [33–35]. *HNF1B* mutations are the most common cause of monogenic CAKUT and are responsible for 5–31 % of cases, depending on the examined cohort [33]. More than 150 different *HNF1B* genetic mutations have been reported, and so far there is no evidence for genotype–phenotype correlation, other than the continuous gene deletion. About 50 % of the genetic abnormalities in *HNF1B* are heterozygous deletions of the entire gene. Those large deletions, which cannot be identified using Sanger sequencing and are also difficult to detect with whole exome sequencing, require copy number variation analysis. The prevalence of *HNF1B* deletions/mutations accruing *de novo* is reported to be as high as 50 % [33]. This explains why often there is no family history of affected individuals. This suggests that molecular analysis should be performed in CAKUT cases with a suggestive phenotype. Those cases can be determined using a clinical "*HNF1B*-score" that was recently proposed as a tool for triggering genetic molecular analysis for *HNF1B* [36].

PAX2—Renal Coloboma Syndrome

Paired Box gene 2 (PAX2) is a transcription factor that plays a central role during early embryonic kidney development. Heterozygous mutations in *PAX2* were first identified in patients with renal coloboma syndrome (also known as "papillorenal syndrome") which involves renal hypodysplasia, optic nerve abnormalities and deafness (Table 15.3) [11]. Nonetheless, *PAX2* mutations can lead to isolated CAKUT without optic nerve or hearing abnormalities and with only subtle features of CAKUT, which clinically can be difficult to detect. *PAX2*-mutations can result in variable kidney phenotypes across the morphologic continuum of CAKUT. Most commonly this includes renal hypodysplasia, renal cysts, multicystic dysplastic kidneys and VUR [37]. Currently, more than 75 disease causing mutations of *PAX2* have been reported, most of which are missense mutations, nonsense mutations or small deletions [37]. Next to *HNF1B*, mutations in *PAX2* probably represent the second most common cause of monogenic CAKUT, accounting for ~5 % of cases [13, 38].

SALL1—Townes–Brocks Syndrome

Spalt-Like Transcription Factor 1 (SALL1) encodes a zinc finger containing transcription factor, that is expressed in the metanephric mesenchyme during early nephrogenesis. Heterozygous mutations in *SALL1* were initially identified in two families with Townes–Brocks syndrome (TBS) (Table 15.3) [39]. This syndrome is characterized by CAKUT, imperforate anus, dysplastic ears with accompanying hearing impairment, and thumb malformations. The reported CAKUT anomalies in patients with *SALL1* mutations include among others: renal hypodysplasia, polycystic kidneys, renal ectopia, and VUR [40]. In addition, in some of the patients, other extrarenal developmental malformations have been described involving the central nervous system, heart, feet, and genitalia [40]. Since the first description of *SALL1* mutations as the genetic cause of TBS, molecular genetic diagnostics have shown that many affected individuals do not fulfill the core clinical features, highlighting the phenotypic variability of this syndrome. Specifically, *SALL1* mutations have been shown in some families to cause isolated CAKUT with no overt extrarenal malformations [14, 15]. More than 75 different mutations and deletions in the *SALL1* gene have been reported [40]. No genotype–phenotype correlation has been detected for *SALL1* mutations. Most *SALL1* mutations are private mutations; some have been reported to occur de novo [40]. No other gene mutation has been described in individuals with TBS. In most cases with a typical TBS phenotype a disease causing *SALL1* mutations can be identified. However, the TBS phenotype overlaps with other genetic syndrome that can have CAKUT as a feature, such as VACTERL syndrome and BOR syndrome (discussed below).

EYA1—Branchio-oto-renal (BOR) Syndrome

Eyes Absent Homolog 1 (EYA1) encodes a transcription factor that is required for normal development of the kidneys, ears, and branchial arches. Heterozygous mutations in *EYA1* cause BOR (i.e., branchio-oto-renal) syndrome that is characterized by structural defects of the ear with hearing loss in most cases (>90 %), branchial fistula or cysts as well as CAKUT (Table 15.3). CAKUT is found in two thirds of the affected patients, and ranges from mild to severe malformations [41, 42]. The clinical variability of BOR syndrome is high and has triggered recommendations for phenotypic criteria for *EYA1* testing in patients with BOR syndrome [43]. Overall *EYA1* disease-causing mutations are identified in about 40% of patients with BOR syndrome [43]. In patients with EYA1-negative BOR syndrome, mutations in the transcriptional factors *SIX1* and *SIX5* have been detected, however, both genes represent by far a more rare cause of BOR syndrome [44, 45]. More than 180 different *EYA1* mutations have been reported, and so far no genotype–phenotype correlation has been documented.

GATA3—Hypoparathyroidism, Sensorineural Deafness, and Renal Disease (HDR) Syndrome

GATA Binding Protein 3 (GATA3) is a zinc-finger transcription factor involved in the embryonic development of the inner ear, parathyroid glands, and kidneys. Genetic abnormalities in *GATA3* cause HDR syndrome, which is characterized by hypoparathyroidism, sensorineural deafness and renal disease (Table 15.3) [46]. The syndrome is also known as "Barakat syndrome" after its first description for this association [47]. Different CAKUT phenotypes have been described in this syndrome (e.g., renal hypodysplasia, single kidney, and VUR). Other associated rare extrarenal clinical features have been reported in several case reports, including ventricular septal defect, polycystic ovaries, Mullerian duct malformations, pyloric stenosis, diabetes, thyroiditis and intellectual disabilities [47–49]. So far, 60 different dominant disease causing mutations in GATA3 have been reported with more than 50% of the cases caused by heterozygous deletions. Not all patients with clinical features compatible with HDR syndrome have identifiable *GATA3* mutations. This may be explained by genetic heterogeneity or by the fact that genetic syndromes have overlapping phenotypic components including the specific combination of hyperparathyroidism and CAKUT, such as DiGeorge syndrome. Interestingly, in several patients a contiguous gene deletion syndrome encompassing a region containing the second DiGeorge syndrome locus (*DGS2*) as well the *GATA3* gene was reported. Those patients presented with variable phenotypes encompassing clinical features of both syndromes [50].

UMOD and MUC1—Medullary Cystic Kidney Disease

Medullary cystic kidney disease (MCKD) is a form of hereditary autosomal dominant tubulointerstitial nephritis that leads to end-stage kidney disease between the third and the sixth decade of life. MCKD can be clinically indistinguishable from other forms of CAKUT, specifically, from renal malformations secondary to hetero-zygous *HNF1B* or *REN* mutations. Moreover, it has recently been stressed that renal cysts are not a typical feature of MCKD, occurring only rarely.

Two types of MCKD were described following genetic mapping of their respective disease causing genes loci. *Uromodulin* (*UMOD*) mutations were identified as the disease causing in MCKD type 2 (Table 15.3) [51, 52]. Only recently *MUC1* was found to be mutated in individuals with MCKD type 1, secondary to an unusual class of mutations in variable number tandem repeats (VNTRs) [53].

The *Uromodulin* (*UMOD*) gene encodes the Tamm–Horsfall protein. Mutations in *UMOD* can also lead to two additional clinical entities named: (1) familial juvenile hyperuricemic nephropathy (FJHN), and (2) glomerulocystic kidney disease (GCKD). Although MCKD represents a subtype of CAKUT, among cases of isolated CAKUT it is estimated that UMOD mutations are very rare [54].

Mucin 1 (*MUC1*) mutations which cause MCKD type 1 lie in a coding GC rich region of a variable number tandem repeat (VNTR) [53]. VNTRs consist of 20–125 copies of a 60 base pairs repeat unit [55]. In all patients with MCKD type 1 a cytosine insertion frameshift mutation in a coding VNTR leads to a premature stop codon. Molecular genetic diagnostics for *MUC1* mutations requires specific methodologies for the detection of these mutations, which cannot be identified by Sanger sequencing, whole-genome, or whole-exome sequencing alone.

HPSE2, LRIG2, and CHRM3—Monogenic Causes of Urinary Bladder Malformations

The phenotypes of most monogenic CAKUT cases in humans involve primarily the kidneys and/or the ureters. However, recently rare monogenic causes of CAKUT with predominant bladder malformations have been reported [56]. Autosomal recessive mutations in either *HPSE2* or *LRIG2* have been identified in patients with urofacial syndrome [57–59] (Table 15.3). This syndrome, also known as Ochoa syndrome, is characterized by typical distorted facial expression with smiling or laughing expression (facial grimace) as well as by a poorly emptying dysmorphic bladder, which appears trabeculated on cystography. Patients usually present in early childhood with voiding dysfunction, but can also have other accompanying features of CAKUT such as hydroureters, hydronephrosis, VUR with recurrent urinary tract infections and secondary renal damage leading to CKD. Both *HPSE2* and *LRIG2* are expressed in the developing bladder. However, the pathomechanisms by which loss of function of their encoded proteins leads to the syndrome is still elusive (55).

Another example for a monogenic bladder malformation phenotype has been described in a family with familial congenital bladder anomalies and a prune-belly-like phenotype. Affected individuals were found to harbor recessive mutations in *CHRM3* (muscarinic acetylcholine receptor M3) (Table 15.3) [60]. A knock out mouse model for *CHRM3* exhibits a similar phenotype. *CHRM3* encodes to the M3 subtype of muscarinic acetylcholine receptors, which mediate urinary bladder contractions. This gene, however, represent an extremely rare genetic cause for prune belly syndrome explaining only a small subset of the patients.

Syndromic CAKUT Genes and Multiple Allelism

More than 200 different rare multiorgan syndromes may feature CAKUT as a phenotypic component [61]. It now appears that for certain genes that cause syndromic CAKUT, different recessive mutations may cause a different spectrum of organ involvement, depending on the severity of the mutated allele involved (i.e., multiple allelism). This mechanism of multiple allelism has been described in CAKUT for the genes that cause Fraser spectrum disorders (Fraser/MOTA/BNAR syndrome) [18]. For instance, the genes *FRAS1*, *FREM2*, and *GRIP1*, cause Fraser syndrome if mutated. While individuals with Fraser syndrome generally have protein-truncating alleles in one of those genes, biallelic missense mutations seem to cause a milder form manifesting as isolated CAKUT [18]. It is possible, that this phenomenon of multiple allelism governing syndromic versus isolated CAKUT exists in other syndromic CAKUT-causing genes as well. Finally, it is important for clinicians to recognize that syndromic forms of CAKUT can initially present as isolated CAKUT. Frequently, extrarenal signs in carriers of CAKUT-causing mutations may be absent or subtle and therefore be overlooked.

Copy Number Variations in CAKUT

Another aspect of the genetic basis of CAKUT involves copy number variations (CNVs). Detection of these genetic abnormalities requires methods of gene dosage analysis such as single-nucleotide polymorphism microarrays. They will usually not be detected by WES. Genetic regions identified by CNV analysis may include a continuous gene deletion syndrome for regions with previously recognized or novel CAKUT-causing gene. In two independent studies, CNVs were identified among 10–16 % of individuals with CAKUT, most commonly involving the *HNF1B* or the DiGeorge/velocarodiofacial locus [62, 63].

Clinical Genetic Approach to Patients with CAKUT

Clinical molecular genetic diagnostics in CAKUT are complicated by the fact that the disease phenotypes vary from "silent traits" with normally appearing kidneys and intact kidney function (i.e., incomplete penetrance) to severe bilateral renal agenesis or hypodysplasia and end-stage kidney disease, even in the presence of identical disease causing alleles. Furthermore, although some of the clinical syndromes mentioned above may be accompanied by characteristic extrarenal features, these are not obligatory.

In clinical practice the evaluation of patients with CAKUT should include: (1) A detailed family history in the form of an annotated pedigree. This will help identify recessive or dominant pattern of transmission in familial cases; (2) meticulous evaluation for extrarenal syndrome-specific signs and symptoms (Table 15.3); (3) thorough evaluation by renal ultrasound for the presence of CAKUT in other family members, because familial CAKUT can be mistakenly considered sporadic when the familial nature of the malformation is overlooked; and (4) referral of the patient to genetic counseling.

Currently, the most common CAKUT-causing genes are *HNF1B* and *PAX2*. Other cases, which often present sporadically, are a result of many different rare diseases causing genes [3, 15, 18]. Identifying a monogenic cause for patients with CAKUT has several implications. First, it provides patients with an etiology-based specific diagnosis to their condition. Second, it allows for early identification of extrarenal features and consequently early treatment interventions when needed. Third, it permits early identification of "apparently unaffected" family members who are affected but are still asymptomatic. Fourth, allow to initiate genetic consulting for future family planning. Finally, it provides a better disease categorization for clinical trials that study outcome of diseases.

Molecular Diagnostic Approach for Patients with CAKUT

CAKUT is usually diagnosed by ultrasound or other imaging studies. CAKUT diagnosis should trigger clinicians to consider genetic analysis for their patients. Molecular analysis of CAKUT-causing genes using experimental known CAKUT genes panels is now available for clinicians worldwide and can be initiated at the following web site www.renalgenes.org. Following identification of CAKUT-causing mutations, the patient should be referred to a CLIA (Clinical Laboratory Improvement Amendments) certified clinical laboratory, as well as genetic counseling. Optimally, the care for patients with CAKUT should be provided by a multidisciplinary team of nephrologists, urologists, and clinical geneticists.

In general, attribution of pathogenicity to a given genetic variant should be subjected to strict criteria and take into consideration several lines of evidence such as amino acid sequence conservation, segregation analysis, tissue specific gene expression, functional studies, and animal models [64]. In addition, the number of families with CAKUT that have been previously reported to have a mutation in the candidate causative gene should also be considered. Some of the CAKUT-causing genes were reported in only few families and therefore any generalizations regarding their role must await the description and characterization of mutations in additional patients.

Future Directions

The progress in high-throughput sequencing will ensure that gene-based disease classification for CAKUT will continue to be introduced into clinical research and practice. This will result in a more accurate etiologic categorization of the different CAKUT entities than can be provided by diagnostic imaging alone. Such assignments will have implications for genetic consulting as well as clinical management in the sense of "personalized medicine" of patients with CAKUT.

References

1. Ichikawa I, Kuwayama F, Pope JC, Stephens FD, Miyazaki Y. Paradigm shift from classic anatomic theories to contemporary cell biological views of CAKUT. Kidney Int. 2002;61:889–98.
2. North American Pediatric Renal Transplant Cooperative Study (NAPRTCS) (2008) 2008 Annual report. The EMMES Corporation, Rockville, MD. 2008.
3. Vivante A, Kohl S, Hwang DY, Dworschak GC, Hildebrandt F. Single-gene causes of congenital anomalies of the kidney and urinary tract (CAKUT) in humans. Pediatr Nephrol. 2014;29:695–704.
4. Chen F. Genetic and developmental basis for urinary tract obstruction. Pediatr Nephrol. 2009;24:1621–32.
5. Weber S. Novel genetic aspects of congenital anomalies of kidney and urinary tract. Curr Opin Pediatr. 2012;24:212–8.
6. Sanna-Cherchi S, Carldl G, Weng PL, Scolari F, Perfumo F, Gharavi AG, et al. Genetic approaches to human renal agenesis/hypoplasia and dysplasia. Pediatr Nephrol. 2007;22:1675–84.
7. Dressler GR. Advances in early kidney specification, development and patterning. Development. 2009;136:3863–74.
8. Rosenblum ND. Developmental biology of the human kidney. Semin Fetal Neonatal Med. 2008;13:125–32.
9. Rasouly HM, Lu W. Lower urinary tract development and disease. Wiley Interdiscip Rev Syst Biol Med. 2013;5:307–42.
10. Altshuler D, Daly MJ, Lander ES. Genetic mapping in human disease. Science. 2008;322(5903):881–8.

11. Sanyanusin P, Schimmenti LA, McNoe LA, Ward TA, Pierpont ME, Sullivan MJ, et al. Mutation of the PAX2 gene in a family with optic nerve colobomas, renal anomalies and vesicoureteral reflux. Nat Genet. 1995;9:358–64.

12. Lindner TH, Njolstad PR, Horikawa Y, Bostad L, Bell GI, Sovik O. A novel syndrome of diabetes mellitus, renal dysfunction and genital malformation associated with a partial deletion of the pseudo-POU domain of hepatocyte nuclear factor-1beta. Hum Mol Genet. 1999;8:2001–8.

13. Thomas R, Sanna-Cherchi S, Warady BA, Furth SL, Kaskel FJ, Gharavi AG. HNF1B and PAX2 mutations are a common cause of renal hypodysplasia in the CKiD cohort. Pediatr Nephrol. 2011;26:897–903.

14. Weber S, Moriniere V, Knuppel T, Charbit M, Dusek J, Ghiggeri GM, et al. Prevalence of mutations in renal developmental genes in children with renal hypodysplasia: results of the ESCAPE study. J Am Soc Nephrol. 2006;17:2864–70.

15. Hwang DY, Dworschak GC, Kohl S, Saisawat P, Vivante A, Hilger AC, et al. Mutations in 12 known dominant disease-causing genes clarify many congenital anomalies of the kidney and urinary tract. Kidney Int. 2014;85:1429–33.

16. Halbritter J, Diaz K, Chaki M, Porath JD, Tarrier B, Fu C, et al. High-throughput mutation analysis in patients with a nephronophthisis-associated ciliopathy applying multiplexed barcoded array-based PCR amplification and next-generation sequencing. J Med Genet. 2012;49:756–67.

17. Halbritter J, Porath JD, Diaz KA, Braun DA, Kohl S, Chaki M, et al. Identification of 99 novel mutations in a worldwide cohort of 1,056 patients with a nephronophthisis-related ciliopathy. Hum Genet. 2013;132:865–84.

18. Kohl S, Hwang DY, Dworschak GC, Hilger AC, Saisawat P, Vivante A, et al. Mild recessive mutations in six Fraser syndrome-related genes cause isolated congenital anomalies of the kidney and urinary tract. J Am Soc Nephrol. 2014;25:1917–22.

19. Mardis ER. The impact of next-generation sequencing technology on genetics. Trends Genet. 2008;24:133–41.

20. Koboldt DC, Steinberg KM, Larson DE, Wilson RK, Mardis ER. The next-generation sequencing revolution and its impact on genomics. Cell. 2013;155:27–38.

21. Hildebrandt F, Heeringa SF, Ruschendorf F, Attanasio M, Nurnberg G, Becker C, et al. A systematic approach to mapping recessive disease genes in individuals from outbred populations. PLoS Genet. 2009;5, e1000353.

22. Lee H, Deignan JL, Dorrani N, Strom SP, Kantarci S, Quintero-Rivera F, et al. Clinical exome sequencing for genetic identification of rare Mendelian disorders. JAMA. 2014;312:1880–7.

23. Yang Y, Muzny DM, Xia F, Niu Z, Person R, Ding Y, et al. Molecular findings among patients referred for clinical whole-exome sequencing. JAMA. 2014;312:1870–9.

24. Devuyst O, Knoers NV, Remuzzi G, Schaefer F, Board of the Working Group for Inherited Kidney Diseases of the European Renal Association and European Dialysis and Transplant Association. Rare inherited kidney diseases: challenges, opportunities, and perspectives. Lancet. 2014;383(9931):1844–59.

25. Hildebrandt F. Genetic kidney diseases. Lancet. 2010;375(9722):1287–95.

26. Saisawat P, Kohl S, Hilger AC, Hwang DY, Yung Gee H, Dworschak GC, et al. Whole-exome resequencing reveals recessive mutations in TRAP1 in individuals with CAKUT and VACTERL association. Kidney Int. 2014;85:1310–7.

27. Humbert C, Silbermann F, Morar B, Parisot M, Zarhrate M, Masson C, et al. Integrin alpha 8 recessive mutations are responsible for bilateral renal agenesis in humans. Am J Hum Genet. 2014;94:288–94.

28. Vivante A, Kleppa MJ, Schulz J, Kohl S, Sharma A, Chen J, Shril S, Hwang DY, Weiss AC, Kaminski MM, Shukrun R, Kemper MJ, Lehnhardt A, Beetz R, Sanna-Cherchi S, Verbitsky M, Gharavi AG, Stuart HM, Feather SA, Goodship JA, Goodship TH, Woolf AS, Westra SJ, Doody DP, Bauer SB, Lee RS, Adam RM, Lu W, Reutter HM, Kehinde EO, Mancini EJ, Lifton RP, Tasic V, Lienkamp SS, Jüppner H, Kispert A, Hildebrandt F. Mutations in TBX18

cause dominant urinary tract malformations via transcriptional dysregulation of ureter development. Am J Hum Genet. 2015;97(2):291–301.

29. Coffinier C, Thepot D, Babinet C, Yaniv M, Barra J. Essential role for the homeoprotein vHNF1/HNF1beta in visceral endoderm differentiation. Development. 1999;126:4785–94.

30. Bellanne-Chantelot C, Chauveau D, Gautier JF, Dubois-Laforgue D, Clauin S, Beaufils S, et al. Clinical spectrum associated with hepatocyte nuclear factor-1beta mutations. Ann Intern Med. 2004;140:510–7.

31. Edghill EL, Bingham C, Ellard S, Hattersley AT. Mutations in hepatocyte nuclear factor-1beta and their related phenotypes. J Med Genet. 2006;43:84–90.

32. Adalat S, Woolf AS, Johnstone KA, Wirsing A, Harries LW, Long DA, et al. HNF1B mutations associate with hypomagnesemia and renal magnesium wasting. J Am Soc Nephrol. 2009;20:1123–31.

33. Clissold RL, Hamilton AJ, Hattersley AT, Ellard S, Bingham C. HNF1B-associated renal and extra-renal disease-an expanding clinical spectrum. Nat Rev Nephrol. 2015;11:102–12.

34. Loirat C, Bellanne-Chantelot C, Husson I, Deschenes G, Guigonis V, Chabane N. Autism in three patients with cystic or hyperechogenic kidneys and chromosome 17q12 deletion. Nephrol Dial Transplant. 2010;25:3430–3.

35. Moreno-De-Luca D, Mulle JG, Kaminsky EB, Sanders SJ, Myers SM, Adam MP, et al. Deletion 17q12 is a recurrent copy number variant that confers high risk of autism and schizophrenia. Am J Hum Genet. 2010;87:618–30.

36. Faguer S, Chassaing N, Bandin F, Prouheze C, Garnier A, Casemayou A, et al. The HNF1B score is a simple tool to select patients for HNF1B gene analysis. Kidney Int. 2014;86:1007–15.

37. Bower M, Salomon R, Allanson J, Antignac C, Benedicenti F, Benetti E, et al. Update of PAX2 mutations in renal coloboma syndrome and establishment of a locus-specific database. Hum Mutat. 2012;33:457–66.

38. Madariaga L, Moriniere V, Jeanpierre C, Bouvier R, Loget P, Martinovic J, et al. Severe prenatal renal anomalies associated with mutations in HNF1B or PAX2 Genes. Clin J Am Soc Nephrol. 2013;8:1179–87.

39. Kohlhase J, Wischermann A, Reichenbach H, Froster U, Engel W. Mutations in the SALL1 putative transcription factor gene cause Townes-Brocks syndrome. Nat Genet. 1998;18:81–3.

40. Kohlhase J. Townes-Brocks Syndrome. In: Pagon RA, Adam MP, Ardinger HH, Wallace SE, Amemiya A, Bean LJH, et al., editors. GeneReviews(R).

41. Abdelhak S, Kalatzis V, Heilig R, Compain S, Samson D, Vincent C, et al. A human homologue of the Drosophila eyes absent gene underlies branchio-oto-renal (BOR) syndrome and identifies a novel gene family. Nat Genet. 1997;15:157–64.

42. Castiglione A, Melchionda S, Carella M, Trevisi P, Bovo R, Manara R, et al. EYA1-related disorders: two clinical cases and a literature review. Int J Pediatr Otorhinolaryngol. 2014;78:1201–10.

43. Chang EH, Menezes M, Meyer NC, Cucci RA, Vervoort VS, Schwartz CE, et al. Branchio-oto-renal syndrome: the mutation spectrum in EYA1 and its phenotypic consequences. Hum Mutat. 2004;23:582–9.

44. Ruf RG, Xu PX, Silvius D, Otto EA, Beekmann F, Muerb UT, et al. SIX1 mutations cause branchio-oto-renal syndrome by disruption of EYA1-SIX1-DNA complexes. Proc Natl Acad Sci U S A. 2004;101:8090–5.

45. Hoskins BE, Cramer CH, Silvius D, Zou D, Raymond RM, Orten DJ, et al. Transcription factor SIX5 is mutated in patients with branchio-oto-renal syndrome. Am J Hum Genet. 2007;80:800–4.

46. Van Esch H, Groenen P, Nesbit MA, Schuffenhauer S, Lichtner P, Vanderlinden G, et al. GATA3 haplo-insufficiency causes human HDR syndrome. Nature. 2000;406(6794):419–22.

47. Barakat AY, D'Albora JB, Martin MM, Jose PA. Familial nephrosis, nerve deafness, and hypoparathyroidism. J Pediatr. 1977;91:61–4.

48. Nesbit MA, Bowl MR, Harding B, Ali A, Ayala A, Crowe C, et al. Characterization of GATA3 mutations in the hypoparathyroidism, deafness, and renal dysplasia (HDR) syndrome. J Biol Chem. 2004;279:22624–34.

49. Muroya K, Hasegawa T, Ito Y, Nagai T, Isotani H, Iwata Y, et al. GATA3 abnormalities and the phenotypic spectrum of HDR syndrome. J Med Genet. 2001;38:374–80.
50. Fukami M, Muroya K, Miyake T, Iso M, Kato F, Yokoi H, et al. GATA3 abnormalities in six patients with HDR syndrome. Endocr J. 2011;58:117–21.
51. Hart TC, Gorry MC, Hart PS, Woodard AS, Shihabi Z, Sandhu J, et al. Mutations of the UMOD gene are responsible for medullary cystic kidney disease 2 and familial juvenile hyper-uricaemic nephropathy. J Med Genet. 2002;39:882–92.
52. Wolf MT, Mucha BE, Attanasio M, Zalewski I, Karle SM, Neumann HP, et al. Mutations of the Uromodulin gene in MCKD type 2 patients cluster in exon 4, which encodes three EGF-like domains. Kidney Int. 2003;64:1580–7.
53. Kirby A, Gnirke A, Jaffe DB, Baresova V, Pochet N, Blumenstiel B, et al. Mutations causing medullary cystic kidney disease type 1 lie in a large VNTR in MUC1 missed by massively parallel sequencing. Nat Genet. 2013;45:299–303.
54. Wolf MT, Hoskins BE, Beck BB, Hoppe B, Tasic V, Otto EA, et al. Mutation analysis of the Uromodulin gene in 96 individuals with urinary tract anomalies (CAKUT). Pediatr Nephrol. 2009;24:55–60.
55. Jeffreys AJ, Wilson V, Thein SL. Individual-specific 'fingerprints' of human DNA. Nature. 1985;316(6023):76–9.
56. Woolf AS, Stuart HM, Newman WG. Genetics of human congenital urinary bladder disease. Pediatr Nephrol. 2014;29:353–60. eScholarID: 203148.
57. Stuart HM, Roberts NA, Hilton EN, McKenzie EA, Daly SB, Hadfield KD, et al. Urinary tract effects of HPSE2 mutations. J Am Soc Nephrol. 2015;26:797–804.
58. Stuart HM, Roberts NA, Burgu B, Daly SB, Urquhart JE, Bhaskar S, et al. LRIG2 mutations cause urofacial syndrome. Am J Hum Genet. 2013;92:259–64.
59. Al Badr W, Al Bader S, Otto E, Hildebrandt F, Ackley T, Peng W, et al. Exome capture and massively parallel sequencing identifies a novel HPSE2 mutation in a Saudi Arabian child with Ochoa (urofacial) syndrome. J Pediatr Urol. 2011;7:569–73.
60. Weber S, Thiele H, Mir S, Toliat MR, Sozeri B, Reutter H, et al. Muscarinic acetylcholine receptor M3 mutation causes urinary bladder disease and a prune-belly-like syndrome. Am J Hum Genet. 2011;89:668–74.
61. Limwongse C. Syndromes and malformations of the urinary tract. In: Avner ED, Harmon WE, Niaudet P, Yoshikawa N, editors. Pediatric nephrology. 6th ed. Berlin: Springer; 2009. p. 122–38.
62. Sanna-Cherchi S, Kiryluk K, Burgess KE, Bodria M, Sampson MG, Hadley D, et al. Copy-number disorders are a common cause of congenital kidney malformations. Am J Hum Genet. 2012;91:987–97.
63. Weber S, Landwehr C, Renkert M, Hoischen A, Wuhl E, Denecke J, et al. Mapping candidate regions and genes for congenital anomalies of the kidneys and urinary tract (CAKUT) by array-based comparative genomic hybridization. Nephrol Dial Transplant. 2011;26:136–43.
64. MacArthur DG, Manolio TA, Dimmock DP, Rehm HL, Shendure J, Abecasis GR, et al. Guidelines for investigating causality of sequence variants in human disease. Nature. 2014;508(7497):469–76.

Chapter 16
Association of Congenital Anomalies of the Kidney and Urinary Tract with Those of Other Organ Systems

Amin J. Barakat

Abbreviations

CAKUT	Congenital anomalies of the kidney and urinary tract
CKD	Chronic kidney disease
CNS	Central nervous system
CV	Cardiovascular
GI	Gastrointestinal
MCA	Multiple congenital anomalies
US	Ultrasound
VUR	Vesicoureteral reflux

An Overview

Congenital anomalies of the kidney and urinary tract (CAKUT) occur in 5–10 % of the population, and represent 25 % of prenatally detected fetal malformations [1, 2]. CAKUT may be single or multiple, and may predispose to pyelonephritis, hypertension, renal calculi, and CKD. About half to two-thirds of CKD in children are secondary to CAKUT.

CAKUT usually occur as isolated malformations, but they are often associated with additional congenital anomalies outside the urinary tract [3–5]. In this chapter, I

A.J. Barakat, M.D., F.A.A.P. (✉)
Department of Pediatrics, Georgetown University Medical Center, Washington, DC, USA

Clinical Professor of Pediatrics, Georgetown University Medical Center,
107 North Virginia Ave, Falls Church, VA 22046, USA
e-mail: aybarakat@aol.com

© Springer International Publishing Switzerland 2016
A.J. Barakat, H. Gil Rushton (eds.), *Congenital Anomalies of the Kidney and Urinary Tract*, DOI 10.1007/978-3-319-29219-9_16

323

Table 16.1 CAKUT associated with abnormalities of other organ systems

Abnormality	%
Ureters	61
Horseshoe kidney	29
Hydronephrosis	29
Bladder	27
Renal dysplasia	26
Renal agenesis	26
Renal arteries	26
Urethra	19
Renal hypoplasia	11
ARPKD[a]	11
Abnormalities of kidney position	7
ADPKD[b]	5

Reprinted with permission from Barakat AJ, Drougas JG, Barakat R. Association of congenital abnormalities of the kidney and urinary tract with those of other organ systems in 13,775 autopsies. Child Nephrol Urol. 1988–89; 9: 271 [5]
[a]Autosomal recessive polycystic kidney disease
[b]Autosomal dominant polycystic kidney disease

discuss the association of CAKUT with anomalies of other organ systems. Table 16.1 presents the CAKUT associated with abnormalities of other organ systems. The appendix lists various conditions, syndromes, and chromosomal aberrations associated with CAKUT.

Up to two-thirds of patients with CAKUT have associated anomalies of other organ systems. In a study of 13,775 autopsies, Barakat et al. [5] found that 47 % of the autopsies with CAKUT have anomalies of other organ systems including cardiovascular (CV), gastrointestinal (GI), central nervous (CNS), skeletal, and genito-reproductive systems as well as abnormalities of the lung and face, chromosomal aberrations, and multiple congenital anomalies (MCA) syndromes (Table 16.2) . This figure was higher (60 %) in autopsies of individuals under age 18 years. Rubenstein et al. [6] found this association in 10 % of all autopsies, and 73 % of autopsies of children under 12. Reviewing over 346,000 consecutive births, Stoll et al. [7] found 0.48 % of newborns have CAKUT. Of these, 34 % had associated congenital anomalies of other organ systems, 7 % had chromosomal abnormalities and 16 % had non-syndromic, non-chromosomal multiple congenital anomalies (MCA). The most common non-urinary anomalies in this study involved the musculoskeletal system, followed by GI, CV and CNS, ear and face.

In a systematic review of 43 cohorts describing over 2600 patients with unilateral renal agenesis, one in every three patients had additional CAKUT. Vesicoureteral reflux (VUR) was the most common urinary tract anomaly, and 31 % had extrarenal anomalies [8]. Of the extrarenal anomalies, GI, cardiac, and musculoskeletal anomalies were identified in 16 %, 14 %, and 13 % of the reported patients, respectively. Miscellaneous anomalies (undescended testes, hypospadias, and CNS anomalies) were reported in 15 % of patients. Female tract anomalies (uterus bicornis, hemiva-

Table 16.2 Abnormalities of other organ systems associated with CAKUT

Organ system	Abnormalities (%)
Heart and cardiovascular system	25
Gastrointestinal tract	18
Central nervous system	10
Skeletal system	9
Lung	7
Face	7
Genito-reproductive system	4
Chromosomal aberrations	4
Others	8
Abdominal wall	4
Syndromes	2
Eyes	1
Miscellaneous	2
Associated abnormalities	47

Reprinted with permission from Barakat AJ, Drougas JG, Barakat R. Association of congenital abnormalities of the kidney and urinary tract with those of other organ systems in 13,775 autopsies. Child Nephrol Urol. 1988–89; 9: 269 [5]

gina, cloaca and MURCS syndrome *MU*llerian agenesis, *R*enal agenesis, and *C*ervicothoracic *S*omite abnormalities) were described in 11 % of female patients.

Prenatal ultrasonography (US) is now routinely performed in many centers between 18 and 20 weeks of gestation. Fetal kidneys can be imaged as early as 9 weeks of gestation. Prenatal US also helps to detect abnormalities of other organ systems. The presence of associated anomalies may worsen the prognosis of patients with CAKUT. Additionally, history of oligohydramnios, low birth weight, prematurity, and first pregnancy should be noted as they appear to be risk factors for neonatal mortality in these patients [9]. Postnatally, CAKUT should be suspected in newborns and children with congenital abnormalities of other organ systems, single umbilical artery, febrile urinary tract infection, significant abnormalities of the ear lobes, supernumerary nipples, chromosomal aberrations, and various malformation syndromes. Children with congenital hypothyroidism have an increased prevalence of CAKUT [10]. Hydronephrosis, including ureteropelvic junction obstruction, followed by renal dysplasia and agenesis are the most common associated anomalies.

The etiology of CAKUT is probably multifactorial and includes chromosomal abnormalities, Mendelian and familial inheritance, known syndromes, teratogenic exposure, and probably an interaction between genetic and environmental factors [7]. Specific mutations can potentially affect the development of the urinary tract, with the final phenotypic outcome depending on modifying factors such as intrauterine, environmental, and occupational factors [11]. The development of the urinary tract is a sequential and integrated process of the primitive renal elements. The pathogenesis of these anomalies is discussed in detail in Chapters 1 and 2. The association of CAKUT and those of other organs represents a malformation sequence which is due to defective formation of tissue that initiates a chain of subsequent abnormalities in the embryo [12]. Malformations usually start prior to the time of normal development. The critical period of embryogenesis of the kidney is believed to be between 15 and 94 days of fetal life, the time which most other organ systems develop [13]. The fifth week of embryonic development is crucial in the development of many organs including the kidneys, heart, and skeletal system. Any insult during this period may result in multiple organ anomalies.

When clinicians are faced with a patient with MCA suggesting a malformation syndrome, the family history should be carefully reviewed and genetic and chromosomal studies performed to try and identify the mode of inheritance and initiate genetic counseling.

Congenital Anomalies of the Heart and Cardiovascular (CV) System

The urinary and CV systems share a common embryologic origin, the mesoderm. Hence, an insult to the mesoderm during embryogenesis may cause defects to both organs. Pod1 (capsulin/epicardin/Tcf21) is a basic helix-loop-helix transcription factor that is highly expressed in the mesenchyme of developing organs including the kidney and the heart [14]. An insult to this factor during embryogenesis may cause defects in both organs. According to the Emilia-Romagna Registry on Congenital Malformations, children with abnormalities of the urinary tract have a ten times greater incidence of cardiovascular malformations than control patients [15].

Up to 25 % [5] to 34 % [16] of patients with CAKUT may have associated CV anomalies. According to Barakat et al. [5] the most common CV defect was patent ductus arteriosus (12 %), followed by ventricular septal defect (8 %) and atrial septal defect (6 %). Adhisivam et al. [16] reported that CV malformations are tenfold higher in children with urinary tract anomalies than in controls. In their series, ventricular septal defect accounted for 60 % of patient with CV anomalies, followed by atrial septal defect and pulmonary stenosis (25 % each). These abnormalities were found mostly in association with ureteral abnormalities including duplication, abnormal renal arteries, horseshoe kidney, hydronephrosis with or without hydroureter, and renal dysplasia. Cardiovascular anomalies seen in patients with CAKUT are presented in Table 16.3.

Buendía Hernández et al. [17] studied 434 patients undergoing angiocardiograms for diagnosis of their congenital heart disease. Fourteen percent of these patients had an associated CAKUT including pyelo-caliectasis (47 %), a duplicated pyelo-caliceal system (26 %), renal hypoplasia (10 %) and duplicated ureters, renal agenesis, pelvic kidney, horseshoe kidney, and others (27 %). The patients were usually urologically asymptomatic. It is evident from all these studies that CAKUT should be considered in any child with abnormalities of the CV

Table 16.3 Heart and cardiovascular (CV) abnormalities seen in patients with CAKUT

Abnormality	% of patients with CAKUT
Patent ductus arteriosus	12
Ventricular septal defect	8
Valvular defects	6
Large vessels	6
Atrial septal defect	6
Patent foramen ovale	3
Coarctation of the aorta	3
Others[a]	6
Heart and CV system	25

Reprinted with permission from Barakat AJ, Drougas JG, Barakat R. Association of congenital abnormalities of the kidney and urinary tract with those of other organ systems in 13,775 autopsies. Child Nephrol Urol. 1988–89; 9: 270 [5]
[a]Tetralogy of Fallot, transposition of great vessels, hypoplastic left heart, truncus arteriosis, common ventricle, others

system. Similarly, a thorough cardiac examination should be performed in patients with CAKUT.

Congenital Anomalies of the Gastrointestinal (GI) Tract

Up to 18 % of patients with CAKUT, mostly abnormal ureters, hydronephrosis, horseshoe kidney, renal agenesis, and dysplasia, may be associated with GI anomalies (Table 16.4). Twenty percent of patients with Hirschsprung's disease (a rare congenital disorder characterized by the absence of ganglion cells in the hindgut with variable distal bowel involvement) are associated with CAKUT, including renal hypoplasia or asymmetry, VUR, hydronephrosis, posterior urethral valve, and duplicated collecting system [18]. It appears reasonable therefore to include a renal US in the routine diagnostic investigation of patients with Hirschsprung's disease. Perlman et al. [19] found that the incidence of anal atresia in patients with CAKUT is 30-fold relative to the general population.

Congenital Anomalies of the Central Nervous System (CNS)

CNS anomalies occur in about 10 % of patients with CAKUT, mostly renal agenesis, bladder abnormalities, and horseshoe kidney. Others include autosomal recessive polycystic kidney disease, hydronephrosis, renal hypoplasia, and abnormal renal vasculature. Bilateral renal dysplasia may be associated with

Table 16.4 Gastrointestinal (GI) abnormalities seen in patients with CAKUT*

Abnormality	% of patients with CAKUT
Imperforate anus	4
Meckel's diverticulum	4
Stomach and intestine	4
Tracheo-esophageal fistula	3
Liver and biliary tract	2
Spleen	1
Pancreas	1
GI tract	18

Reprinted with permission from Barakat AJ, Drougas JG, Barakat R. Association of congenital abnormalities of the kidney and urinary tract with those of other organ systems in 13,775 autopsies. Child Nephrol Urol. 1988–89; 9: 270 [5]

Table 16.5 Central nervous system (CNS) abnormalities seen in patients with CAKUT*

Abnormality	% of patients with CAKUT
Brain	6
Meningomyelocele/spina bifida	4
Hydrocephalus	2
Spinal cord	0.3
CNS	10

Reprinted with permission from Barakat AJ, Drougas JG, Barakat R. Association of congenital abnormalities of the kidney and urinary tract with those of other organ systems in 13,775 autopsies. Child Nephrol Urol. 1988–89; 9: 271 [5].

anencephaly, hydronephrosis, spina bifida, and encephalocele [20]. The CNS anomalies associated with CAKUT are shown in Table 16.5. Lu et al. [21] described five patients with CNS malformations (thin, hypoplastic, or absent corpus callosum, hydrocephalus or ventriculomegaly, Chiari type I malformation, and tethered spinal cord), associated with ureteral and renal defects (VUR, ureteropelvic and ureterovesical junction abnormalities, as well as bifid and megaureter). These patients had haploinsufficiency for the NFIA transcription factor gene due to chromosomal translocation or deletion.

Congenital Anomalies of the Skeletal System

Congenital skeletal anomalies occur in up to 9 % of patients with CAKUT and consist of abnormalities of upper extremities and hands (4 %), vertebral column and ribs (4 %), lower extremities and feet (3 %), and hips and pelvis (2 %) [5]. These abnormalities were mostly associated with anomalies of the ureter and bladder and hydronephrosis, followed by horseshoe kidney, renal agenesis, and abnormal urethra. The co-occurrence of renal and limb anomalies is referred to as the acro-renal syndrome, which occurs in 1 in 20,000 births [22]. Common limb defects include oligodactyly, ectrodactyly, syndactyly, or brachydactyly of the carpal and tarsal bones. Common renal anomalies include unilateral renal agenesis, bilateral renal hypoplasia, renal ectopia, hydrone-phrosis, VUR, and duplication anomalies. Acro-renal anomalies also occur in various syndromes including Acro-renal-ocular (AROS), Townes–Brocks, Pallister–Hall, Hajdu–Cheney, acro-renal-mandibular, Fraser, short rib polydactyly, VACTERL association, MURCS, and Poland syndromes (Refer to the Appendix).

Congenital Anomalies of the Lung and Diaphragm

Congenital anomalies of the lung were seen in 6 % of patients with CAKUT, and those of the diaphragm in 2 % [5]. Hypoplastic lungs, abnormal lung lobes, and abnormal diaphragm were associated with abnormalities of the ureters, bladder, and renal arteries, renal dysplasia, and agenesis. Pulmonary hypoplasia occurs in patients with severe renal anomalies that result in reduced amniotic fluid volume [23]. Pulmonary hypoplasia may result from thoracic compression due to reduced amniotic fluid. Fetal breathing movements are essential for normal antenatal lung growth, and these movements are significantly lower in patients with oligohydramnios. Other factors may also be responsible for abnormal lung growth such as reduction in renal proline production by the kidney. The association of fetal pulmonary hypoplasia with bilateral renal agenesis is known as the Potter's syndrome which consists of oligohydramnios, characteristic facial abnormalities (low set floppy ears, small chin, flattened nose, hypertelorism) and limb defects. Extralobular sequestration of the lung has also been described in association with renal aplasia. The most serious anomalies threatening fetal survival are bilateral renal agenesis and bladder outlet obstruction, followed by bilateral renal dyplasia/hypoplasia, and bilateral multicystic kidney. Despite perinatal and prolonged morbidity, fetal vesicoamniotic shunts in fetuses with urinary tract obstruction can offer patients with a poor prognosis an improved chance of survival [24].

Congenital diaphragmatic hernia especially when bilateral, may be associated with aplastic, polycystic, horseshoe, double, and ectopic kidney, hydronephrosis, hydroureter, and ectopic intrathoracic kidney.

Congenital Anomalies of the Reproductive Organs

Abnormalities of the Mullerian system, ovaries, and kidney may result from a common embryologic defect since the Wolffian and Mullerian ducts develop in anatomical proximity. Since the gonads are formed from the genital ridge and mesonephros, a defect in that region could account for the multiple organ defect. The association of Mullerian and renal agenesis could be an autosomal dominant disorder. Four percent of patients with CAKUT have associated anomalies of the reproductive organs with or without those of the external genitalia [5]. These are usually found in association with renal agenesis and dysplasia, horseshoe kidney, and ureter and bladder abnormalities. One out of every three patients with unilateral renal agenesis has a significant anomaly of the uterus, ovary or vagina [25, 26]. Renal anomalies have been reported in 40 % of patients with Mullerian aplasia and 40 % of women with unicornuate uterus. Mullerian anomalies occur in up to 37–60 % of females and 12 % of males with unilateral renal agenesis [26]. Abnormalities in females include agenetic, duplicated, rudimentary, unicornuate, or bicornuate uterus, double or absent vagina, absent or hypoplastic ovary, absent fallopian tube, and abnormal external genitalia. Abnormalities in males include cryptorchidism, seminal vesicle cyst, hypoplastic vas, unilateral prostatic agenesis, cystic testicular dysplasia, and hypospadias. Prenatal detection of unilateral renal agenesis should prompt the physician to look for associated genital abnormalities.

Chromosomal Aberrations

The association of chromosomal aberrations with multiple congenital anomalies is well known. The incidence of CAKUT is much higher in many forms of chromosomal aberrations than in the general population [27]. Chromosomal abnormalities occur in about 4–7 % of infants with CAKUT [5, 7]. The actual incidence of these abnormalities is probably higher than what is reported in the literature since many reports do not include investigation of the urinary tract. Autosomal trisomies (trisomy 8, 13, 18, and 21) have a very high incidence of CAKUT (75 % of trisomy 8, 33–70 % of trisomy 18, 50–60 % of trisomy 13, and 7 % of trisomy 21). CAKUT also occur in autosomal monosomies including 33 % of patients with chromosome 4 short arm deletion (4p–), 40 % of chromosome 5 short arm deletion (5p– or Cri-du-chat syndrome), and 40 % of chromosome 18 long arm deletion (18q–). CAKUT also occurs in 60–80 % of patients with Turner syndrome, with horseshoe kidney being the most commonly reported anomaly (20–40 %). CAKUT, especially cystic renal dysplasia and hydronephrosis occur in over 50 % of patients with triploidy (69 chromosomes) and tetraploidy (92 chromosomes), as well as in 60–100 % of patients with the "cat-eye" syndrome. Nicolaides et al. [28] found chromosomal abnormalities in 23 % of fetuses with obstructive uropathy. Karyotyping should be performed in patients with a major anomaly or those where intervention is considered, to rule out a chromosomal aberration. CAKUT should also be suspected in patients with chromosome aberrations associated with multiple congenital anomalies.

A specific syndrome is usually identified in about 24 % of patients with multiple malformations [29]. Since 27–50 % of these malformations are due to chromosomal aberrations and since CAKUT represents 50 % of fetal malformations, a karyotype study should be seriously considered in fetuses with CAKUT associated with other malformations.

Congenital Anomalies of the Face and Ears

Congenital facial anomalies and cleft palate with or without cleft lip occur in 7 % of patients with CAKUT, particularly abnormalities of the ureters and bladder, as well as renal agenesis and hypoplasia [5].

Both urogenital and auditory systems develop around the 5th to 8th week of gestation. Thus any insult to the fetus at this time may result in an anomaly of both organs. The severity of the auditory system defects often parallels those of the urogenital system [30].

Preauricular ear tags (small, skin-colored nodules that can be found anywhere along a line drawn between the tragus to the angle of the mouth) occur in 1.7 per 1000 newborns, and pits (small openings at the anterior margin of the crus of the helix) in 1–5 % [31]. Deshpande and Watson [32] studied 13,136 consecutive newborns over a 41-month period. 7.3/1000 of these newborns had minor external ear anomalies (preauricular skin tags, preauricular sinuses, ear pits, and misshapen pinnae). Both ear tags and pits can be found in isolation or as part of a genetic syndrome.

Individuals with ear anomalies are more associated with CAKUT than the general population, probably due to the fact that they are often a part of specific multiple congenital anomaly (MCA) syndromes that have high incidence of renal anomalies [33]. CHARGE association occurs in 1/10,000 and encompasses a wide spectrum of anomalies including coloboma of iris or retina, retarded growth and development, heart anomalies, coanal atresia, genital hypoplasia and ear defects (auricular dysmorphology—low set ears, deficient cartilage, and absent lobules). Renal anomalies occur in 25 % of CHARGE patients and include renal ectopia, malrotation, and dysgenesis, horseshoe kidney, hydronephrosis, and vesicoureteric reflux [34].

Townes–Brocks syndrome is an autosomal dominant disorder with multiple malformations and variable expression. Major findings include external ear anomalies, hearing loss, preaxial polydactyly and triphalangeal thumbs, imperforate anus, and renal malformations. CAKUT occur in about 27 % of these patients and include aplastic, hypoplastic or dysplastic kidneys, multicystic kidney, posterior urethral valve, VUR, meatal stenosis, and hypospadias [35].

Beckwith–Wiedemann syndrome is characterized by somatic overgrowth, macroglossia, anterior abdominal wall defects, and macrosomia. The ear lobes have creases and pits. CAKUT occurs in over 50 % of these cases and includes nephromegaly, renal cysts, duplicated collecting system, VUR, and hydronephrosis.

Because of the association of ear and renal anomalies, it was recommended in the past that all patients who have ear pits or tags undergo routine renal US because of the association of ear and renal anomalies. However, evidence is mounting that it is unnecessary to obtain routine renal US in patients who have isolated preauricular ear pits or tags. Kugelman and associates [36] evaluated the need of renal US in newborns who had isolated preauricular ear pits or tags. The incidence of renal abnormalities among infants who had isolated ear pits or tags was 2.2 % compared with 3.1 % among healthy newborns. The authors suggested that routine renal US is not indicated for patients who have isolated ear pits or tags, but should be considered in patients who have three or more minor anomalies that include ear pits or tags and in patients in whom a genetic syndrome is suspected. Wang et al. [33] also suggested to perform a renal US in patients with preauricular pits, cup ears, or any other ear anomaly that is accompanied by one or more of the following: other malformations or dysmorphic features, a family history of deafness, auricular and/or renal malformations, or a maternal history of gestational diabetes. Renal anomalies associated with those of the ears include hydronephrosis, horseshoe kidney, and renal aplasia or hypoplasia. 5.3 % of children with unilateral renal agenesis have associated auditory abnormalities [30].

Single Umbilical Artery

Single umbilical artery, the most common developmental abnormality of the umbilical cord, is frequently associated with an increased incidence of atresia of hollow visceral organs, gastrointestinal, urogenital, musculoskeletal, CV, CNS, and limb abnormalities [37] CAKUT including cystic renal dysplasia, posterior urethral valve, urethral atresia, urethral diverticulum, hypoplastic or absent bladder, urethral atresia, Potter's sequence, and Meckel's syndrome may also occur in patients with single umbilical artery [38].

Meckel's syndrome, which is transmitted as an autosomal recessive trait, has a highly variable phenotype with cystic renal dysplasia being the most consistent associated abnormality. The other more common anomalies include posterior encephalocele, cleft palate, polydactyly, syndactyly, ambiguous genitalia, hypoplastic urinary bladder, and cysts in the liver and lungs. The association of Meckel's syndrome with single umbilical artery may have a common pathogenesis, probably urinary outflow obstruction secondary to bladder hypoplasia or vascular insufficiency resulting in cystic renal dysplasia [38]. The association may also be entirely coincidental. In addition to CAKUT, anomalies of the GI, CV, musculoskeletal, and central nervous systems and limb reduction defects may also occur. The presence of a single umbilical artery is a marker that should suggest to the clinician the possible association of CAKUT.

Supernumerary Nipples

Supernumerary nipples occur in 0.22–6 % of the population [39]. They are usually solitary arising in the milk lines, but they can also be multiple and occur in other parts of the body. These nipples are benign, but rarely may undergo hormonal changes and disease. Treatment is not needed, but surgical removal is considered for cosmetic reasons or discomfort. They may be familial with an autosomal dominant inheritance.

Supernumerary nipples may be associated with CAKUT, including duplicated collecting system, hypoplastic, microcystic and polycystic kidneys, hydronephrosis, ureteropelvic junction stenosis, and Wilms' tumor. While there is discrepancy in the literature regarding the frequency of association of supernumerary nipples and renal anomalies, most authors seem to agree that the random finding of isolated supernumerary nipples probably does not justify renal investigation [40, 41]. However, investigation seems to be justified when urinary tract infection or MCA are present.

Conclusion

Awareness of the association of CAKUT with anomalies of other systems and syndromes is essential in the management of affected patients, especially when the anomaly is not evident on routine physical examination and when early intervention can contribute to prevention of renal damage and CKD. CAKUT should be suspected in patients with multiple congenital anomalies particularly in those with chromosomal aberrations, as well as in newborns and children with single umbilical artery, urinary tract infection, significant abnormalities of the ear lobes, supernumerary nipples, congenital abnormalities of other organ systems, and congenital hypothyroidism.

References

1. Barakat AY, Drougas JG. Occurrence of congenital abnormalities of the kidney and urinary tract in 13,775 autopsies. Urology. 1991;38:347–50.
2. Barakat AJ, Chesney RW, editors. Pediatric nephrology for primary care. Elk Grove Village, Illinois: American Academy of Pediatrics; 2009.
3. Sanna-Cherchi S, Caridi G, Weng PL, Scolari F, Perfumo F, Gharavi AG, et al. Genetic approaches to human renal agenesis/hypoplasia and dysplasia. Pediatr Nephrol. 2007;22:1675–84.
4. Woolf AS, Price KL, Scambler PJ, Winyard PJ. Evolving concepts in human renal dysplasia. J Am Soc Nephrol. 2004;15.998–1007.
5. Barakat AJ, Drougas JG, Barakat R. Association of congenital abnormalities of the kidney and urinary tract with those of other organ systems in 13,775 autopsies. Child Nephrol Urol. 1988–89; 9:269–72.
6. Rubinstein M, Meyer R, Bernstein J. Congenital abnormalities of the urinary system. I. A postmortem survey of developmental anomalies and acquired congenital lesions in a children's hospital. J Pediatr. 1961;58:356–66.
7. Stoll C, Dott B, Alembik Y, Roth MP. Associated non-urinary congenital anomalies among infants with congenital anomalies of the kidney and urinary tract (CAKUT). Eur J Med Genet. 2014;57:322–8.
8. Westland R, Schreuder MF, Ket JCF, van Wijk JAE. Unilateral renal agenesis: a systematic review on associated anomalies and renal injury. Nephrol Dial Transplant. 2013;28(7):1844–55. doi:10.1093/ndt/gft012.

9. Melo BF, Aguiar MB, Bouzada MCF, Aguiar RL, Pereira AK, Paixão GM, et al. Early risk factors for neonatal mortality in CAKUT: analysis of 524 affected newborns. Pediatr Nephrol. 2012;27:965–72.

10. Kumar J, Gordillo R, Kaskel FJ, Druschel CM, Woroniecki RP. Increased prevalence of renal and urinary tract anomalies in children with congenital hypothyroidism. J Pediatr. 2009;154:263–6.

11. Renkema KY, Winyard PJ, Skovorodkin IN, Levtchenko E, Hindryckx A, Jeanpierre C, et al. Novel perspectives for investigating congenital anomalies of the kidney and urinary tract (CAKUT). Nephrol Dial Transplant. 2011;26:3843–51. doi:10.1093/ndt/gfr655.

12. Jones KL, Jones MC, del Campo M. Smith's Recognizable Patterns of Human Malformation, 7th edition, Elsevier Health Sciences; 2013.

13. Tondury G. Aetiological factors in human malformation. Triangle. 1965;7:90–100.

14. Cui S, Schwartz L, Quaggin SE. Pod1 is required in stromal cells for glomerulogenesis. Dev Dyn. 2003;226:512–22.

15. Cocchi G, Magnani C, Morini MS, Garani GP, Milan M, Calzolari E. Urinary tract abnormalities (UTA) and associated malformations: data of the Emilia-Romagna Registry. IMER Group. Emilia-Romagna Registry on Congenital Malformations. Eur J Epidemiol. 1996;12:493–7.

16. Adhisivam B, Prahlad N, Vijayakumar M, Nammalwar BR, Muralinath S. Cardiovascular malformations associated with urinary tract anomalies. Indian J Nephrol. 2005;15:8–9.

17. Buendía Hernández A, Vázquez J, Fuentes J, Attié F, Ovseyevitz J. Anomalies of the urinary tract associated with congenital heart diseases. Arch Inst Cardiol Mex. 1987;57:207–11.

18. Prato AP, Rossi V, Mosconi M, Holm C, Lantieri F, Griseri P, et al. A prospective observational study of associated anomalies in Hirschsprung's disease. Orphanet J Rare Dis. 2013;8:184–96. http://www.ojrd.com/content/8/1/184.

19. Perlman S, Bilik R, Leibovitch L, Katorza E, Achiron R, Gilboa Y. More than a gut feeling – sonographic prenatal diagnosis of imperforate anus in a high-risk population. Article first published online: 22 Aug 2014. doi:10.1002/pd.4472

20. Rimoin DL, Pyeritz RE, Korf B, editors. Emery and Rimoin's Principles and Practice of Medical Genetics. 2013, Elsevier Ltd. Chapter 62, p. 17.

21. Lu W, Quintero-Rivera F, Fan Y, Alkuraya FS, Donovan DJ, Xi Q, et al. NFIA haploinsufficiency is associated with a CNS malformation syndrome and urinary tract defects. PLoS Genet. 2007;3, e80.

22. Natarajan C, Jeyachandran D, Subramaniyan B, Thanigachalam D, Rajagopalan A. Congenital anomalies of the kidney and hand: a review. Clin Kidney J. 2013;6:144–9. doi:10.1093/ckj/sfsl86.

23. May C, Greenough A. Pulmonary hypoplaqsia and congenital renal anomalies. Arch Med Sci. 2006;1:6–9.

24. Ethun CG, Zamora IJ, Roth DR, Kale A, Cisek L, Belfort MA, et al. Outcomes of fetuses with lower urinary tract obstruction treated with vesicoamniotic shunt: a single-institution experience. J Pediatr Surg. 2013;48:956–62. doi:10.1016/j.jpedsurg.2013.02.011.

25. Barakat AJ. Association of unilateral renal agenesis and genital anomalies. Case Rep Clin Pract Rev. 2002;3:57–60.

26. Thompson DP, Lynn HB. Genital anomalies associated with solitary kidney. Mayo Clinic Proc. 1966;41:538–48.

27. Barakat AY, Butler MG. Renal and urinary tract abnormalities associated with chromosome aberrations. Int J Pediatr Nephrol. 1987;8:215–26.

28. Nicolaides KH, Rodeck CH, Gosden CM. Rapid karyotyping in non-lethal fetal malformations. Lancet. 1986;1:283–7.

29. Polani PE. Delineation of malformation syndromes. In: Littlefield JW, de Grouchy J, editors. Birth defects. Amsterdam: Excerpta Medica; 1977. p. 422–5.

30. Huang H-M, Yeh R-M, Tan C-T, Chao M-C, Lin K-N. Auditory abnormalities associated with unilateral renal agenesis. Int J Pediatr Otorhinolaryngol. 2001;60:113–8.

31. Adam M, Hudgins L. The importance of minor anomalies in the evaluation of the newborn. The importance of minor anomalies in the evaluation of the newborn Neo reviews 2003; 4;99. doi: 10.1542/neo.4-4-e99. Downloaded from http://neoreviews.aappublications.org by JoDee Anderson on 20 June 2008.
32. Deshpande SA, Watson H. Renal ultrasonography not required in babies with isolated minor ear anomalies. Arch Dis Child Fetal Neonatal Ed. 2006;91:F29–30.
33. Wang RY, Earl DL, Ruder RO, Graham Jr JM. Syndromic ear anomalies and renal ultrasounds. Pediatrics. 2001;108, E32.
34. Blake KD, Davenport SLH, Hall BD, Hefner MA, Pagon RA, Williams MS, et al. CHARGE Association: an update and review for the primary pediatrician. Clin Pediatr. 1998;37:159–73.
35. Powell CM, Michaelis RC. Townes-Brocks syndrome. J Med Genet. 1999;36:89–93. doi:10.1136/jmg.36.2.89.
36. Kugelman A, Tubi A, Bader D, Chemo M, Dabbah H. Preauricular tags and pits in the newborn: the role of renal ultrasonography. J Pediatr. 2002;141:388–91.
37. Heifetz SA. Single umbilical artery: a statistical analysis of 237 autopsy cases and review of literature. Perspect Pediatr Pathol. 1984;8:345–78.
38. Sur M, Nayler S, Muc R. Association of single umbilical artery with common and rare congenital malformations. Internet J Pediatr Neonatol. 2003;4:1–7.
39. Brown J, Schwartz RA. Supernumerary nipples: an overview. Pediatr Derm. 2003;71:344–6.
40. Mimouni F. Association of supernumerary nipples and renal anomalies. AJDC. 1986;142:591.
41. Hoyme HF. Minor malformations: significant or insignificant? AJDC. 1987;141:947.

Appendix

Conditions and Syndromes Associated with Congenital Anomalies of the Kidney and Urinary Tract

Amin J. Barakat

Abbreviations

AD	Autosomal dominant
AR	Autosomal recessive
CV	Cardiovascular
GI	Gastrointestinal
GU	Genitourinary
PUV	Posterior urethral valves
UP	Ureteropelvic
UPJ	Ureteropelvic junction
UVJ	Ureterovesical junction
VU	Vesicoureteral
VUR	Vesicoureteral reflux
XL	X-linked
XLD	X-linked dominant
XLR	X-linked recessive

A.J. Barakat M.D., F.A.A.P. (✉)
Department of Pediatrics, Georgetown University Medical Center, Washington, DC, USA

Clinical Professor of Pediatrics, Georgetown University Medical Center, 107 North Virginia Ave, Falls Church, VA 22046, USA
e-mail: aybarakat@aol.com

© Springer International Publishing Switzerland 2016
A.J. Barakat, H. Gil Rushton (eds.), *Congenital Anomalies of the Kidney and Urinary Tract*, DOI 10.1007/978-3-319-29219-9

This section is intended to help the readers to suspect and diagnose kidney and urinary tract anomalies associated with various conditions and syndromes, and help them initiate diagnostic studies and genetic counseling, or refer patients to the appropriate specialist. The conditions are presented alphabetically using the OMIM terminology and including the OMIM reference number. This is followed by a brief presentation of the main features of the condition, associated kidney and urinary tract anomalies, and mode of inheritance. A more comprehensive list of conditions associated with kidney and urinary tract anomalies is available [1–6].

The mode of inheritance and gene map locus of the genetic disorders can be found on OMIM "Online Mendelian Inheritance in Man" [1], which is a comprehensive authoritative compendium of information on genetic disorders and genes. OMIM is updated daily and is freely available at (http://www.ncbi.nlm.nih.gov/omim/). Editorial decisions take place at Johns Hopkins University School of Medicine. Authors are located at Johns Hopkins and around the world. Distribution of OMIM and software development are provided by the National Center for Biotechnology Information (NCBI) at the National Library of Medicine. It is recommended to refer to OMIM to review the updated mode of inheritance and genetic information since this is a fast growing field and this information may change.

A list of many chromosomal aberrations associated with renal and urinary tract anomalies is also provided. A more detailed list is available [7, 8].

Syndrome/condition OMIM reference no.	Main features	Renal/urinary tract anomalies	Inheritance
Aase-Smith 1 147800	Joint contractures, cleft palate, Dandy-Walker malformation	Axial rotation of the kidneys	AD
Abdominal muscles, absence of, with urinary tract abnormality and cryptorchidism (Prune Belly) 100100	Congenital absence of abdominal musculature, urinary tract abnormalities, cryptorchidism	Dilated urinary tract, dysplastic, aplastic, multicystic and hydronephrotic kidneys, hypoplastic or absent urethra, PUV	AR
Abruzzo-Erickson 302905	Cleft palate, coloboma, deafness, short stature, radial synostosis	Horseshoe kidney, hypospadias	XLR
Achondrogenesis 200610	Micromelic dwarfism, short trunk, fetal hydrops	Hydronephrosis, hydroureter, double collecting system	AR AD
Acrocephalopolydactylous dysplasia (Elejalde) 200995	Acrocephaly, hexadactyly of hands, gigantism, thick skin, visceromegaly, connective tissue hyperplasia	Cystic renal dysplasia	AR
Acrofacial dysostosis 1 (Nager type) 154400	Craniofacial, limb and musculoskeletal anomalies, hearing loss	Unilateral renal agenesis, double ureters, VUR	AD AR

Syndrome/condition OMIM reference no.	Main features	Renal/urinary tract anomalies	Inheritance
Acrorenal 102520	Acral anomalies of hands and feet, urinary tract abnormalities	Ectopic, aplastic, and hypoplastic kidneys; bladder neck obstruction ureteral hypoplasia, trigone deformity VUR, horseshoe kidney	AR
Acrorenal-mandibular 200980	Ectrodactyly, hypoplastic mandible, renal disease	Dysplastic, polycystic and agenetic kidneys	AR
Adams-Oliver 1 100300	Growth deficiency, absence defects of limbs, scalp, and skull	Double collecting system	AD
Adrenal hyperplasia (2l-hydroxylase deficiency) 201910	Virilization, adrenal insufficiency	Unilateral renal agenesis, UPJ obstruction, double collecting system	AR
Alagille 1 118450	Unusual facies, vertebral and eye anomalies, chronic cholestasis, peripheral pulmonary stenosis	Unilateral renal agenesis and dysplasia, horseshoe kidney, renal artery stenosis, VUR	AD
Alcohol embryopathy (Fetal alcohol syndrome)	Prenatal and postnatal growth retardation, microcephaly, short palpebral fissures, joint contractures, mental retardation, chronic arthropathy	Unilateral renal agenesis and hypoplasia, hydronephrosis, duplication of urinary tract, horseshoe kidney	–
Anencephaly 206500	Same	Hydronephrosis, horseshoe kidney, polycystic kidney, renal agenesis and hypoplasia, urethral atresia	?AR
Aniridia, partial, unilateral renal agenesis, psychomotor retardation 206750	Same	Unilateral renal agenesis	?AR
Antley-Bixler (Trapezoidocephaly-Synostosis) 207410	Cranio- and humeroradial synostosis, midface hypoplasia, abnormal ears, narrow chest and pelvis, digital abnormalities	Ectopia, duplication of kidney and ureter, renal agenesis	AR AD
Apert 101200	Irregular craniosynostosis, midfacial hypoplasia, syndactyly, broad distal phalanx of thumb and big toe	Polycystic kidneys, hydronephrosis	AD

(continued)

(continued)

Syndrome/condition OMIM reference no.	Main features	Renal/urinary tract anomalies	Inheritance
ARIMA 243910	Agenesis of the cerebellar vermis, ocular abnormalities, cystic kidney disease, possible liver disease	Polycystic and medullary cystic and multicystic kidneys, nephronophthisis	AR
Arthrogryposis, distal, type IIA 193700	Mask-like "whistling" face, ulnar deviation of hands, talipes equinovarus	Renal hypoplasia with contralateral hydronephrosis	AD
Arthro-osteo-renal dysplasia	Bone and joint abnormalities, renal and congenital heart disease, hearing loss	Renal cystic dysplasia	?
Baller-Gerold 218600	Craniosynostosis, radial aplasia or hypoplasia, other skeletal abnormalities, psychomotor delay	Crossed renal ectopia, pelvic kidney, renal agenesis, VUR	AR
Bifid nose with or without anorectal and renal anomalies 608980	Bifid nose, renal and anorectal anomalies	Unilateral or bilateral enal agenesis	AR
Beckwith-Wiedemann EMG (Exomphalos-macroglossia-gigantism) 130650	Somatic overgrowth, macroglossia, anterior abdominal wall defects, macrosomia, ear helix anomaly	Affects 59 %. Nephromegaly, renal cysts, double collecting system, Wilms' sporadic tumor, VUR, hydronephrosis	AD
Biliary atresia, extrahepatic 210500	Biliary atresia, renal and cardiac malformations	Renal aplasia or hypoplasia, polycystic kidneys, megaureter, atresia of ureter	?AR
Bloom 210900	Growth failure, facial telangiectasia, defective immunity	Wilms' tumor	AR
Bowen-Conradi 211180	Microcephaly, prominent nose, micrognathia, joint deformities	Horseshoe kidney, double collecting system	AR
Branchiootorenal 1 113650	Preauricular pits, cervical fistulae, hearing loss	Ectopic, aplastic, hypoplastic, dysplastic, and polycystic kidneys	AD
C (Opitz trigonocephaly) 211750	Trigonocephaly, polysyndactyly, mental retardation, dysmorphic	Unilateral renal agenesis, hypospadias facies, cardiac defects	AR
Campomelic dysplasia 114290	Congenital bowing of long bones, abnormal facies, dwarfism, other defects	Hydronephrosis, hydroureter, hypoplastic and cystic kidneys	AD

Syndrome/condition OMIM reference no.	Main features	Renal/urinary tract anomalies	Inheritance
Caroli disease, isolated 600643	Segmental cystic dilatation of intrahepatic bile ducts, cholelithiasis, hepatic and pancreatic fibrosis, congenital anomalies, failure to thrive	Medullary sponge, and polycystic kidney disease	AD AR
Carpenter 1 201000	Acrocephaly, peculiar facies, brachysyndactyly of hands, mental retardation	Hydronephrosis, hydroureter	AR
Cayler cardiofacial 125520	Asymmetric crying facies, cardiovascular and other anomalies	Unilateral agenetic, ectopic, cystic, and dysplastic kidney, fetal lobulation	AD
Cerebrocostomandibular 117650	Cerebral maldevelopment, micrognathia, severe costovertebral abnormalities	Renal ectopia, medullary cysts	AD
Cerebro-hepato-renal (Passarge)	Hypotonia, abnormal ears, hepatomegaly, renal cysts, failure to thrive	Cortical cysts, hypospadias	?AR
Cerebrooculofacio-skeletal (COFS) 214150	Microcephaly, ocular, facial and skeletal abnormalities, mental retardation	Horseshoe kidney, bilateral renal agenesis, double collecting system, absent ureter and bladder	AR
CHARGE 214800	Coloboma, cardiac, genital, inner ear and retinal anomalies, choanal atresia	Unilateral renal agenesis, ectopia, double collecting system, posterior urethral valves, UPJ obstruction, hypospadias, duplication	AD
Chromosome aberrations	See p 355		
Cleft lip/palate with abnormal thumbs and microcephaly 216100	Same	Horseshoe kidney, renal agenesis	?AR
Cohen 216550	Hypotonia, obesity, characteristic facial features, psychomotor delay	UPJ obstruction	AR
Coloboma of macula with type B brachydactyly 120400	Pigmented macular coloboma, type B brachydactyly, others	Unilateral renal agenesis	?AD

(continued)

(continued)

Syndrome/condition OMIM reference no.	Main features	Renal/urinary tract anomalies	Inheritance
Congenital hemidysplasia with ichthyosiform erythroderma and limb defects (CHILD) 308050	Congenital hemidysplasia, unilateral ichthyosiform erythroderma, ipsilateral limb defects	Ipsilateral renal agenesis	XLD
Cornelia de Lange 122470	Pre- and postnatal growth deficiency, dysmorphic facies, hirsutism, mental retardation	Renal cystic dysplasia and hypoplasia, hydronephrosis, hypospadias	Sporadic ?AD
Denys-Drash 194080	Pseudohermaphroditism, nephropathy, and Wilms' tumor in various combinations	Wilms' tumor, ectopic kidney	Sporadic
Diaphragmatic hernia, congenital 142340	Congenital diaphragmatic hernia, respiratory distress at birth	Aplastic, polycystic, horseshoe, double and ectopic kidney; hydronephrosis, hydroureter	?AR
Diethylstilbestrol, exposure in utero	Abnormalities and neoplasm of genital tract	Urethral stenosis, hypospadias	–
DiGeorge 188400	Hypocalcemia, absence of thymus and parathyroid glands, immunodeficiency, congenital heart defect, characteristic facies	Hydronephrosis, malrotation of kidneys	Sporadic AD
Donnai-Barrow (Faciooculoacousticorenal) 222448	Ocular and craniofacial anomalies, sensorineural deafness, proteinuria	VUR	AR
Duane-radial ray (Acrorenoocular) 607323	Mental retardation, microcephaly, cardiac and urinary tract anomalies	Unilateral renal agenesis, VUR, renal hypoplasia, malrotation and ectopia, horseshoe kidney	AD
Dubowitz 223370	Short stature, microcephaly, peculiar facies, mental retardation	Hypospadias, small penis, VUR, hydronephrosis	AR
Dyskeratosis congenita 305000	Abnormal pigmentation, nail dystrophy, leukoplakia of oral mucosa, pancytopenia	Ureteral and urethral stenosis, small penis	XLR
Dyssegmental dysplasia Rolland-Desbuquois type 224400	Short trunk and limbs, narrow chest, vertebral defects, reduced joint mobility, death in neonatal period	Hydronephrosis, hydroureter	AR

Syndrome/condition OMIM reference no.	Main features	Renal/urinary tract anomalies	Inheritance
Ectrodactyly-ectodermal dysplasia and cleft lip/palate 1 (EEC 1) 129900	Ectrodactyly, ectodermal dysplasia, cleft lip/palate	Unilateral renal agenesis and dysplasia, hypospadias, ureterocele, hydronephrosis, ureter atresia	AD
Ehlers-Danlos 130050 and others	Hyperelasticity and fragility of skin and blood vessels, hypermobility of joints	UPJ abnormality, polycystic/medullary sponge kidney, bladder neck obstruction	AD, AR XL Sporadic
Ellis-van Creveld (Chondroectodermal dysplasia) 225500	Acromelic dwarfism, polydactyly, hypoplasia and dystrophy of nails and teeth, cardiac malformations	Renal agenesis and dysplasia, multicystic kidneys, hypospadias, megaureter, epispadias	AR
Epidermolysis bullosa dystrophica 131750 226600	Subepidermal blisters, ulceration of mucosae, flexion contractures of fingers, osteoporosis	Hydronephrosis, hydroureter, meatal stenosis, ureteral strictures, bladder hypertrophy	AD AR
Faciocardiorenal 227280	Characteristic facies, severe mental retardation, cardiac and renal defects	Horseshoe kidney, hydroureter	AR
Familial adenomatous polyposis 1 175100	Colon polyposis, epidermal cysts, osteomas	Hydronephrosis	AD AR
Fanconi anemia, complementation Group D2 (Fanconi pancytopenia) 227646	Pancytopenia, hyperpigmentation, skeletal deformities, absent or hypoplastic thumb	33 % Affected. Aplastic, ectopic, and horseshoe kidney, duplication of urinary tract, hydronephrosis, renal cysts	AR
Femoral-facial 134780	Femoral hypoplasia, unusual facies, cleft palate	Hemangioma of urinary tract, polycystic kidneys, renal agenesis and hypoplasia, abnormal collecting system	Sporadic
FG 300422 and others	Congenital hypotonia, macrocephaly, mental retardation, imperforate anus, partial agenesis of corpus callosum	Dilatation of urinary tract, urolithiasis	XL
Focal dermal hypoplasia 305600	Atrophy and linear pigmentation of skin, dysplastic nails, anomalies of eyes, hands, and vertebrae	Horseshoe kidney, unilateral renal agenesis	XLD

(continued)

(continued)

Syndrome/condition OMIM reference no.	Main features	Renal/urinary tract anomalies	Inheritance
Fraser 219000	Unilateral or bilateral absence of palpebral fissures with other abnormalities	25 % Affected. Renal and ureteral aplasia, hypospadias, urethral meatal stenosis	AR
Frontometaphyseal dysplasia 305620	Prominent supraorbital ridges, metaphyseal dysplasia, joint limitations, conductive deafness	Double collecting system, UV obstruction, hydronephrosis, pelvicalyceal junction obstruction	XL
Frontonasal dysplasia 136760	Findings limited to face and head. Median facial cleft, ocular hypertelorism	Unilateral renal agenesis, renal hypoplasia	Sporadic ?AR
Fryns 229850	Coarse facies, corneal opacities, cleft lip/palate, diaphragmatic defect, distal limb deformities	Renal cystic dysplasia, duplication of urinary tract, hypospadias, renal cysts, hydronephrosis, urethral stricture, hypoplastic renal arteries	AR
Genitopatellar 606170	Absent patella, scrotal hypoplasia, renal anomalies, dysmorphic facies, mental retardation	Multicystic kidney, hydronephrosis	AR fused renal ectopia
Hajdu-Cheney 102500	Acro-osteolysis, generalized osteoporosis, joint laxity, small stature, skeletal dysplasia, early loss of teeth	Polycystic, dysplastic and hypoplastic kidneys, VUR	AD
Hand-foot-genital 140000	Small feet, abnormal toes and thumbs, duplication of genital track in females	Hypospadias, ectopic ureteral orifice, VUR	AD
Hypoparathyroidism, sensorineural deafness, and renal disease (HDR, Barakat) 146255	Hypoparathyroidism, nerve deafness, renal disease	Renal dysplasia, hypoplasia or aplasia cystic kidney, pelvicalyceal deformity, VUR	AD
Heart, congenital malformations	Cardiac murmur and other findings depending on nature of malformation	Renal agenesis, dysgenesis, ectopia, and hypoplasia. 25 % of VSD have renal abnormalities particularly hypoplasia	?
Hemifacial microsomia 164210	Unilateral deformity of external ears, eye and vertebral anomalies	Unilateral renal agenesis and crossed ectopia, ureteral duplication, renal artery abnormality, cystic kidney	Sporadic AR

Syndrome/condition OMIM reference no.	Main features	Renal/urinary tract anomalies	Inheritance
Hennekam lymphangiectasia-lymphedema 235510	Intestinal and renal lymphangiectasia, dysmorphic facies, mental retardation	VUR, crossed renal ectopia, renal lymphangiectasis	AR
Hemihyperplasia, isolated 235000	Total or partial asymmetry, hemihypertrophy, hemiareflexia, scoliosis	Wilms' tumor, enlarged kidneys, medullary sponge kidneys, hypospadias	?AR ?AD
Hirschsprung disease, susceptibility to, 1 142623	Absence of ganglion cells in parts of intestine, other congenital anomalies	Hydronephrosis, renal hypoplasia, hydro-nephrosis, VUR, PUV, double collecting system	Sporadic AD
Hyperprolinemia, type I 239500	Elevated plasma levels of L-proline, nephropathy, photogenic epilepsy	Renal hypoplasia	AR
Hypertelorism, microtia facial clefting 239800	Hypertelorism, microtia, clefting, psychomotor retardation, atretic auditory canals	Ectopic kidneys	AR
Hypoglossia-hypodactylia (Hanhart) 103300	Aglossia, micrognathia, hypodactyly, cranial nerve palsy	Unilateral renal agenesis	Sporadic
Hypothyroidism, congenital, nongoitrous, 2 218700	Thyroid dysgenesis, cretinism if treatment is not initiated first 2 months	Hydronephrosis, UPJ obstruction, renal dysplasia and agenesis	Sporadic AR AD
IFAP syndrome with or without Bresheck syndrome 308205	Ichthyosis follicularis, atrichia, photophobia, short stature, seizures	Renal dysplasia, hypospadias	XLR Sporadic AD
Inflammatory bowel disease 1 (Crohn and ulcerative colitis included) 266600	Abdominal pain, diarrhea, weight loss, growth retardation	Nephrolithiasis, hydronephrosis, hydroureter, ileovesical fistulae	?AR
IVIC 147750	Radial ray hypoplasia, hearing impairment, internal ophthalmoplegia, thrombocytopenia	Renal aplasia, hypoplasia, ectopia and malrotation	AD
Johanson-Blizzard 243800	Hypoplastic alae nasi, hypothyroidism, congenital deafness, pancreatic achylia	Hydronephrosis, single urogenital orifice, VUR	AR
Joubert 1 213300	Aplasia of cerebellar vermis, psychomotor retardation, coloboma of eye	Nephronophthisis	AR

(continued)

(continued)

Syndrome/condition OMIM reference no.	Main features	Renal/urinary tract anomalies	Inheritance
Kabuki 1 147920	Mental retardation, postnatal dwarfism, peculiar facies, skeletal anomalies	Affects 25 %. Hydronephrosis ectopic, horseshoe, dysplastic, and agenetic kidney, ureteral duplication	?AD
KAL 1 gene (Kallmann) 300836	Anosmia, color blindness, hypogonadism	Unilateral renal agenesis, VUR	XLR AD, AR
Kaufman oculocerebrofacial 244450	Growth and mental retardation, microcephaly, hypotonia, hypertelorism, other eye abnormalities	Caliectasis, ureterectasia, bifurcation of renal pelvis	AR Sporadic
Klippel-Trenaunay-Weber 149000	Asymmetric limb hypertrophy, hemangiomas	Diffuse bilateral nephroblastoma, hemangioma of urinary tract, renal artery aneurysm	Sporadic ?AD
Lacrimoauriculo- dentodigital 149730	Nasolacrimal duct obstruction, cup-shaped pinnas, enamel dysplasia, digital malformations	Unilateral or renal agenesis, cystic kidneys	AD
Larsen 150250	Osteochondrodysplasia, craniofacial anomalies, multiple joint dislocations	Hydronephrosis, polycystic kidney disease, unilateral renal agenesis	AD AR
Laurence-Moon 245800	Retinitis pigmentosa, mental retardation, obesity, short stature, hypogonadism, polydactyly	Cystic, dysplastic, hypoplastic, and hydronephrotic kidneys; VUR	AR
Leopard 1 151100	Multiple lentigines, pulmonary stenosis, deafness	Hypospadias	AD
Lipodystrophy, congenital generalized, type 2 269700	Generalized loss of fat, hypertrichosis, increased pigmentation, hepatosplenomegaly, acceleration of somatic growth, enlarged genitalia, insulin-resistant nonketotic diabetes	Nephromegaly, hydronephrosis, hydroureter	AR
Lymphedema- hypoparathyroidism 247410	Congenital lymphedema, hypoparathyroidism, nephropathy, mitral valve prolapse, brachytelephalangy	Hypoplastic kidneys, congenital nephropathy	?AR ?XLR

Syndrome/condition OMIM reference no.	Main features	Renal/urinary tract anomalies	Inheritance
Marden-Walker 248700	Blepharophimosis, microphthalmia, cleft palate, congenital joint contractures, failure to thrive	Microcystic renal disease, dilated collecting system	AR
Marfan 154700	Tall stature, ectopia lentis, mitral valve prolapse, aortic root dilatation, aortic dissection	Hydronephrosis, hydroureter; polycystic, ectopic and medullary sponge kidney; unilateral renal agenesis; nephrolithiasis; ureteral stenosis; duplication of urinary tract	AD
Marshall-Smith 602535	Failure to thrive, accelerated skeletal maturation, craniofacial dysmorphism, psychomotor retardation	Hydronephrosis, hydroureter	Sporadic
Mayer-Rokitansky-Kuster-Hauser 277000	Uterovaginal atresia in otherwise normal females, urogenital adysplasia primary amenorrhea	Occurs in 36%. Unilateral/bilateral renal agenesis, renal dysplasia/hypoplasia, double renal pelvis and ureters, pelvic and solitary fused kidney, caliectasis, hypospadias	Sporadic ?AD
McKusick-Kaufman 236700	Hydrometrocolpos, polydactyly, congenital heart malformation	Polycystic kidneys, hydronephrosis, bladder neck obstruction	AR
Meckel type 7 267010	Dandy-Walker malformation; cerebellar malformations; renal, hepatic and pancreatic dysplasia	Multicystic dysplastic and cystic kidneys	AR
Meckel, type 4 (Meckel-Gruber) 611134	Occipital encephalocele, microcephaly, abnormal facies, cleft lip/palate, polydactyly	Dysplastic, polycystic, hypoplastic, horseshoe, hydronephrotic and medullary sponge kidney; dilated ureters; renal vascular abnormalities	AR

(continued)

(continued)

Syndrome/condition OMIM reference no.	Main features	Renal/urinary tract anomalies	Inheritance
Megalourethra, scaphoid	Absence of corpus spongiosum, dilated anterior urethra, urologic, GI skeletal and cardiac abnormalities	Renal dysplasia or hypoplasia, hydronephrosis, horseshoe kidney, VUR, PUV	–
Melorheostosis, isolated 155950	Hyperostosis, bone pain, limb anomalies, vascular malformation	Renal artery stenosis, hypoplastic kidney	Sporadic
Menkes disease 309400	Ceruloplasmin deficiency, copper malabsorption, peculiar hair, progressive neurological impairment	Hydronephrosis, hydroureter, VUR, neurogenic bladder, bladder diverticula	XLR
Metatropic dysplasia 156530	Short-limbed dwarfism, narrow thorax with short ribs, progressive kyphoscoliosis	Bilateral hydroureter	AR AD Sporadic
Microphthalmia, syndromic 1 309800	Microphthalmia, anophthalmia, anomalies of digits, teeth, and ears	Hydroureter, hypospadias, renal dysplasia	?Sporadic
Miller-Dieker Lissencephaly 247200	Microcephaly, incomplete brain development, vertical ridge in forehead, mental deficiency, seizures	Unilateral renal agenesis, cystic renal dysplasia	AR
Mulibrey nanism 253250	Progressive growth failure, hydrocephalus, ocular abnormalities, hypotonia, hepatomegaly	Wilms' tumor	AR
Mullerian duct aplasia, unilateral renal agenesis, and cervicothoracic somite anomalies; MURCS 601076	Short stature, mullerian duct aplasia, renal anomalies, cervical defects	Renal agenesis, dysplasia and ectopia, renal cysts	Sporadic
Myotonic dystrophy 160900	Myotonia, muscle wasting, cataract, hypogonadism	Polycystic kidneys	AD
N 310465	Mental retardation, visual impairment, deafness, spasticity	Hypospadias	XLR
Nephrosis with deafness and urinary tract and digital malformations 256200	Same	Ureteral constriction, double collecting system, UV and bladder neck obstruction	AR XLD
Neu-Laxova 256520	Intrauterine growth retardation, microcephaly, abnormal facies	Unilateral renal agenesis	AR

Syndrome/condition OMIM reference no.	Main features	Renal/urinary tract anomalies	Inheritance
Neurofibromatosis, type 1 162200	Cafe au lait spots, neurofibromatosis CNS involvement	Neurofibromatosis of lower urinary tract	AD
Neural tube defects 182940	Asymptomatic or neurologic symptoms, urinary incontinence	Ureteral duplication, neurogenic bladder	AR AD
Nevus, epidermal 162900	Midfacial nevus, seizures, mental deficiency	Renal hamartoma, nephroblastoma, renal artery stenosis	?Sporadic
Nipples, supernumerary 163700	Accessory nipples, and sometimes breast tissue	Double collecting system, hypoplastic, microcystic and polycystic kidneys, hydronephrosis, UPJ stenosis, ureteral prolapse, Wilms' tumor	AD
Noduli cutanei, multiple, urinary tract abnormalities 163850	Same	Hydronephrosis, double collecting system	?
Noonan 1 163950	Short stature, webbed neck, pulmonary stenosis, mental retardation	Polycystic, malrotated and hydronephrotic kidneys; double collecting system	AD
Omphalocele, autosomal 164750	Abdominal wall defect	Horseshoe kidney, patent urachus	AR
Opitz GBBB 145410	Ocular hypertelorism, dysphagia, hoarse cry, hypospadias	Unilateral duplication of renal pelvis and ureters, VUR	AD
Orofacial cleft 1 119530	Same	Renal agenesis, horseshoe kidney	–
Orofaciodigital VIII 300484	Malformation of oral cavity, face and digits, anomalies of anterior teeth, mental retardation	Polycystic kidney disease	XL
Melnick-Needles 309350	Bowing of long bones, short upper limbs, ribbon-like ribs, typical facies, sclerosis of base of skull	Hydronephrosis, hydroureter, ureteral stenosis, dysplastic kidneys	XLD Sporadic
Otopalatodigital, type I 311300	Short stature, characteristic craniofacial features, cleft palate, conductive deafness, bone dysplasia	Renal hypoplasia	XLD
Pallister-Hall 1 146510	Polysyndactyly, hypothalamic hamartoma, seizures	Horseshoe, agenetic, dysplastic, and ectopic kidney	AD

(continued)

(continued)

Syndrome/condition OMIM reference no.	Main features	Renal/urinary tract anomalies	Inheritance
Papillorenal syndrome 120330	Ocular and renal anomalies, less common CNS and genital anomalies	Oligomeganephronia, multicystic dysplastic aplastic, hypoplastic kidney, horseshoe kidney, VUR	AD
Perlman 267000	Large birth size, unusual facies, death in neonatal period, tendency to neoplasia	Large kidneys, hydronephrosis, renal dysplasia and hamartomas, nephroblastomatosis	AR
Peroxisome biogenesis disorder 1A (Zellweger) 214100	Failure to thrive, cerebral, renal and skeletal abnormalities; severe hypotonia, liver disease, distinctive facies, death in early infancy	Renal cysts and dysplasia, hypospadias, hydroureter	AR
Peters anomaly 604229	Anterior segment anomalies of the eye: abnormalities of the iris and clouding of corneal	Occur in 10–19 %. Multicystic renal dysplasia, renal hypoplasia, hydronephrosis, duplication of kidney and ureter	AR AD
Peutz-Jeghers 175200	Intestinal polyposis, mucocutaneous pigmentation	Ureteral and bladder polyposis	AD
Pituitary adenoma, ACTH-secreting 219090	Obesity, osteoporosis, growth	Renal dysplasia, urolithiasis, retardation, hypertension	Sporadic ?AR
Pneumothorax, primary spontaneous 173600	Same	Obstructive uropathy, polycystic kidneys	AD
Poland 173800	Unilateral aplasia of pectoralis major with ipsilateral symbrachydactyly and hypo/aplasia of breast and nipples	Renal aplasia or hypoplasia, double collecting system	Sporadic AD
Polycystic kidney, cataract, and congenital blindness 263100	Same	Polycystic, medullary cystic, atrophic and microcystic kidneys	?
Polycystic kidney disease, autosomal recessive 263200	Same, pulmonary hypoplasia, liver involvement	Duplication of urinary tract, ureteral atresia or stenosis, urethral valves, hypospadias, hypoplastic bladder	AR

Syndrome/condition OMIM reference no.	Main features	Renal/urinary tract anomalies	Inheritance
Polydactyly with neonatal chondrodystrophy type III (Naurnoff type)	Thoracic narrowing, hypoplastic lungs, short cranial base, death in perinatal period	Dysplastic kidneys	AR
Proteus 176920	Hemihypertrophy, scoliosis, overgrowth of lower extremities, partial macrodactyly, lipomas, pigmented nevi	Hypoplastic kidney	?
Pyloric stenosis, infantile hypertrophic, 1 179010	Hypertrophic pylorus, projectile vomiting at age 2–6 weeks	Polycystic, horseshoe and hypoplastic kidney; double collecting system; hydronephrosis	?AD
Radial-renal 179280	Radial ray aplasia, short stature, renal anomalies	Unilateral renal agenesis, crossed ectopia, VUR	?
Renal cyst and diabetes 137920	Maturity onset diabetes of the young, nondiabetic renal disease, genital abnormalities	Renal cysts, abnormal collecting systems, enlarged renal pelvis, hypoplastic, aplastic and horseshoe kidney	AD
Renal, genital, and middle ear anomalies 267400	Abnormal facies, low folded ears, renal abnormalities, vaginal atresia, deafness secondary to middle ear anomalies	Renal agenesis or hypoplasia, hemiatrophy of urinary bladder	?
Renal-hepatic-pancreatic dysplasia 1 208540	Hepatomegaly, hepatic, pancreatic and renal dysplasia	Polycystin and dysplastic kidneys	AR
Renal hypodysplasia/ aplasia 1 191830	Potter facies, pulmonary hypoplasia, limb deformity	Aplastic, dysplastic, hypoplastic multicystic and polycystic kidney, hypospadias, absent ureters/bladder, absent penis	AR
Rhizomelic chondrodysplasia punctata, type 1 215100	Flat face, cataract, spasticity short femur/humerus, dwarfism, mental retardation	Micromulticystic kidneys	?AR
Right atrial isomerism (Ivemark) 208530	Congenital asplenia; cardiac, GI, GU and skeletal abnormalities	Agenetic, hypoplastic, dysplastic, horseshoe, ptotic and cystic kidneys; ureteral and urethral valves; hydronephrosis; double collecting system	Sporadic AR

(continued)

(continued)

Syndrome/condition OMIM reference no.	Main features	Renal/urinary tract anomalies	Inheritance
Roberts 268300	Hypomelia, midfacial defect, severe growth retardation	Polycystic and horseshoe kidney, hydronephrosis, ureteral stenosis	AR
Robinow, autosomal dominant 180700	Mesomelic dwarfism, hemi-vertebrae, characteristic facies, hypoplastic external genitalia	Duplication of urinary tract, hydronephrosis, short urethra, VUR	AD
Rubella, congenital	Small for date, microcephaly, cataracts, heart defects, hepatosplenomegaly	Polycystic and unilateral agenetic kidney, double collecting system, hypospadias	–
Rubinstein-Taybi 1 180849	Broad thumbs and great toes, characteristic facial abnormalities, mental retardation	Affects 50 %. Renal calculi, ectopic, aplastic or extra kidney, double renal pelvis, dilated ureter, posterior urethral valves, VUR	Sporadic ?AD
Rudiger 268650	Coarse facial features, lack of ear cartilage, bifid uvula, brachydactyly	UPJ obstruction, VU stenosis, microphallus	?AR
Sacral defect with anterior meningocele 600145	All degrees of severity, from imperforate anus to sirenomelia, spina bifida, limb fusion	Agentic, dysplastic, and horseshoe kidney; duplication of urinary tract, polycystic kidneys, hydronephrosis absent bladder	AD AR XL
Schinzel-Giedion midface retraction 269150	Distinctive facial features, mental retardation, multiple congenital	Hydronephrosis, hypospadias, ectopic kidney, megaureter malformations, seizures	AD
Schwartz-Jampel, type 1 255800	Myotonia, short stature, blepharophimosis, joint contractures, myopia, pigeon chest	Microcystic kidney disease	?AD
Seckel 210600	Severe short stature, microcephaly, narrow face, beak-like nose	Renal ectopy and hypoplasia	AR
Senior-Loken 1 266900	Tapetoretinal degeneration, renal anomalies	Nephronophthisis, renal dysplasia	AR
Short-rib thoracic dysplasia 1 (Jeune) 208500	Rib cage and bone abnormalities, short stature, respiratory distress	Cystic and dysplastic kidneys	AR

Syndrome/condition OMIM reference no.	Main features	Renal/urinary tract anomalies	Inheritance
Short-rib thoracic dysplasia 3 with/without polydactyly 613091	Hydrops fetalis, polydactyly, short limbs, metaphyseal dysplasia of tubular bones, neonatal death	Cystic, dysplastic and hypoplastic kidneys, cystic or hypoplastic ureters	AR
Short-rib thoracic dysplasia 4 (asphyxiating thoracic dystrophy) 613819	Hypoplastic thorax, respiratory difficulty, protruding abdomen, polydactyly, tapetoretinal degeneration	Cystic renal dysplasia, VUJ stenosis, nephronophthisis, hypoplastic ureters	AR
Short-rib thoracic dysplasia 6 with/without polydactyly 263520	Medial cleft lip, polydactyly, short limbs, genital abnormalities, death in perinatal period	Cystic kidneys	AR
Short-rib thoracic dysplasia 9 with/without polydactyly 266920	Cone-shaped epiphyses of phalanges, bone dysplasia, anomalies of major organs, retinitis pigmentosa, ataxia	Medullary cystic disease, renal dysplasia, hypospadias	AR
Silver-Russell 180860	Prenatal-onset short stature, skeletal asymmetry, minor malformations, classical facial phenotype	UPJ obstruction, VUR, hypospadias	AD
Smith-Lemli-Opitz 270400	Growth retardation, microcephaly, mental retardation, abnormal facies, hypospadias, microphallus	Rotated, hypoplastic, dysplastic or multicystic kidney; cortical cysts; hypospadias	AR
Sotos 1 (cerebral gigantism) 117550	Acceleration of growth, acromegalic appearance, characteristic facies, variable mental retardation	Urethral stricture, Wilms' tumor	Sporadic AD
Spondylocostal dysostosis 1 277300	Vertebral and rib defects, short trunk, scoliosis	Unilateral renal agenesis, duplicated ureters, renal ectopia, horseshoe kidney	AR
Spondylocostal dysostosis 5 122600	Vertebral anomalies, barrel-shaped chest, rib defects, short neck	Unilateral agenesis and ectopia of kidney, hydronephrosis	AD
Syndactyly, type V 186300	Metacarpal and metatarsal 3–4 or 4–5 fusion	Renal hypoplasia, bladder exstrophy	AD
Telangiectasia, hereditary hemorrhagic, of Rendu, Osler and Weber 187300	Vascular dysplasia, generalized telangiectasias, bleeding, liver disease	Telangiectasias of urinary bladder	AD

(continued)

(continued)

Syndrome/condition OMIM reference no.	Main features	Renal/urinary tract anomalies	Inheritance
Thalidomide embryopathy	Limb defects	Renal agenesis, cystic dysplasia, hydronephrosis	–
Thanatophoric dysplasia, type I 187600	Short-limb dwarfism, narrow thorax, large cranium, respiratory distress, hypotonia	Hydronephrosis, horseshoe kidney	AD AR
Torticollis, keloids, cryptorchidism, and renal dysplasia 314300	Congenital muscular torticollis, multiple keloids, cryptorchidism, renal disease	Renal dysplasia and hypoplasia, urethral meatal stenosis, UPJ obstruction	XL
Townes-Brocks 107480	Imperforate anus, dysplastic ears, digital, renal, and cardiac anomalies	Polycystic, aplastic, hypoplastic, and dysplastic kidneys, hypospadias, VUR, PUV	AD
Tracheoesophageal fistula with or without esophageal atresia 189960	Same, dysmorphic facial features, cardiac anomalies	Horseshoe kidney, ureter duplication, cystic kidneys, VUR, pelvic or solitary kidney, hypospadias	Sporadic
Trichorhinophalangeal syndrome, type II 150230	Thin, sparse hair, bulbous nose, multiple exostoses, mental retardation, microcephaly	VUR, prune belly	Sporadic ?AD
Tuberous sclerosis 1 191100	Epilepsy, mental retardation, adenoma sebaceum, retinal phakomas	40–80 % affected. Renal angiomyolipomas, cystic kidneys, adenomas, or renal cell carcinoma	AD
Ulnar-mammary 181450	Abnormal development of ulnar rays, axillary apocrine glands, and vertebral column	Unilateral renal agenesis, malrotation	AD
Umbilical artery, single	Same	Duplicated or dilated renal pelvis, hydronephrosis, VUR, horseshoe kidney, unilateral renal agenesis, cystic renal dysplasia, PUV, hypoplastic or absent bladder, urethral atresia	–
Urofacial 1 236730	Hydronephrosis, peculiar facial expression, congenital urinary bladder dysfunction	Hydronephrosis, hydroureter, posterior urethral valves, VUR, neuropathic bladder	AR
Uterine anomalies 192000	Uterovaginal duplication, hematocolpos	Unilateral renal agenesis	Sporadic ?AD

Syndrome/condition OMIM reference no.	Main features	Renal/urinary tract anomalies	Inheritance
VATER association 192350	Vertebral anomalies, Anal atresia, T-E fistula, Radial dysplasia	Agenesis, ectopia, horseshoe kidney, hydronephrosis, UPJ stenosis, hypospadias, recto-urethral, and vesical fistulae	Sporadic ?
Visceral myopathy 155310	Megacystis, dilated small bowel, severe abdominal pain, abnormal intestinal motility	Megacystis, hydronephrosis, hydroureter	AD
Visceral neuropathy, familial 243180	Intermittent episodes of obstruction, familial abdominal pain or distention, megaduodenum, smooth muscle degeneration	Hydronephrosis, VUR, megacystis	AR
Von Hippel-Landau 193300	Cerebellar with retinal or spinal cord hemangioblastomas, pancreatic cysts, and renal lesions. Symptoms related to cerebellar or retinal tumors	66 % Affected. Renal adenoma, carcinoma or cysts; pheochromocytoma; ureterocele	AD
Weyers acrofacial dysostosis 193530	Ulnar ray defects with oligodactyly, antecubital pterygia, sternal anomalies, cleft lip/palate	Horseshoe kidney, ureteral duplication	AD
Williams-Beuren 194050	Typical facies, CV disease, developmental delay, learning disability	Solitary, small, asymmetric and pelvic kidney, renal artery stenosis, VUR	AD Sporadic
Wolfram 222300	Diabetes insipidus and mellitus, sensory deafness, optic atrophy	Hydronephrosis, hydroureter, neurogenic bladder, sclerosis of bladder neck	AR

Chromosomal aberrations	Renal and urinary tract anomalies
Autosomal trisomies	
Trisomy 8	75 % Affected. Hydronephrosis, horseshoe and nonfunctioning kidney, bifid pelvis, VUR
Trisomy 13	50–60 % Affected. Cystic, aplastic, horseshoe, and hydronephrotic kidney, duplication of urinary tract, megacystis, UVJ obstruction, bladder neck stenosis
Trisomy 18	Duplication of urinary tract (33–70 %); ectopic, horseshoe, cystic, hydronephrotic, aplastic, and hypoplastic kidney, Wilms' tumor, hamartoma, fetal lobulation, and rotational anomalies of the kidney

(continued)

(continued)

Chromosomal aberrations	Renal and urinary tract anomalies
Trisomy 21	7 % Affected. Aplastic, hypoplastic, dysplastic, cystic, and horseshoe kidney, hydronephrosis, hydroureter; ureteral stenosis, persistent fetal lobulation, hypoplastic or large bladder, urethral valves and stricture, renal artery stenosis
4q2 or 3	Cystic, hypoplastic, aplastic, or horseshoe kidney; VUR, hydronephrosis, hydroureter
10q2	Hypoplastic, dysplastic, cystic, hydronephrotic, and double kidneys; double collecting system
18q2	Polycystic and ectopic kidneys, VUR, hydroureter, unspecified renal malformations
2q21-> qter	Ectopic, dysplastic, and horseshoe kidneys, ureteral atresia
3q2	Cystic dysplasia, duplication of kidney, accessory kidney
6p21-> pter	Horseshoe and hypoplastic kidney, triple renal artery, double renal vein
9p	Hydronephrosis, horseshoe kidney
10p11-> pter	Rotated, aplastic, cystic, dysplastic, and double kidneys; megaureter, aplastic ureter
10q2	Hypoplastic, dysplastic, cystic, hydronephrotic, and double kidneys; double collecting system
11q2	Renal agenesis, VUR
12q2	Hydronephrosis, ureterocele, pelvic kidney
12q24.1-> qter	Ureterocele, hydronephrosis, ectopic, and aplastic kidney
17q21-> qter	Hypoplastic and cystic kidneys, hyperplastic urinary bladder
18q2	Polycystic and ectopic kidneys, VUR, hydroureter, unspecified renal malformations
19q13-> pter	Hydronephrosis, hydroureter, ectopic, malrotated and cystic kidneys
20p	Hydronephrosis, polycystic kidneys, double collecting system
Autosomal monosomies	
5p- (Cri-du-chat)	40 % Affected. Ectasia of distal tubules, cystic and horseshoe kidney, duplication of urinary tract, hypospadias, hypoplasia of penis
18 q-	40 % Affected. Polycystic, aplastic, ectopic, and horseshoe kidney, hydronephrosis, hydroureter, hypoplastic penis and scrotum, hypospadias
4p-	33 % Affected. Agenetic, hypoplastic, hydronephrotic, and nonfunctioning kidney, VUR, dilated collecting system, hypospadias
17p11.2	22 % Affected. Enlarged or solitary kidney, hydroureter, hydropelvis, malpositioned UVJ
4q3	Double collecting system, hydronephrosis, lobulated kidneys
7q13-> p21	Hydronephrosis, renal dysplasia, ureteral diverticula, ureterocele, double collecting system
10p13-->pter	Cystic and segmental renal dysplasia, double collecting system, hydronephrosis, hydroureter
11q2	Multicystic kidneys, double collecting system, hydronephrosis
13q-	Hypospadias, epispadias, hydroureter, ambiguous genitalia
18p	Unspecified renal malformations

Chromosomal aberrations	Renal and urinary tract anomalies
21q	Aplasia, dysplasia, and abnormal shape of kidney
22q12	Dysplastic and cystic kidneys
Sex chromosomes	
Turner syndrome (XO)	60–80 % Affected. Horseshoe kidney (commonest); duplications and rotational anomalies; hydronephrotic, ectopic, ptotic, aplastic, hypoplastic, and cystic kidney, urethral meatal stenosis, hypertension, double renal artery, UPJ and UVJ stenosis
Fragile X syndrome	UPJ stenosis
Klinefelter syndrome (XXY)	Renal cysts, hydronephrosis, hydroureter, ureterocele
49, XXXXX	Renal hypoplasia and dysplasia
Other chromosomal aberrations	
Cat-eye syndrome	60–100 % Affected. Renal agenesis, hypoplasia and cystic dysplasia, horseshoe and pelvic kidney, UPJ obstruction, VU stenosis and reflux, hypoplastic urinary bladder
Tetraploidy (92 chromosomes)	50 % Affected. Renal hypoplasia or dysplasia, megaureter, VUR, urethral stenosis
Triploidy (69 chromosomes)	Cystic renal dysplasia and hydronephrosis (50 %), fetal lobulations, pelvic kidney
18p Tetrasomy	Malrotated or horseshoe kidney, double ureter
r (13)	Aplastic, hypoplastic, or ectopic kidney
r (18)	Hydronephrosis, megaureter, VU obstruction

References

1. Online Mendelian Inheritance in Man, OMIM (TM). McKusick-Nathans Institute for Genetic Medicine, Johns Hopkins University (Baltimore, MD) and National Center for Biotechnology Information, National Library of Medicine (Bethesda, MD) http://www.ncbi.nlm.nih.gov/omim/.
2. Barakat AY, editor. Renal disease in children: clinical evaluation and diagnosis. New York: Springer; 1990.
3. Barakat AJ, Chesney RW, editors. Pediatric nephrology for primary care. Elk Grove Village, IL: American Academy of Pediatrics; 2009.
4. Jones KL, Jones MC, del Campo M. Smith's recognizable patterns of human malformation. 7th ed. Philadelphia, PA: Elsevier Health Sciences; 2013.
5. Rimoin DL, Connor JM, Pyeritz RE, Korf BR. Emory and Rimoin's principles and practice of medical genetics edition. 5th ed. Philadelphia, PA: Churchill Livingstone; 2007.
6. Avner ED, Harmon WE, Niaudet P, Yoshikawa N, editors. Pediatric nephrology. 6th ed. New York: Springer; 2010.
7. Barakat AY, Seikaly MG, Der Kaloustian VM. Urogenital abnormalities in genetic disease. J Urol. 1986;136:778–85.
8. Barakat AY, Butler MG. Renal and urinary tract abnormalities associated with chromosome aberrations. Int J Pediatr Nephrol. 1987;8:215–26.

Index

© Springer International Publishing Switzerland 2016
A.J. Barakat, H. Gil Rushton (eds.), *Congenital Anomalies of the Kidney
and Urinary Tract*, DOI 10.1007/978-3-319-29219-9

Printed in Great Britain
by Amazon

87573689R00217